Cambridge History of Medicine

Science and empire

Cambridge History of Medicine

Editors

CHARLES WEBSTER, *All Souls College, Oxford*
CHARLES ROSENBERG, *Professor of History and the Sociology of Science, University of Pennsylvania*

Science and empire

EAST COAST FEVER IN RHODESIA AND THE TRANSVAAL

PAUL F. CRANEFIELD
The Rockefeller University, New York

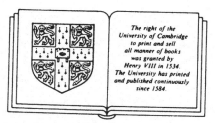

The right of the
University of Cambridge
to print and sell
all manner of books
was granted by
Henry VIII in 1534.
The University has printed
and published continuously
since 1584.

CAMBRIDGE UNIVERSITY PRESS

CAMBRIDGE
NEW YORK   PORT CHESTER
MELBOURNE   SYDNEY

PUBLISHED BY THE PRESS SYNDICATE OF THE UNIVERSITY OF CAMBRIDGE
The Pitt Building, Trumpington Street, Cambridge, United Kingdom

CAMBRIDGE UNIVERSITY PRESS
The Edinburgh Building, Cambridge CB2 2RU, UK
40 West 20th Street, New York NY 10011–4211, USA
477 Williamstown Road, Port Melbourne, VIC 3207, Australia
Ruiz de Alarcón 13, 28014 Madrid, Spain
Dock House, The Waterfront, Cape Town 8001, South Africa

http://www.cambridge.org

First published 1991
First paperback edition 2002

A catalogue record for this book is available from the British Library

ISBN 0 521 39253 5 hardback
ISBN 0 521 52449 0 paperback

*To the memory of far too
many friends I had
hoped would read this book:*

*Erwin H. Ackerknecht
Drew Middleton
Michael L. Powell
Charles B. Schmitt*

Contents

Illustrations

Preface

The appearance of a new disease is a rare event, as is the identification of a previously unrecognized disease. A serious new disease, whether it affects human beings or affects animals of economic importance, presents challenges to the public, to its government and to scientists. East Coast fever, which can wipe out a herd of cattle in three weeks, was first identified in Rhodesia between 1901 and 1903. It caused problems for various governments, it caused something close to panic in the Rhodesian public, and it presented a challenge to the scientists who investigated it in the hope of finding its cause and a way to treat it or to prevent it by immunization. The scientists did discover the parasite that causes East Coast fever and they did discover the tick that transmits that parasite, but no one has yet discovered a cure or a preventive vaccine.

East Coast fever appeared at an interesting time. Modern methods of publication and communication were in place, but they had not been in place for very long. It was the age of the telegram, when long discussions, detailed analysis and thoughtful letters had their final effect only after being condensed to a few dozen words.[1] Although the foundations of modern bacteriology and parasitology were in place, East Coast fever appeared early enough to be studied by the first or second generation of bacteriologists, by the Cape of Good Hope's first government entomologist, and by one of the two founders of scientific bacteriology, Robert Koch. And yet it occurred at a time when its spread and the investigation of it were so extensively documented that it is possible to study its history in considerable detail.

No great scientific systems were overthrown in the course of the study of East Coast fever. But that study does provide a well-documented example of what Butterfield called "those cases in which men not only solved a problem but had to alter their mentality in the process." It is also a "detailed study of . . . scientific workers whose names have been comparatively unknown." The best work on East Coast fever was done by two scientific workers, Charles Lounsbury and Arnold Theiler, who are far less well known than Robert Koch and their work was hampered by their reliance on the earlier work of that "great figure." I have tried, again in Butterfield's words, "to discuss the particular intellectual knots that had to be untied" by Lounsbury and Theiler, knots that had been tied by Koch.[2]

The fact that East Coast fever is a disease of cattle rather than of human beings adds to its interest, as does the fact that it is a disease of the tropical and subtropical parts of the world. What Kenneth Warren[3] has called "the great neglected diseases of mankind" are, by and large, diseases caused by parasites. They are also particularly common in tropical and subtropical areas and in developing countries. As John A. Pino points out,[4] the "neglected diseases of livestock" are of equal or greater economic importance. Not only have those diseases been neglected, so has the study of their history.

Historians of medicine will note another feature of the history of this disease of cattle. By 1900 nearly all studies of diseases that affect human beings were published in scientific or medical journals. But that was not true of the publication of the results of studies of diseases of animals. The classic study of Texas fever by Smith and Kilborne appeared, in 1893, as a report of the U.S. Department of Agriculture. East Coast fever, another disease of cattle, was also studied under the auspices of governmental departments of agriculture. As a result, although most of the early studies of East Coast fever eventually appeared in scientific journals, they were initially published as government documents or as annual reports, which are much harder to locate than are most scientific journals.

Although several of the men who played a role in the early story of East Coast fever later played an important role in advancing scientific agriculture in Great Britain, the title *Science and Empire* should not lead the reader to expect a profound enquiry into the social and economic implications of the role of the British Empire in the conduct of scientific research.[5] That title does, however, capture some essential features of the story of East Coast fever. Although the disease had long been present in German East Africa (now Tanzania) it was first seen by a European scientist when Robert Koch observed it in Dar-es-Salaam while on a tour of duty for the German government. The massive outbreak which is the subject of this book began in 1901 when cattle were shipped from Dar-es-Salaam to restock the herds of Rhodesia, where colonial settlers had begun to arrive only eleven years earlier. The discovery of the disease and of its cause took place in three British colonies, Rhodesia, the Transvaal and the Cape of Good Hope. Important decisions had to be taken in London, either by the Colonial Office or by the British South Africa Company. None of the twenty or so government officials, scientists and practical veterinarians who played an important role in the story of East Coast fever was educated or trained in either Rhodesia or South Africa, and only one was born in South Africa. Even J. G. Kotzé, who was born in South Africa, studied law in London. The rest were immigrants, or like Koch and his assistants, visitors. The men who coped with East Coast fever were born and educated in Ireland, Scotland, England, Germany and Switzerland; one, educated in Massachusetts, was actually born in Brooklyn, N.Y. Many of them thought of and referred to the United Kingdom as "home." Even in the post-colonial era East Coast fever has attracted international interest: the most important internationally supported center for research on diseases of animals in Africa, the International Laboratory for Research in Animal Diseases (I.L.R.A.D.), directs much of its attention to the study of East Coast fever. As that suggests, the history of East Coast fever is of interest for yet another reason, which is that the disease is still a major burden on the economy of large parts of Africa.

In 1982 the government of Zimbabwe published two stamps to commemorate the centenary of Robert Koch's discovery of the tubercle bacillus. When I bought a first-day cover in Harare in 1984, I found that the official insert[6] contained a brief history of the importance of tuberculosis, of the importance of Koch's research on it, *and*, in passing, a remark that Koch had conducted research in Rhodesia. That remark made me wonder what had brought Koch to Rhodesia: the present book is the result. If I had, at that time, known of Dr. Deborah Dwork's excellent article[7] on some aspects of Koch's visit to Rhodesia my curiosity might have been satisfied, but by the time that Dr. Vivian Nutton called it to my attention I was already surrounded by photocopies of various source materials.

Because I have tried to write both a study and a story, I have included not only things that struck me as being either interesting or important but also a few things that seemed to me to be amusing. I have not hesitated to document the foibles and idiosyncracies of some of the individuals who played a role in the story. I have also resorted to fairly extensive direct quotation to convey the views of the scientists and the officials of the various governments in their own words and to convey the flavor of the time and place.

Most of this book deals with events that occurred in 1902, 1903 and 1904; I have followed Arnold Theiler's work on certain parasites through to 1910. The chapter on the eradication of East Coast fever in South Africa and Rhodesia deals with events between 1904 and the 1950s. Chapter 11 reviews one aspect of the scientific study of East Coast fever between 1910 and 1988 and shows that animals that suffer from East Coast fever develop both a condition that resembles leukemia and a condition that resembles AIDS.

I ordinarily use the place name that was in use during the colonial period, and often add the present-day name in parentheses. In this I have followed D. N. Beach:[8] "for colonial centres and colonial titles, colonial terminology has been retained." The place names of the colonial period that appear most frequently are Rhodesia (Zimbabwe), Salisbury (Harare), Fort Victoria (Masvingo), Gwelo (Gweru), Melsetter (Chimanimani), and Umtali (Mutare). I sometimes use "South Africa" loosely to describe the four colonies that did not, in fact, become the Union of South Africa until 1910, and I sometimes refer to Rhodesia as a colony. In early reports each initial letter in the name of a disease was often capitalized, as in Redwater, Rhodesian Redwater or Texas Fever. I have followed the style of the source in direct quotations and in passages where it is clear that an indirect quotation is being made. Elsewhere I retain initial capitals only for geographical names, e.g. Rhodesian redwater, Texas fever, East Coast fever.

Most of the material that I cite from the National Archives of Zimbabwe is from the extensive records of the British South Africa Company, often incorrectly said to have been destroyed during the Second World War. As Baxter pointed out, most of the departmental records of the B.S.A.C. remained in Rhodesia after it became independent of the Company in 1923 and a large quantity of additional material was returned from London in 1936.[9] It was the 23,000 files that remained in London that were destroyed by an air raid in 1941. Much of the material in the files of the British South Africa Company is also found in the Colonial Office files at the Public Record Office, but some material of crucial importance is found only in the National Archives of Zimbabwe. For that reason I am much indebted to the staff of that archive, as well as to those who created it and those who have done an excellent job of maintaining it and its facilities since Zimbabwe became independent in 1980.

I have consulted two bibliographies which are not cited elsewhere in the text, one by B. A. Matson[10] and one by Robert Uskavitch[10]. Another useful secondary source has been P. J. Posthumus's compilation of biographies of South African veterinarians.[11]

I have been helped by the patient and expert typing and retyping of a frequently revised manuscript by Ms. Nalayini A. Fernando. I am deeply obligated to The Rockefeller University and I cannot close without mentioning that my office and laboratory at that University are in Theobald Smith Hall. It was Theobald Smith who discovered that the serious disease of cattle known as Texas fever is caused by a parasite and transmitted by ticks: the first problem that confronted the early investigators of East Coast fever was to decide whether it was a new disease or merely a virulent form of Texas fever. In addition, one of the great figures in the study of East Coast fever was Arnold Theiler, and it was in Theobald Smith Hall that his son, Max Theiler, developed the vaccine against yellow fever.

Acknowledgments

My special thanks go to Mrs. Paddy Vickery, head of the Historical Reference Collection of the Bulawayo Public Library. I wrote to her in July 1985 to enquire whether there was any material on Koch in the Bulawayo Public Library. Her three-page long, single-spaced reply, the result of hours of work, listed enough material to convince me that my project was worthwhile. Without Mrs. Vickery's letter of August 2, 1985, I might have gone no further.

Without the unstinting help and advice of Professor William Trager on abstruse parasitological matters, I might well have given up, and would certainly have made many more mistakes than I have; my thanks to him.

I am equally indebted to Miss Benita Horder, Librarian of The Royal College of Veterinary Surgeons, 32 Belgrave Square, London. Miss Horder and her staff repeatedly helped me to find otherwise inaccessible material and Miss Horder herself often called my attention to important material that I might otherwise have overlooked.

Mrs. Elsa W. Kostick and Miss Pat Mackey, of the library of The Rockefeller University, have been helpful far beyond the call of duty in seeking out, through inter-library loans, many books and articles that were by no means easy to track down and obtain; Mrs. Sonya W. Mirsky, Librarian of The Rockefeller University, has been equally helpful. I thank them, and I thank the almost invariably helpful staffs of many other libraries and all of those persons unknown to me who created those libraries or helped to preserve them over the years.

I am particularly indebted to Charles Webster, the late Charles B. Schmitt and the late E. H. Ackerknecht for their encouragement. I also thank Louis Bolze, who called my attention to Stanley Portal Hyatt's *The Old Transport Road*; Miss Sue Bramley, who provided me with copies of letters to David Bruce from G. Stanley Bruce; Professor David W. Brocklesby and Dr. C. G. D. Brown, who provided me with invaluable help with respect to chapter 11; the late William Coleman, who provided encouragement and advice; Lesley Cripps, for her help in arranging my visit to Hereward Cripps; Hereward Cripps and his family for sharing with me their memories of the early aftermath of East Coast fever; Basil Davidson, for calling my attention to Apollon Davidson's biography of Rhodes; Chris Doubleday, for his thoughtful and meticulous sub-editing of my text; Professor Donald W. Fawcett, for his advice on recent studies of East Coast fever and for his permission to publish the electron micrograph that appears on the jacket; Professor F. Fehrenbach of the Robert Koch-Institut des Bundesgesundheitsamtes and Mr. Klaus Gerber, Chief Librarian of that institute, for information about F. K. Kleine and Fred Neufeld; J. P. Fraser-McKenzie, for his advice about the cattle industry of modern Zimbabwe; Eric J. Freeman, Librarian of the Wellcome Institute for the History of Medicine, and his staff, for many courtesies; Mr. Robin Fryde of Thorold's bookstore in Johannesburg, for so promptly locating and sending me a copy of the long out-of-print biography of Arnold Theiler by Thelma Gutsche; John Garnett, for information about F. B. Smith; Professor Werner M. Graf, for advice on certain translations from German; Stuart Hargreaves, for directing me to Sinclair's article on the history of East Coast fever; the late D. A. Lawrence, for calling my attention to Gutsche's biography of Theiler; Professor John A. Lawrence, for valuable discussions of East Coast fever and advice on many specific problems; J. B. Loudon, M.D., for his advice on the role of cattle in African society; Professor Maclyn McCarty for many valuable discussions and for commenting on chapters 10 and 11; the late Drew Middleton, for many helpful discussions; Douglas and Monica Parham for their generous hospitality in Zimbabwe; Dr. Iain Pattison, for his advice on John McFadyean and on veterinary research in Great Britain; Professor T. O. Ranger, for reading and commenting on chapter 9; Professor Maria Rudzinska, for helpful discussions about the parasites that cause Texas fever and East Coast fever; Julia Sheppard, for help with the archives of the Contemporary Medical Archives Centre of the Wellcome Institute for the History of Medicine and for helpful suggestions as to other sources; Ms. Jill Sherratt and Mr. P. M. Thwaite of Charter

Consolidated for permission to reprint Figure 3; Professor Ralph Steinman, for reading and commenting on chapter 11; Professor Hao Wang, for many stimulating discussions; Professor Victor J. Wilson, for his advice on various translations of articles written in French; Dr. Michael Worboys, for lending me a copy of his doctoral dissertation; Dr. Conrad E. Yunker, for advice on tick-borne diseases in modern Zimbabwe; and three anonymous referees whose comments on an earlier draft of the book provided many helpful suggestions.

Since I do not know which libraries supplied the inter-library loans that have been so helpful, I cannot thank them by name, but only collectively. I can and do thank by name the libraries that I have used: they include, in New York: the library of The New York Academy of Medicine; the library of The Rockefeller University; the Central Research Library of the New York Public Library; the Mid-Manhattan branch of the New York Public Library; the General Society Library; and the library of the Century Association.

In London: the Public Record Office, Kew; the library of the Royal College of Veterinary Surgeons; the British Library (including the main library, the Official Publications Library, the Newspaper Library at Colindale, the Science and Reference Information Service, and the India Office Library and Records); various libraries of the British Museum, Natural History (the general library, the Entomology library and the Zoology library); the library of the Royal Botanic Gardens, Kew; the library and the archives of the Wellcome Institute for the History of Medicine; the library and the archives of the Wellcome Tropical Institute; the library of the Royal Society; the library of the London School of Hygiene and Tropical Medicine; the library of the Royal Commonwealth Society; the library of the Foreign and Commonwealth Office; the General Register Office, St Catherines House; the library of the Athenaeum Club; the library of the United Oxford and Cambridge University Club; and the library and archives of the Savile Club.

In Edinburgh: the National Library of Scotland and the library of the University of Edinburgh.

In Zimbabwe: the library and the archives of the National Archives of Zimbabwe, where I have always received friendly assistance and access to very important material; the Historical Reference Collection of the Bulawayo Public Library; the Queen Victoria

Memorial Public Library, Harare; the library of the Bulawayo Club; and the library of the Harare Club.

In Cape Town: the Cape Archives Depot; in Pretoria: the Transvaal Archives Depot; in Windhoek: the State Archives Windhoek and the Ludwig von Estorff Reference Library.

In Copenhagen: the University Library (Science section and Humanities section) and the Royal Library. In Oslo: the combined National and University Library. In Zurich: the Central Library of the City, Canton and University of Zurich.

For their hospitality during many visits to Zimbabwe, I am indebted to the Harare Club, the Bulawayo Club and the Umtali Club (now the Mutare Club). For extending the hospitality of the Umtali Club to me I am particularly grateful to Dr. Boyd Gillam.

1

Prologue

Almost all of the cattle in Rhodesia died in 1896: "total annihilation of the cattle by rinderpest – no milk, no beef in a few days – but lots of lovely smells from dead cattle." Thus Earl Grey, writing to his son from Bulawayo, Rhodesia, May 8, 1896.[1]

Less than six years later, after a slow and costly replacement of the cattle that had been wiped out by rinderpest, another almost invariably fatal disease of cattle broke out in Rhodesia. Originally thought to be a virulent form of an already well-known disease, Texas fever or redwater, it was, in fact, a disease never before seen in Rhodesia, a disease unknown to veterinary science, a disease that we now call East Coast fever.

Stanley Portal Hyatt, who made a living by operating ox-drawn wagon trains, and who was bankrupted by the death of his oxen, later wrote:[2]

Rinderpest was the Act of God. The spread of African Coast Fever was due entirely to the criminal folly of men . . . The Chartered Company's government was bombarded with requests, prayers, petitions to take prompt measures . . . The only answer was . . . that the plague did not exist . . . the reason was obvious – Rhodes had just died, and to admit the existence of a new cattle disease would have sent down Rhodesian shares.

Months afterwards, when all the cattle on the high veld were dead, the government found itself compelled to admit that mistakes had been made . . . I attacked them so strongly in the columns of one of the great London financial dailies, that they were compelled to do something. What they did was send Dr. Koch out to investigate. He could not stop the disease, because there were practically no more oxen to die; but he could tell them the cause of it.

Hyatt's letter, dated Hartley, Mashonaland, October 1, 1902, appeared anonymously in the *Financial News* on November 28, 1902, a few days after the great German bacteriologist, Robert

Koch, had been asked to undertake an investigation. Hyatt was wrong in his belief that his letter provoked the employment of Koch, he overvalued the results of Koch's work, and he was probably wrong in believing that the spread of the disease could have been prevented. But he was not wrong about the British South Africa Company's concern over the price of its shares. The day that his letter appeared a copy was sent by the Company's managing director in London to the Company's administrator in Salisbury with a covering letter:[3] "Some idiot sent the enclosed letter to the Financial News and it appeared this morning. Fortunately it is so obviously biased and extravagant that it produced no effect on the market . . . Do you think you can spot the writer?"

East Coast fever was not a new disease, but it was unknown to veterinary practice or veterinary science until it appeared in epidemic form[4] in Rhodesia late in 1901. The spread of the disease produced an angry public reaction directed against the local representatives of the British South Africa Company and an equally stubborn refusal by the public to follow sound expert advice. Urgent requests for help and advice went to Australia, Cape Town, Buenos Aires, London, Paris, Toulouse, Berlin, Baton Rouge and even the famous Texas cattle ranch, the King Ranch. The progress of the disease, and of the investigation of it, were followed closely by veterinary scientists throughout the world. The colorful and controversial Colonial Secretary, Joseph Chamberlain, furiously opposed the employment of a famous bacteriologist to investigate the disease because that bacteriologist was a German. In spite of Chamberlain's objections, Robert Koch, who was one of the founders of modern bacteriology, was brought from Berlin to Bulawayo at great expense (including a personal fee equivalent to £200,000 today), spent more than a year in Bulawayo and contributed little that was useful. While Koch was at work in Bulawayo, in South Africa a salaried government entomologist, Charles Lounsbury, and a salaried government veterinary bacteriologist, Arnold Theiler, sorted out the facts and got most of them right. It took more than fifty years to bring the epidemic fully under control in Rhodesia and South Africa. And all this may have been caused by a single infected tick or infected animal that managed to find its way, by sea and land, from Dar-es-Salaam to Umtali.

The spread of the disease

The annual Umtali Agricultural Show, in late April and early May, 1901, was a great success. Twenty prizes were awarded for cattle and the local newspaper, the *Rhodesia Advertiser*,[5] commented on May 9, 1901: "The cattle exhibits were really extraordinary for such a place as Umtali both as regards to quality and variety. We have no hesitation in saying that there are few places in Africa that could compete with Umtali for the quality of its cattle." On May 16, the *Advertiser* reported that a speaker at the Agricultural Dinner on May 3 had said that "the class of cattle now in Rhodesia . . . were much better than what was here before the rinderpest." After votes of thanks, the band struck up *God Save the King* and "there terminated one of the pleasantest social functions ever held in Umtali."

Less than a year later, on March 18, 1902, Lionel Cripps, whose farm was in the hills of the Vumba, well outside Umtali, made an entry in his diary:[6] "Large numbers of cattle are dying and have died during the past few months – the [illegible] have lost nearly all their spans [of oxen] and losses heavy in town. In Melsetter the disease is spreading and it is now bad in Salisbury."

Nothing had appeared in the *Rhodesia Advertiser* from May 1901 through September 1901 to suggest any problem. Although three cattle belonging to the Sanitary Board were quarantined for red-water in late June, the *Advertiser* published no reports of serious cattle disease in July or August, or even as spring approached, as it does in the southern hemisphere, in September. But on October 10 the *Advertiser* reported that the Sanitary Board had lost six more cattle and its issue of October 24 contained an official proclamation listing five areas in which "Red-Water" had broken out. It said: "By virtue of the provisions of the Animals Diseases Act of 1881, I hereby declare the said areas to be infected . . . no animals shall be allowed to stray or to be removed into any uninfected area from the said infected areas." One of the areas was the Quarantine Station of the Umtali Sanitary Board (19 cases) and another was the Water-works Farm, Umtali (29 cases). But the other three areas, with a total of 112 cases, were in Melsetter, which is nearly sixty miles south of Umtali and considerably further along ox-cart trails.

The spread was relentless. The *Rhodesia Advertiser* for November 14, 1901 reported that the Sanitary Board had been put to heavy expense in hiring cattle to replace those affected by the disease. On

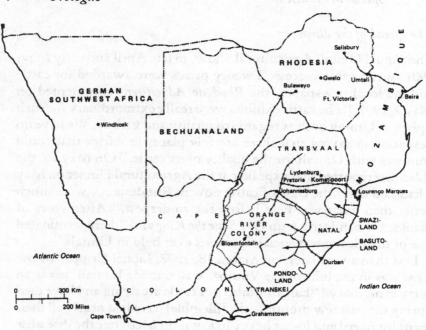

Fig. 1   Southern Africa: map showing places mentioned in the
text and showing railroads as of late 1901. Dar-es-Salaam is not
shown; it is on the coast of German East Africa (Tanzania)
about 1,000 miles north and 500 miles east of Beira. Based on a
map in R. I. Rotberg, *The Founder: Cecil Rhodes and the Pursuit
of Power*, New York, Oxford University Press, 1988.

December 5, the *Advertiser* carried another infected area proclamation, this time dealing with the Penhalonga Valley a few miles
north of Umtali, although there was still no comment in the news
columns. By January 23, 1902, we find another official notice in the
Advertiser: "Transport Riders and Cattle Owners in the Umtali
district are warned that by reason of the thorough infection of the
Umtali commonage with the 'RED-WATER TICK' Outspanning
or Grazing Animals on this ground is dangerous, as by so doing
there is considerable risk of losing unacclimatized cattle, and of
spreading the disease throughout the district."

That notice appeared again on January 30, 1902, but it was
probably far too late to check the spread of the disease, even if that
had ever been possible, for in the same issue we find that "the
disease is now unusually prevalent in the Salisbury, Umtali and

Melsetter districts." Within three months of the October outbreak the disease had reached Salisbury, 165 miles west of Umtali and was on its way south to Bulawayo, 275 miles south-west of Salisbury.

The *Bulawayo Chronicle* for April 25, 1902 noted that the disease had reached Gwelo, halfway from Salisbury to Bulawayo, where the "outbreak has been the sole topic of conversation in town for the past two days, for its serious nature cannot be underestimated." The same issue of the *Chronicle* contained a Government Notice: "during the prevalence of the Redwater in the Salisbury and Umtali districts, permits will not be granted to allow stock to move in the direction of Salisbury beyond Enkeldoorn." (Enkeldoorn, now Chivhu, is about 90 miles south of Salisbury and 85 miles north-west of Gwelo.) On April 29, the *Chronicle* reported that no cattle were to proceed from Gwelo towards Bulawayo, or to cross the Shangani river in the opposite direction (the Shangani is about two-thirds of the way from Bulawayo to Gwelo). But, on May 7, we read in the *Chronicle* that "a disease – whether redwater or not does not seem to be ascertained – has broken out . . . at Khami [a mere seven miles south-west of Bulawayo]," that "farmers in general view the situation with gloomy foreboding and fear that many cattle will be carried off," and that "the price of donkeys has risen further." The *Chronicle* of May 12 reported that "the much dreaded pest has made its appearance in Bulawayo." Much dreaded indeed:[7] "there was a stampede on account of it, in all directions, of white men fleeing with their cattle from the African Coast fever which had worked its way from Beira via Salisbury to Bulawayo."

Many Government Notices had appeared, designed to prevent the spread of the disease. A very different notice appeared on July 24, 1902, advising the public that "Farmers, Transport-Riders and others" would be given assistance in purchasing donkeys.[8] On August 5, 1902 the Board of Directors of the British South Africa Company appropriated £10,000 for that purpose and soon began attempts to buy donkeys in India and Spain,[9] thus conceding that oxen could no longer be relied on for transport in Rhodesia.

The annual Umtali Agricultural Show was held again the next year; it began on May 2, 1902. The *Rhodesia Advertiser* for May 8 described it as "a brilliant success," but there were no prizes for cattle. The cattle disease had appeared in Umtali in October, 1901; by May, 1902, there were no cattle left to compete for prizes. And if there were a few cattle still alive, their owners were certainly not going to risk bringing them to or anywhere near Umtali.

In the chapters that follow I will tell how the public reacted (usually by blaming the government while not cooperating with it); tell how several governments (that of the British South Africa Company, which governed Rhodesia, that of Great Britain, and those of South Africa) responded; tell of a prolonged and complicated search for expert advice; tell why, for purely local political reasons, the British South Africa Company insisted that Robert Koch work in Bulawayo instead of Pretoria and why that mattered so much; tell of the work of veterinarians and of scientists (especially Robert Koch and Arnold Theiler); tell how difficult it is to prove that a new disease is a new disease and to identify its cause; tell of the long struggle to contain the disease by quarantine, dipping to kill ticks, fencing and even the eradication of herds; tell what we know about East Coast fever today; and tell why Joseph Chamberlain, outraged at being asked to secure the services of Robert Koch, scribbled:[10] "if the Royal Society has another candidate I would suggest to Rhodesian Government that Bacteriology is not entirely 'made in Germany'. Then if they still want *Koch* they may ask him themselves." They did want him and they did ask him themselves – much good it did them.

2

The places and the players

It is not easy to set the stage on which our story was played. It is a story of two diseases, of two kinds of parasite, of two kinds of tick, of many governments and of many people. The diseases were redwater (Texas fever) and Rhodesian redwater (East Coast fever). The parasites were those that cause those diseases. The ticks were the blue tick and the brown tick, which have very different habits. As many as eight governments played a role: those of Great Britain, Germany, Rhodesia and Australia, as well as the governments of the four provinces of what is now the Republic of South Africa. (When East Coast fever first invaded South Africa, two of those provinces were British colonies: the Cape Colony and Natal. The other two provinces, about to lose the Boer War and become British colonies, were the still independent Orange Free State and the Transvaal.) As to people, they ranged from the Secretary of State for the Colonies (Joseph Chamberlain) and a future winner of the Nobel Prize (Robert Koch) to bankrupt European settlers and African communal farmers whose store of wealth and way of life were at risk.

The country that is now known as Zimbabwe was, for many centuries, protected from the outside world by being remote from the Indian Ocean and by being, along much of its eastern border, separated from that ocean by a mountain range. Thus protected, it largely escaped the attention of the slave trade. Its eastern regions were the object of Portuguese exploration and trading at market centers ("trade fairs" or "feiras") in the sixteenth, seventeenth and eighteenth centuries and even into the nineteenth century. Although Zimbabwe escaped actual colonization by the Portuguese, the Portuguese influence remained strong as late as the 1880s, particularly in the regions now known as eastern Mashonaland and Manicaland. Apart from that, the original peoples of what is now Zimbabwe were not seriously disturbed from outside their territory until 1838, when a group of Zulu origin, led by Mzilikazi, invaded the south-west. The main settlement of that group was named Bulawayo as two of Chaka's towns had been some years earlier. The region occupied by Mzilikazi and his followers (the Ndebele or Matabele) became known as Matabeleland; the rest of the country, still occupied by the Shona, became known as Mashonaland, at least for the administrative purposes of the British South Africa Company.[1]

Livingstone's Zambezi expeditions occurred between 1853 and 1863. Europeans seeking elephant ivory, including the famous hunter F. C. Selous (known in fiction as Allan Quartermain), ranged far and wide across the region in the late 1870s and 1880s. Although the discovery of gold by Hartley and Mauch in the late 1860s had attracted what C. D. Rudd called a "rum lot" of adventurers to the country, it remained reasonably autonomous until Mzilikazi's successor, Lobengula, signed the fateful Rudd concession in 1888. The Rudd concession gave its grantees "complete and exclusive charge over all metals and minerals" in Lobengula's kingdom. The ownership of the Rudd concession was soon transferred to an organization called the Central Search Association, which continued to own it until the formation of the British South Africa Company. Rhodes and his partner, Alfred Beit, having amassed a huge fortune from the diamond and gold mines of South Africa, now proposed to extend the British empire in Africa to the north. That extension of the empire was to cost the taxpayers nothing, because it would be funded by a private company, the British South Africa Company, which, once formed, would be in a position to sell shares because it owned the Rudd concession with its promise of rich new gold fields.[2]

The British South Africa Company, the B.S.A.C. or Chartered Company, was granted a Royal Charter in October, 1889. That Charter gave, or appeared to give, the British South Africa Company extensive powers over the region that makes up the countries now known as Zimbabwe and Zambia, "including powers necessary for the purposes of government, and the preservation of public order" (subject, however, "to the approval of one of our Principal Secretaries of State," i.e. the Colonial Secretary). The charter thus appeared to give the directors of a shareholder-owned, profit-making company full governmental powers, powers ranging all

the way from the right to hang people to the right to print postage
stamps.[3]

The Chartered Company soon took advantage both of the Rudd
concession and of its charter, to send a small army, the "Pioneer
Column," north to "Fort Salisbury" (now Harare). This began the
occupation and colonial settlement of what was to become Rhodesia. A bewildering series of proclamations and legal maneuvers
designed to bring the government of the country under the control
of the Colonial Office occurred in 1891, but by 1892 the government of Rhodesia was, for all practical purposes, in the hands of the
Chartered Company and its Administrator, L. S. Jameson. In 1894
a complex agreement was reached which gave the Colonial Office's
High Commissioner for South Africa extensive powers to confirm
or overrule various actions, but the Chartered Company continued
to retain all day-to-day power.

In 1898, partly as the result of African uprisings and partly as the
result of the Jameson raid, which is discussed below and in chapter
6, the Colonial Office strengthened its control over Rhodesia by
restricting the power of the Chartered Company's Administrator
and by increasing the power of its own Resident Commissioner.
The Resident Commissioner was given "full power to call for
reports or information from the Administrator [and], on information furnished by him, the High Commissioner would act in
confirming, reserving or disallowing ordinances."[4] The decree of
1898 also created a local Executive Council and a local Legislative
Council but, in practice, the B.S.A.C. and its Administrator
remained in full control. However, although the Chartered Company's Administrator had full *local* power, he was subordinate to
the London office of the B.S.A.C. The Resident Commissioner
also had extensive *local* powers of oversight, but he too was subordinate, not only to the High Commissioner for South Africa but
also to the Colonial Office in London. And both the Administrator
and the Resident Commissioner had to deal with the colonial
settlers.

Between 1890 and 1898 Rhodesia had produced a little gold,
many problems and no dividends for the shareholders of the
B.S.A.C. But it had succeeded in one of Rhodes' goals, that of
attracting settlers, who increasingly demanded a role in the government. They did obtain seats on the Legislative Council in 1898. By
1902, the economic dislocation caused by the Boer War, combined

with the death of Rhodes, led to increased demands by the settlers for an even greater voice in the government, a voice which they obtained in 1903. East Coast fever thus appeared in a country that had two sources of governmental authority, the Chartered Company and the Colonial Office, and a settler population that was demanding more and more self-government. The Chartered Company and the Colonial Office had many reasons to distrust each other and the settlers were only too ready to distrust the Chartered Company and were not ready to take its view of the new cattle disease on faith.

The ticks

Both Texas fever (redwater) and East Coast fever are transmitted by the bite of a tick. There are four stages in the life of a tick. It begins life as an egg; that egg hatches to yield a "larva." The larva, having sucked blood from a host, retires for a time to grow, shed its skin, and emerge as a "nymph." The nymph, after it too has sucked blood from a host, in turn retires for a time, which it also dedicates to growing and to shedding its skin. Having shed its skin (or "moulted") the nymph emerges as an adult tick, either male or female. Adult ticks, having again fed on the blood of a host, mate. The fertilized female, engorged with blood, lays thousands of eggs.

The larval forms, the nymphs, the adults and the mating adults of the blue tick remain on the same animal. The female finally drops off that animal to lay her eggs on the ground. A tick that spends all of its life on one animal cannot transmit a disease by feeding on another animal. But the female blue tick, if she has fed upon an animal infected with Texas fever, acquires its causal parasite and passes it on to her eggs. The generation that is born from those eggs then infect the animal they feed upon. The brown tick, which transmits East Coast fever, passes through the same stages of egg, larva, nymph and adult, but each time it sheds its skin, it moves from one animal to another, and can thus, in a single generation, carry the disease from one animal to another. But the parasites do not appear in its eggs and thus do not pass from one generation to the next.[5]

Rinderpest

Rinderpest, the "cattle plague," is a lethal disease of cattle, of antelope and of some other wild animals.[6] It is not transmitted by ticks. It is caused by a virus and passes directly from one animal to another. The cattle plague moved from north to south over the continent of Africa, beginning along the east coast opposite Aden in 1889 and ending at the Cape in 1897. That plague killed virtually all of the cattle in southern Africa, including most of the cattle in Rhodesia. Efforts to prevent its spread included the killing of apparently healthy cattle belonging to the Africans, to whom the killing seemed to be done without reason. That apparently arbitrary slaughter unquestionably played a role in causing the uprising of 1896 (for other causes of that uprising, including mismanagement by the Chartered Company, see Ranger;[7] for an analysis of some of the other social, economic and political results of rinderpest in South Africa, see van Onselen).[8]

The cattle plague had other effects on the story of East Coast fever. Robert Koch was summoned to investigate it; his success in producing a partially and temporarily effective vaccine was one of the reasons why he seemed to the Rhodesian authorities to be the right man to investigate "Rhodesian redwater." Many of the scientists or veterinarians who figured in the rinderpest story, such as Gray, Hutcheon, Watkins-Pitchford, Robertson and Theiler, also figured in the later study of East Coast fever. Finally, it was the destruction of the cattle by rinderpest that necessitated the subsequent importation of cattle, including the cattle that brought East Coast fever into Rhodesia.

Redwater

Redwater (Texas fever) is a disease of cattle in which "pear-shaped" parasites appear in the red blood cells and destroy them. The pigment of the red blood cells, released into the blood stream, appears in the urine and makes it red, hence red urine or "red water." In Texas fever, when infected blue ticks feed upon an uninfected animal, the parasite that causes the disease infects the animal by way of the tick's saliva. An uninfected tick that feeds on an animal suffering from Texas fever in turn becomes infected by the parasite. Mature, infected female ticks drop off the animal after they have fed, and lay as many as 3,000 eggs. About half of those eggs, and of the larvae to which they give birth, remain infected with the parasite. The resulting infected offspring infect any animal they feed upon. Since a single infected female tick can produce at least two thousand infected offspring, each of which can infect a healthy animal, the ability of the tick to spread this disease is enormous.

Texas fever (redwater) was, by 1901, a well-known disease of cattle. It had long been prevalent in the south-western part of the United States (hence "Texas fever"). The role of the tick in spreading the disease, and the fact that the parasite could be carried forward to future generations of ticks by the egg of the tick, was demonstrated by Theobald Smith and F. L. Kilborne, and published by them in 1893.[9] Their study is regarded as a great classic for many reasons, not the least being that it gave the first proof of transmission of any disease from one animal to another by an arthropod. Texas fever had appeared in southern Africa by 1870 and was well established there by the 1890s. It concerns us because the outbreak of cattle disease that began in Rhodesia in October, 1901, was for many months regarded as being merely an unusually severe outbreak of Texas fever (redwater), severe enough to warrant a new name, "Rhodesian Redwater." The insistence of the government, advised by its veterinarians, that the disease was not new but was only a severe form of redwater not only delayed the study of the disease, it also infuriated the farmers, many of whom were convinced almost from the beginning that the disease was indeed a new one.

Gall sickness

Gall sickness or anaplasmosis is another tick-borne disease, caused by a parasite that invades and destroys red cells. It is carried by the same tick that carries redwater, it destroys red blood cells, and cattle can suffer from redwater and gall sickness at the same time. This explains the occasional reference to gall sickness as a possible cause of the death of the cattle that began to die in 1901, but in 1901 the term gall sickness was, as it still is, used loosely to mean any disease of cattle that is accompanied by jaundice. We will hear more of "true" gall sickness, or anaplasmosis, in chapter 10.

East Coast fever

Rhodesian redwater was renamed African Coast fever by Robert Koch because he believed that it was not redwater but a different disease, one that, although new to Rhodesia, had long been entrenched along the east coast of Africa. The term African Coast fever was soon replaced by the term East Coast fever. Like redwater, East Coast fever is transmitted by ticks. Both diseases appear in the warm and rainy season, during which ticks multiply profusely. Since the brown tick, which transmits the disease, was already widespread in Rhodesia, all that was needed to produce a serious outbreak was the introduction of the parasite.

Cattle infected with East Coast fever do not develop anemia, jaundice or red urine even though the parasite that causes the disease is present in the red blood cells. The parasite that causes East Coast fever is very different in appearance from the "pear-shaped" parasite of redwater, but when Robert Koch observed it in 1897 and described it in 1898, he regarded it as being only an immature stage or variant form of the pear-shaped parasite that causes redwater. He also thought that the disease he had seen was only a form of redwater.

The parasite that invades the red blood cells in East Coast fever does not multiply within those red blood cells nor does it destroy them; it multiplies within certain white blood cells (the lymphocytes), and in lymphoid tissues. The parasites within lymphoid cells were mentioned by Koch in 1903 and are known as Koch's blue bodies, but all of the early students of the disease regarded it as being characterized by an abnormal condition of the red blood cells. Moreover, an attack of East Coast fever can cause redwater to reappear in an animal that had previously recovered from redwater, and can cause the redwater parasite to reappear in that animal's blood.

Animals infected with East Coast fever develop a high fever, swollen lymph nodes and enlargement of other lymphoid tissues, including the spleen and the lymphoid patches in the intestine (Peyer's patches). The immediate cause of death is usually emaciation combined with massive edema (waterlogging) of the lungs. The clinical picture is very different from that of redwater yet, as we will see, Koch in 1898, and Gray and Robertson in 1902, looked on the new disease as being merely an unusually severe form of redwater.

Not only is the parasite that causes East Coast fever different from the parasite that causes Texas fever, it is transmitted by a different tick, the brown tick. The parasite that causes East Coast fever does not appear in the eggs of the brown tick. The new-born larvae are thus harmless, but, if they feed on an infected animal, they acquire the parasite. Having fed, they drop off the animal to moult and then, as nymphs, find a new animal to feed upon and to infect. Similarly, if an uninfected nymph feeds on an infected animal, it will, after it drops off and moults, become an adult tick capable of infecting the animal on which it feeds. The brown tick thus transmits the disease only if its larvae or nymphs, having fed on an infected animal, drop off and develop into the next stage, which infects a new animal. The parasite that causes Texas fever multiplies within the tick but need not multiply within the infected animal. The parasite that causes East Coast fever *must*, if it is to survive, multiply both within the tick *and* within the infected animal. The blue tick can transmit Texas fever (redwater) but cannot transmit East Coast fever. The brown tick can transmit East Coast fever but it cannot transmit Texas fever.

There are similarities between redwater and East Coast fever. Both are transmitted by ticks; in both a parasite can be found in the red blood cells; both cause a high fever in cattle; and emaciation and death can result from either disease. But there are striking differences between the diseases. In redwater, the red blood cells are destroyed, causing jaundice, anemia and hemoglobinuria (red water). In East Coast fever there is *no red water*! There are parasites in the red blood cells but they do not destroy the red cells, there is no jaundice, there is no anemia and, above all there is no red urine. The lungs are severely affected in East Coast fever but not in Texas fever. Moreover, cattle that have survived redwater and have thus become immune to it ("salted") can die very quickly from East Coast fever. Thus, as we will see, to argue that the new disease was only a severe form of redwater, the government veterinarians had to explain why it did not produce red urine, why it could strike down "salted" cattle, and why it affected the lungs.

The Chartered Company and East Coast fever

Four men figured prominently in the response of the British South Africa Company to the new cattle disease. They were by no means non-entities. W. H. Milton played a major role, since, as its "Administrator," he was the Chartered Company's senior figure in Rhodesia. J. G. Kotzé was Attorney-General, and was, from May 1902 to October 1902, Acting Administrator. J. M. Orpen was the Surveyor-General, responsible for all titles to land, and was also Minister of Agriculture; Charles E. Gray was the Government Veterinary Surgeon. Most of the conflict between the government and the farming, ox-transport and mining communities arose from the policies of Gray as enforced by Orpen, who was Gray's immediate superior.

Milton was born in England in 1854 and emigrated to the Cape Colony in 1878.[10] In 1891 he became Private Secretary to Rhodes when Rhodes was Prime Minister of the Cape Colony. Milton was sent to Rhodesia after the Jameson raid and soon became Chief Secretary for Native Affairs (in September 1896, at the end of the 1896 "uprising"). He became Acting Administrator in 1897 and Administrator in 1898. Credited with a complete reorganization of the government of Rhodesia and of its civil service, he was obviously very capable but he began as Rhodes' man and his allegiance was definitely to the B.S.A.C., and *not* to the Colonial Office. For better or worse, he was out of the country during a crucial period of the East Coast fever problem. (On April 15, 1902, the London-based directors of the Chartered Company appointed the Attorney-General of Rhodesia, J. G. Kotzé, to serve as Acting Administrator while Milton was on leave in London.[11] Milton must have left Salisbury before the middle of May, since he sailed for London from Cape Town on May 21. He did not return to Salisbury until late October; thus during a crucial period of our story he was on leave and Kotzé acted in his place.)

Kotzé was a member of an old and prosperous Afrikaner family that had settled in the Cape in 1691.[12] Born on November 5, 1849, he was baptized Johannes Gijsbert Kotzé but he later changed his name to John Gilbert Kotzé. He qualified for the Bar in London and soon became a judge. It is said that when he was appointed as a judge in the then British-controlled Transvaal in 1877 he was, at the age of 27, the youngest man ever to have been a judge in any British territory. His personal clerk, later to become his long-time friend, was H. Rider Haggard. Kotzé was Chief Justice of the High Court of the Transvaal from 1881 to 1898; at the end of his career he was a member of the Appellate Court in the Cape Province; he died in Cape Town in 1940. Kruger dismissed Kotzé from his post as Chief Justice of the Transvaal in 1898 because Kotzé had insisted that the court had a right to review legislation and to determine that it was unconstitutional. When he was sworn in for his fourth term as President of the Transvaal on May 12, 1898, Kruger denounced Kotzé for having assumed the "testing right" which is "the principle of the Devil" and compared him to Korah, Dathan and Abiram, who had also assumed the "testing right" until God destroyed them. (According to the sixteenth chapter of the Book of Numbers, the earth swallowed up Korah, Dathan and Abiram; Kotzé only had to move to Rhodesia.) The whole episode did its bit towards causing the Boer War since it helped to convince Alfred Milner that Kruger was "irredeemable and inaccessible to reason."

After Kruger dismissed him, Kotzé spent a couple of years in the Cape Colony and then, in 1900, became Attorney-General of Rhodesia, a post he held until some time in 1903, when he returned to South Africa (Kotzé's successor took office on April 7, 1903). Kotzé was obviously very able, but his commitment to Rhodesia was presumably tentative and temporary. He no doubt began to plan a return to South Africa as soon as the Boer War ended; moreover, his powers were only those of an Acting Administrator. He nevertheless played a decisive role during the search for outside expert advice.

On a day-to-day basis the problem of East Coast fever was in the hands of Joseph M. Orpen and Charles E. Gray. Orpen was not a young man in 1902: he was born in Dublin on November 5, 1828.[13] The son of a physician, he arrived in South Africa in 1846 and qualified as a surveyor in 1849. As a pioneer settler of the Orange Free State he was a member of its first Volksraad in 1853 and helped form its constitution in 1854. Between 1872 and 1896 he represented various constituencies in the Cape parliament and became known as the "father" of the Cape parliament and of the Cape civil service. He was appointed Surveyor-General, Minister of Lands and Minister of Agriculture of Rhodesia in January, 1897. Orpen, who had met Rhodes as early as 1877,[14] was described as "adventurous, tough, versatile, exceptionally active and intelligent." But he met his match in East Coast fever. Orpen regarded himself as having "for a layman unusual knowledge of chemistry, physiology and medicine."[15] He was convinced, both on the basis of his own experience as a "practical farmer" and on the basis of Gray's advice, that there was no new disease present, only a recrudescence of "Tick Fever." Somewhat unpersuasively, at least to readers of our time, he wrote, on May 22, 1902,[15] that "In the present stage of the World's advancement in science, the discovery of a new contagious disease would be almost as remarkable as the discovery of a new continent." That conviction, and Gray's advice, were to bring Orpen into angry conflict with the community at large and to cost him his position as Minister of Agriculture.

Charles E. Gray was a key figure in the history of East Coast fever. His career typifies the unsatisfactory status of the veterinary profession around 1900. Gray, who was born in Edinburgh on April 10, 1864, was originally a Post Office telegraphist and, as a telegraphist with the British army, was present at the relief of Khartoum. He qualified as a veterinarian (Member of the Royal College of Veterinary Surgeons, i.e. M.R.C.V.S.) in 1890 and, according to Posthumus,[16] went to America,

but found employment very scarce . . . he found work as an assistant to an M.R.C.V.S. colleague in Philadelphia, but after earning sufficient money to return home, he sailed for England. After a three week visit to his family he sailed for South Africa at the end of 1895, hoping to obtain work as a veterinary surgeon. Veterinary work was however unobtainable, so he reverted to his original training and became a telegraphist [in Rhodesia] on Jan. 1, 1896 . . . When rinderpest broke out in Rhodesia two months later the Rhodesian authorities approached Duncan Hutcheon (Chief Veterinary Officer of the Cape of Good Hope) for assistance, but he referred them to Gray's presence in their country.

Gray's work on rinderpest was interrupted by the 1896 uprising, so he joined the Army; after the uprising he still could not find work as a veterinary surgeon, so he once again became a telegraphist and a postmaster. Later in 1896 he was finally appointed "Acting Government Veterinary Surgeon"; he remained head of the veterinary department until 1905. L. E. W. Bevan, who met Gray in 1904, described him[17] as "a little Scot with shaggy eyebrows and moustache, a pair of twinkling eyes – for him everything was the best in the best of all possible worlds." Having struggled with East Coast fever for three years, Gray, almost certainly with a sigh of relief, became Principal Veterinary Surgeon of the Transvaal in 1905. In 1911 he became the first Principal Veterinary Surgeon of the Union of South Africa, a post he held until he retired in 1921. An obituary in the *Veterinary Record*[18] says that he had qualified in Edinburgh "with exceptional brilliancy" and that "His great work in fighting rinderpest and other cattle diseases has evoked many enthusiastic tributes." Yet he was all but unable to find employment as a veterinarian until six years after he had qualified. (This was not an uncommon story for the period: Arnold Theiler, who was to figure prominently in the history of East Coast fever, left Switzerland for lack of employment, and his early years in South Africa were very difficult.)

The Colonial Office

In 1902 the Resident Commissioner, who represented the Colonial Office in Rhodesia, was Marshall Clarke. He reported directly to the High Commissioner for South Africa, Alfred Milner, then based in Johannesburg. Milner in turn reported to the Colonial Office in London, sometimes directly to the Colonial Secretary, Joseph Chamberlain, and sometimes to other officials of the Colonial Office. I will discuss Milner at the beginning of chapter 4 and Chamberlain in chapter 6. Marshall Clarke was a professional administrator who had served with distinction in Basutoland and Zululand. He was Resident Commissioner in Rhodesia from 1898 to 1905, having been appointed soon after the reorganization of the Colonial Office's oversight of Rhodesia that followed the Jameson raid and the 1896 uprising.[19]

The Jameson raid

The Jameson raid, which is also discussed in chapter 6, affected everything that happened in South Africa and Rhodesia during the next few years, including the response to East Coast fever. In 1895, Rhodes, his partner Alfred Beit, and other men who represented gold-mining interests in or around Johannesburg, conspired to overthrow the government of the Transvaal. A "spontaneous" protest in Johannesburg was to be followed by a summons to a small army waiting on the border. That army, formed and led by the Administrator of Rhodesia, L. S. Jameson, was to ride in to help the protesters. The protesters were to seize the Johannesburg arsenal and they and Jameson's army were to seize Johannesburg itself. The High Commissioner for South Africa was then to intervene as a "mediator" and raise the British flag over the Transvaal. The plan was cancelled at the last minute but Jameson and his army rode in anyway. Their capture exposed the conspiracy, which came to be referred to as the Jameson raid even though the raid was only a small part of it.[20] As a result of the Jameson raid, the Colonial Office moved towards greater control over the B.S.A.C., Alfred Milner became the new High Commissioner, Earl Grey replaced Jameson as Administrator of Rhodesia, Milton was sent to Rhodesia and soon replaced Grey as Administrator, and Marshall Clarke became the new Resident Commissioner.

The transport riders

Before the building of the railroads, all movement of goods and materials in Rhodesia was in the hands of the "transport riders," who drove wagons or wagon trains hauled by donkeys, mules or trek-oxen. According to Stanley Portal Hyatt,[21] the full-sized bullock wagon was 18 feet long, and, if it had a $3^{1}/_{2}$-inch axle, could carry a load of 9,500 pounds. These were not fully covered wagons; they usually had only a half-tent, under which the driver lived. A fully-loaded 18-foot-long wagon was drawn by sixteen strong oxen; Hyatt himself preferred a 16-foot wagon that was drawn by sixteen lighter oxen: more mobile and moving faster, it could, in the course of a year, earn its owner more money than a heavy wagon, even though it could carry a load of only 8,000 pounds. Hyatt said that "The mines were dependent on the transport riders for their very existence." The transport riders went on rough roads or created roads where none had existed. As Hyatt put it, "in South Africa, a road is anything along which a wagon has once passed." The transport riders were the sole movers of goods before the railroads were built, and they remained almost as important for some time after the railways were built. They competed with the railways for long-distance transport and they remained indispensable for transport of goods from the railways to regions near the railways, and for transport in regions not served by the railways.

Buying and selling cattle and trading in other goods were the favorite sidelines of the transport riders. And the ordinary farmer had his own ox-drawn wagon, which he used to go from his farm to the nearby market town and back again. All of Rhodesia was infested with the brown tick, as were all of its oxen. Thus, as soon as East Coast fever was introduced, it was spread, via the brown tick and the transport riders' ox-drawn wagon trains. It spread first along the main routes and later along the byways. In many ways the story of the spread of East Coast fever is the story of the transport riders. And, by killing the oxen, East Coast fever destroyed the investment and the income of the transport riders. At his high point, just before the disease broke out, Hyatt reckoned that he and his two brothers "owned some six thousand pounds worth of property." At that time, between his income as a transport rider and his profits as a cattle trader, Hyatt hoped to become a rich man within two or three years. Instead, he soon found himself bankrupt, all four of his wagons "abandoned on the veld, abandoned beside the bones of their dead cattle." And, "a few months later we were just able to pay our fares out of that miserable country."

The Rhodesian veterinarians

In the section on Southern Rhodesia in *A History of the Overseas Veterinary Services,*[22] D. A. Lawrence suggests that Gray had seven young veterinarians at his disposal in 1902, all of them under thirty; namely O. A. O'Neill, J. J. Gorman, J. M. Sinclair, C. R. Edmonds, G. N. Tomlinson, E. M. Jarvis and G. S. Bruce. But I can find no evidence in the Southern Rhodesia Civil Service Lists[23] that Tomlinson was on Gray's staff in 1902; moreover, O'Neill left Rhodesia for South Africa early in 1902. That leaves J. J. Gorman, who joined the service early in 1897; J. M. Sinclair, who qualified in 1895 and joined the service in 1899; E. M. Jarvis, who qualified in 1894 and joined the service in January, 1901; C. R. Edmonds, who joined the service on October 26, 1901, and G. S. Bruce, who did not join the service until June 14, 1902 and arrived in Rhodesia only in July, 1902. This means that between early October, 1901, and July 1, 1902, while East Coast fever was spreading throughout the country, Gray had the help only of O'Neill, who was about to leave, and of Gorman, Sinclair, Jarvis and Edmonds. In the middle of 1903, with East Coast fever well entrenched and still spreading, the staff consisted of Gray, Jarvis, Sinclair, Gorman, Edmonds and G. S. Bruce. But by then, Gray and Sinclair were in Bulawayo assisting Koch, and Edmonds was on general veterinary duty in Bulawayo, which left the rest of the country in the hands of Jarvis, Gorman and Bruce.

There was also a staff of some fifteen laymen who worked as cattle inspectors, but Gray and his staff were badly overworked, trying as they were to cope with many serious diseases of livestock. None of them had been trained in microbiology and they were suddenly confronted with the swift spread of a previously unknown and lethal disease of cattle, one with which they were ill-equipped to deal.

The South African experts

Various veterinarians and scientists in the South African colonies were drawn into the East Coast fever problem; they included the veterinary bacteriologists Alexander Edington, William Robertson and Arnold Theiler, the veterinarians Herbert Watkins-Pitchford and Stewart Stockman, and the entomologist Charles Lounsbury. They are identified more fully in the text or notes. The Chief Veterinary Surgeon of the Cape of Good Hope, Duncan Hutcheon, played a special role, both as the most experienced veterinarian in southern Africa and as head of a well-staffed department.[24] Gray and Hutcheon exchanged letters about the new disease as early as March, 1902; Hutcheon sent Robertson to Salisbury in May 1902 and came to Salisbury himself in August, 1902. He was a key advisor in the search for expert advice, he joined Arnold Theiler in important investigations in the Transvaal in early 1903 and he constantly supported the work of Charles Lounsbury.

3

A new disease?

The first false trail in the history of East Coast fever arose from the belief that it was a virulent form of redwater introduced into Rhodesia by cattle that were imported by Cecil Rhodes at the end of 1900 to replenish the herds that had been destroyed by rinderpest. On May 26, 1900, while on a visit to Rhodesia, Rhodes wrote to the High Commissioner for South Africa, Alfred Milner, as follows:

> The bearer, Mr. Ross, one of our native commissioners, is going to Australia to buy cattle; kindly advise him and give him a letter of introduction. I am already preparing for settling the Colonial or Englishman choosing to remain. I have added to irrigating ideas, dry farms with cattle, and am sending Ross to Australia to buy the first 1,000 head ... The Colonials are very pleased with this country [Rhodesia] and they must remain, at any rate some ...
>
> I want to settle the Colonials, start the railway to the Victoria Falls, see the mines personally and form my judgment as to gold prospects, help Milton to start his North-Eastern Rhodesia and see to the telegraph to Egypt, besides many other minor details.[1]

The cattle (999 of them) arrived at the port of Beira in Mozambique in December, 1900. (We will hear of Beira again: as the seaport closest to Rhodesia, it was an important point of entry; it still is of vital importance to Zimbabwe.) Some 200 of the Australian cattle died at Beira; the rest were moved to Umtali, where they were quarantined in January, 1901. By March, 1901, all but three of the cattle were dead: on March 14, the *Rhodesia Advertiser* published a letter which complained of "the unsanitary state of the town," the result of "the death of nearly a thousand head of cattle, many being unburied." Since most of the Australian cattle died in Umtali, the disease that appeared there the following October was blamed on the imported cattle by many early observers. As we have seen in chapter 1, there was no sign of disease among the local cattle when the Umtali Agricultural Show was held in late April and early May, 1901, which is hardly what one would have expected if the Australian cattle had introduced a new and lethal disease to the local herds as early as January of that year. In fact, the Australian cattle almost certainly died of various diseases already present in Beira and Umtali, diseases (including redwater and anaplasmosis) to which they had no immunity.

The conviction of the farmers and transport riders that the disease had been brought into the country by the Australian cattle was so strong that on May 29, 1902, the Resident Commissioner at Mafeking urged the High Commissioner to ask the Governor–General of Australia for information about Rhodes' cattle.[2] On May 30, Milner telegraphed Kotzé

I am informed cattle disease . . . probably introduced by . . . a thousand cattle . . . imported . . . from Australia . . . if you think that any information could be obtained from Australia which might help . . . I am prepared to communicate with the Governor-General by telegraph, but I should require full details as to the circumstances under which the cattle were purchased and as to the reasons for attributing the infection to them.[2]

Kotzé replied at length the next day, May 31, 1902, that the Agricultural Department was certain that the disease was tick fever or redwater, and that a bacteriologist from the Cape (Robertson) had confirmed that opinion.[2] "It has not been any professional authorities who doubted the nature of the disease but uninformed persons who would not accept the decisions of professional authorities . . . [and who] have assumed that the disease was imported from Australia." Nevertheless, Kotzé thought, it might be useful to find out whether any such disease existed in the part of Australia where the cattle came from "in order to satisfy the South African public mind."

On June 5, the Governor of Natal also warned Milner about the Australian cattle,[3] but by then Milner had already made the first appeal for advice from outside southern Africa. On June 2, 1902, he telegraphed to the Governor-General of Australia, Lord Hopetoun:[2]

A virulent form of cattle disease is now prevalent in Rhodesia which is stated to be Tick Fever called locally Redwater. It has been suggested that the disease may have been imported by a shipment of cattle purchased in Sydney for the Chartered Company . . . Little value is attached to the suggestion by the Rhodesian Authorities but I should be glad if the history of the cattle in question could be traced and if you could inform me authoritatively whether this or any other disease existed among them or in the districts from which they came. It would be of great assistance to know what treatment is found most successful in dealing with tick fever in Australia.

Hopetoun replied on July 14 that there was no reason to believe that the disease was imported into Rhodesia by cattle from New South Wales or Queensland. Hopetoun's reply was accompanied by persuasive documentation. The Government Veterinary Surgeon, J. D. Stewart, reported from Sydney, on June 18, 1902, that the cattle were purchased by Ross in districts where neither tick fever nor the cattle tick had been known to exist. Moreover, "before embarkation the cattle were inspected by an Inspector of Stock and declared free of contagious and infectious diseases. They were also very carefully inspected by Mr. Ross. No enzootic or epizootic diseases have been reported from the districts where the cattle were selected, with the exception of isolated cases of tuberculosis and actinomycosis."[4] A statement from the Chief Inspector of Stock, P. R. Gordon, dated June 14, 1902 said "It would have been impossible for the Tick fever to have been introduced into Rhodesia from New South Wales, for the reason that it has never existed in that State." As to Queensland, no cattle had been shipped from there. Gordon enclosed reports and articles on protective inoculation against tick fever, an architectural plan for a dipping station, and a copy of Lignières' review of redwater, the definitive study available at the time.[5] On August 16, 1902, Milner forwarded the report and its enclosures to Marshall Clarke, the Colonial Office's Resident Commissioner in Salisbury.[6]

The belief that the "new disease" had been imported along with the Australian cattle caused endless confusion and poisoned the debate between the government and the settlers throughout 1902 and 1903. The government veterinarian, Gray, knew that the Australian cattle were not the cause of the outbreak, but the settlers were convinced that the Australian cattle had introduced and spread the disease, and they blamed the government for having failed to begin to control the spread of the disease the moment the Australian cattle had died.

Although many people believed for many years after the first outbreak of the new disease that it had been introduced by the

Australian cattle, J. M. Sinclair stated as early as 1910[7] that "There is no doubt whatever that these Australian cattle died of Redwater, pure and simple, which they contracted on Beira flats, Coast fever being introduced into Beira subsequent to the arrival and departure of the Australian cattle." Two of the three Australian cattle that survived in Umtali were sent to Salisbury where they did in fact die of East Coast fever. Around 1908, R. F. Stirling[8] was shown an animal on the farm of a member of the government veterinary services that was said to be the sole survivor of the original 999.

It is easy to imagine how shocked the local farmers must have been by the death of a large herd of cattle brought at great cost all the way from Australia by Rhodes himself and it is not surprising that so many settlers persisted in their belief that the outbreak that occurred many months after the arrival of those cattle had something to do with the new plague. It is all but certain that it did not, but there remains some small doubt about just when East Coast fever did arrive in Rhodesia and how it was spread from Beira to Umtali and to Salisbury. It must have arrived after the cattle-proud Umtali Agricultural Show that ended on May 3, 1901. If the outbreaks in October, 1901, were caused by East Coast fever, the disease must have arrived by early October. On the other hand Sinclair[7] blamed it on "a lot of cattle shipped at Dar-es-Salaam . . . some were landed at Beira, several truckloads were sent by rail to Umtali, two of which went on to Salisbury. Disease broke out among both lots, but its true nature was not recognized." The rest of those cattle stayed on the ship and went to the port of Lourenço Marques (Maputo) on Delagoa Bay in Portuguese East Africa (Mozambique), from where the disease was later introduced into the Transvaal.

Unfortunately Sinclair, who suggested that this may have happened as late as December, 1901, did not specify exact dates; if this was the first introduction of East Coast fever the disease should have broken out in Salisbury at almost the same time that it broke out in Umtali. It is a small point: either the disease was introduced to Umtali and then spread via the ox-transport route to Salisbury or it was introduced to both Salisbury and Umtali in the way that Sinclair thought. There is a very faint possibility that the outbreak in October, November and December of 1901 was redwater and that the new disease, East Coast fever, really did appear more or less simultaneously in Umtali and Salisbury in January, 1902. In any event, Gray, Sinclair and other later students of the subject eventually agreed that East Coast fever was introduced into Rhodesia by cattle imported from German East Africa (now Tanzania), where it remains prevalent today.[9]

Although the Umtali Agricultural Show, held in late April and early May, 1901, was notable for the quality and variety of its exhibits of cattle, an angry exchange about the Australian cattle had already occurred. A letter signed "an Australian" had appeared in the (Salisbury) *Rhodesia Herald* in March, 1901 saying that "This country is not stocked because all the stock that were here in 1896 are dead from rinderpest." An editorial in the *Rhodesia Advertiser* of March 28, 1901, rejoined:

The stock raiser in Rhodesia has had the following things to contend with during the ten years' occupation of this country: Two native wars; one Boer war; rinderpest (killing 99% of all stock in Rhodesia); anthrax; lung-sickness; red-water; ticks (real ticks – not the Australian harmless tick, but a real poisonous crab-tick, requiring a blow from a sledge hammer to kill it); embolism; pleuro-pneumonia; dysentery among calves . . . locusts; wild animals; floods and droughts; unhealthy climate for man and beast; scarcity of competent veterinary surgeons; high – extremely high – prices of veterinary services and medicines; and other difficulties too numerous to mention.

These remarks, which appeared six months *before* the new outbreak, reveal a climate of public opinion that would become much more accusatory as East Coast fever ran out of control, the opinion of a public that was by no means prepared to accept reassurance from its government.

Whether the disease reached Rhodesia in October, 1901 or January, 1902 it certainly forced itself on Gray's attention on January 14 and 15, 1902, when he received four ominous telegrams from Umtali. Two were from the government veterinary surgeon, E. M. Jarvis:[10] "Urgently desire your opinion . . . serious outbreak occurring here. Can you come at once utmost importance you should do so without delay" and "Disease new to me. Do not believe it Rinderpest . . . might bring Serum & syringes." The other two were from the Resident Magistrate: "re Jarvis wire . . . it is urgent that you come down at once" and "It has the symptoms of anthrax, gall sickness & rinderpest."

The first systematic review of the outbreak is found in Charles E. Gray's report for the year ending March 31, 1902.[11] Although that

report was not published until 1903, Gray sent most of it in a letter
to Duncan Hutcheon on April 11, 1902. Gray also sent a copy of
that letter to Alexander Edington in Grahamstown. At the beginning of the letter Gray thanked Hutcheon for sending him his views
and those of others on the nature of the outbreak. Gray said he was
inclined towards Edington's view[12] but he added that he saw no
reason not to suppose that "we are simply passing through an
unusually severe Redwater season with extensive invasion of areas
hitherto only slightly infected." If so, he said, he must have been
mistaken in his belief that the Salisbury and Umtali areas had
previously been thoroughly infected with redwater.

Gray rejected the possibility that the disease had been imported
from Australia. He said that some of the Australian cattle had died
from acute redwater, typically accompanied by severe constipation
and hemoglobinuria, some had died from a lingering chronic form
of redwater, typically characterized by emaciation and anemia, and
that the rest had died from gall sickness. He added that he had no
record of any marked mortality amongst local stock from the
disorder at that time. Moreover, "the present wet season [roughly
November, 1901 through February or March, 1902] was characterized by . . . an abnormal number of ticks everywhere . . . [and] by a
severe outbreak of typical cases of redwater at Salisbury . . . [and]
almost simultaneously . . . a still more severe one . . . at Umtali."
But, as time went on, he began to see cases of redwater that were
less typical; not only were the animals not constipated but they died
without having developed red urine (hemoglobinuria). Gray discounted that finding by citing a report from Queensland that said
that hemoglobinuria is not an invariable finding in redwater.
However, "about the middle of January [1902] when these atypical
cases appeared in Salisbury I received a pressing telegram . . . asking
me to come through [to Umtali] as sickness amongst stock was
very prevalent and seemed to be of an undecided character . . . and
presented symptoms suspicious of anthrax, gall-sickness and rinderpest." The first group of twelve animals he examined in Umtali
were "in a bad state" but none of them showed hemoglobinuria.
While in Umtali, Gray examined three groups of animals (about
fifty in all), conducted a complete autopsy of a dead animal, made
microscopic studies of the spleen and blood which appeared to rule
out anthrax, and found that the injection of rinderpest serum did
not improve the condition of the two animals in which it was tried.

But he and Jarvis agreed that the sickness was simply redwater, sometimes perhaps complicated by an additional infection.

On January 16, 1902, two stories appeared in the *Rhodesia Advertiser*. One said that Gray and Jarvis "believe that the present outbreak is largely due to the abundant presence . . . of the redwater tick whose numbers are so great that animals . . . which might reasonably be supposed [to be immune] have developed a modified form of the disease complicated by a septic infection." A column headed "Farm Notes" called for "some definite pronouncement from the veterinary experts as to the nature of the sickness which is carrying off cattle which the country can ill spare" and complained that "the authorities are not taking sufficiently stringent measures to stop the spread of a disease that may be highly contagious . . . more energy ought to be infused into those who have the working of our laws."

After Gray left Umtali he reassured the farming community in a 1,500-word pamphlet entitled "Redwater, Tick Fever, Texas Fever or Bovine Malaria" that was published in Salisbury[13] and was reprinted in full in the *Advertiser* on January 30, 1902. (The *Bulawayo Chronicle* paid no attention to it until May 1, 1902, less than two weeks before the disease reached Bulawayo.) The pamphlet began "A few notes on the nature of the above disease, and hints as to simple precautions which may be adopted with a view to its prevention, may prove of service, seeing it is now unusually prevalent in the Salisbury, Umtali and Melsetter districts." Gray went on to say that "Bovine malaria is known and recognized in almost every quarter of the globe . . . [and] a fairly clear understanding of . . . its causation and the manner in which it spreads has been arrived at . . . red or highly coloured urine . . . is a usual but not invariable symptom." Since "redwater is spread, not directly from animal to animal, but by way of the cattle tick . . . any measure [which] . . . reduces the number [of ticks] attached to an animal increases that animal's chances of escaping the disease." Gray went on to give a formula for tick dip and a formula for preventing the disease by administering a concoction of carbolic acid, quinine and linseed oil. A similar concoction, containing calomel along with the other ingredients, was recommended for treatment of the disease. Rest, palatable food and oatmeal gruel were also recommended. Later in his pamphlet Grey remarked that: "Mr. H. Hayes . . . says of this disease: 'formerly it was known . . . as redwater disease . . . [but]

haematuria (blood-coloured urine) has no necessary connection with this malady, and is not a constant symptom of it'." Gray added, much less persuasively, that "Smith and Kilborne (American investigators) found haematuria in 33 out of 46 cases."

The "Farm Notes" column of the *Advertiser* for February 6, 1902 commented:

Public confidence has been somewhat restored, thanks to the efforts of the veterinary staff and to their diagnosis of what was first thought to be a new disease among cattle. It is now pronounced to be our old friend 'red-water' under a new guise. Tick-fever would be a better name for the disease, as red-water is not a symptom of the present outbreak. It is gratifying to note that the Manica Farmers' Association passed a vote of thanks to Messrs. Gray and Jarvis for their good work done. Men of their stamp are needed in this country.

This was the last praise Gray was to get.

Reverting to Gray's annual report:[11] after he returned to Salisbury, in January, 1902, Gray found "typical cases of redwater occurring everywhere, here and there interspersed with cases of an atypical nature." Gray also found cases that showed a condition that is far from typical of redwater, waterlogging (edema) of the lungs associated with coughing up "masses of ... albuminous froth." That condition is, in fact, a characteristic finding in East Coast fever and Grey even noted that

nowhere in any redwater literature to which I have had access have I found any reference to changes in the lungs, save a casual remark made by M. Lignière [*sic*] who says he has found but little the matter with the lungs, save in some cases a tendency to a condition of oedematous pneumonia, but I inferred from the tone of his remark that someone else had described lung lesions associated with redwater.

Gray noted, on autopsy, marked infiltration of the mesenteric lymph glands, which is not found in redwater, and massive enlargement of the spleen, which is characteristic of redwater but not of East Coast fever. He also reported that he had found the typical redwater parasite in blood smears.

Puzzled by the massive pulmonary edema, Gray took two calves "previously immunized to redwater" and inoculated them with blood from a case "which showed emphysema of the lungs at post-mortem." The animals remained in perfect health but, as was learned later, East Coast fever cannot be transmitted by a single inoculation of the blood of an infected animal into an uninfected

animal. In further justification of his conclusion that the outbreak
was one of redwater, Gray noted that

it seems improbable that animals grazing on the same veldt and associated
closely with each other should fall victims to two distinct infections, and
that some of these should present all the typical indications of ordinary
redwater, including the demonstrated presence of the pyrosoma [the
Texas fever parasite] while others showing post-mortem appearances
more or less identical to those of the typical cases should be considered to
be suffering from a different disease because no haemoglobinuria is evident at post-mortem, or because there is pronounced pulmonary disturb-
ance of a type, which, so far as I know, has not been previously described.

Gray went on to attribute the waterlogging of the lungs to the
excessive labor of breathing caused by the anemia and by the
altitude, Umtali and Salisbury being well above sea level. He thus
explained away both the absence of red urine (hemoglobinuria) and
the presence of pulmonary edema.

The argumentative tone of Gray's report suggests that he had
some doubts about the "atypical" cases. If he did, he suppressed
them, which is a pity because he was the first person to observe and
report the clinical and post-mortem characteristics of East Coast
fever. According to Gray, as of March 31, 1902, "In Umtali over
400 animals have died during the past five months, . . . in Salisbury
the loss now stands at about 500; mortality having gone up with a
bound . . . during the last three weeks of fine weather."

The farmers and the transport riders may have been reassured by
Gray's pamphlet of January, 1902, but they did not stay reassured
for long. An editorial in the *Rhodesia Advertiser* of March 13, 1902
urged the government to seek further expert advice. On March 18
Lionel Cripps had become sufficiently concerned to make the entry
in his diary that is quoted in chapter 1, and on March 29, at Cripps'
invitation, Gray again addressed the Umtali Farmers Association.
The importance of the matter can be judged by the amount of space
that the *Advertiser* devoted to Gray's remarks. Cecil Rhodes, the
founder of Rhodesia, regarded as a benefactor and hero by most of
the Rhodesian settlers, had died on March 26: the *Advertiser* of April
3 devoted a column and a half to the death of Rhodes and almost as
much space to a report of Gray's address to the farmers. Gray said
that he had no hesitation in describing the present outbreak as
redwater and recommended that all the young stock be inoculated
with blood from an animal which had recovered. He added that

"the disease was redwater with the addition of a pyaemia tick to give extra trouble ... Mr. Strickland mentioned that salted [i.e. immune] redwater animals had died. Mr. Gray said this was quite possible as they may succumb to another form of the disease."

Having again reassured the farmers of Umtali, Gray returned to Salisbury on April 7, only to find that on April 5 the Rhodesian Landowners and Farmers Association had sent a telegram[14] from Bulawayo to Surveyor-General Orpen, demanding that the government "take immediate steps to prevent disease reaching this province. Association request you to proclaim broad closed area between Mashonaland and Matabeleland otherwise stock farmers and mining companies threaten to dispose of all stock held by them owing to their fear of the disease, which would be a terrible blow to this country." The Secretary of the Association sent a longer telegram to the same effect.[15] Since Orpen was, in fact, visiting Bulawayo, Gray had to send two long telegrams to deal with the situation, one to Orpen and one to the Landowners and Farmers Association.[16] Gray assured Orpen that the disease had subsided since the weather became cooler and that it had not extended to native cattle. Gray said that he had directed cattle inspectors everywhere to detain wagons with sick oxen until the spans were clean and to report detention by wire, so that he could ascertain the extent to which the disease prevailed throughout the country. As to the "suspension of ox transport over a wide belt between Gwelo and Bulawayo ... I have replied ... that ... disease is result of Redwater infection."

To the Landowners and Farmers Association Gray telegraphed[16] that

there is no immediate cause for alarm as the sickness ... which is apparently subsiding ... is ... Redwater ... disseminated indirectly by ticks as malaria is said to be by mosquitoes ... Instructions have been issued to all cattle inspectors to detain any sick cattle ... and cattle inspectors have been requested to warn any transport rider that this disease has been prevalent at Umtali and Salisbury and if they load for those parts they run the risk of losing stock and being detained indefinitely. There are good grounds for believing that all the main transport routes in Rhodesia are already more or less infected with Redwater.

The Association was not satisfied, because on April 14, Veterinary Surgeon Gorman wired to Gray from Bulawayo[16] saying that its President, Colonel Napier, had been making enquiries of him:

"Farmers here intend holding meeting on Friday [April 18] when the matter will be discussed. Please let me have all useful information concerning the disease by next mail or if too late by wire."

On April 17 Orpen sent a long telegram[16] to the Civil Commissioner in Bulawayo, in reply to a telegram of April 16, reaffirming the position that the disease was not a new disease imported by the Australian cattle but was only redwater, now abundant because of the unusual abundance of ticks. Animals formerly infected with redwater might have lost their immunity and were thus now likely to show a relapse. Since such animals were present throughout the country, no legislation could check the spread of the disease. Orpen added that, although the movement of stock from Salisbury to the south had been checked, the general infection of Rhodesia by redwater had taken place so long ago that the disease would most assuredly break out anywhere when favorable conditions existed.

From then on, public dissatisfaction intensified almost from day to day and began to attract attention in South Africa. The *Rhodesia Herald* for April 19, 1902, reported that the Landowners and Farmers Association, had, at a meeting held in Salisbury, requested the government to procure extra veterinary assistance and "censured the government for not being sufficiently alive to the situation." That story was picked up in Salisbury by Reuter and the *Cape Times* printed it on April 23. On April 26, the *Cape Times*[17] reported (from Reuter, Bulawayo) that the Chamber of Mines had addressed a long wire to the government pointing out that "the mining industry will be paralyzed, as it will be impossible to get supplies to the mines. Transport riders, who loaded for Selukwe, have turned back. The disease seems to be exceedingly virulent." Not only did Reuter and the *Cape Times* pick up the story, the clippings were sent from Cape Town to the London office of the B.S.A.C. on April 30.[18] A later Reuter dispatch appeared in the *Cape Times* on May 2; the Cape Town representative of the B.S.A.C. (J. A. Stevens) sent it to Salisbury and received a reassuring reply. "Reuters Report exaggerated and so far as at present known mortality amongst cattle which have been confined to Salisbury and Umtali districts is due to Redwater, a disease which has existed in Africa for generations." This too was duly forwarded to London.[19]

On April 30, Stevens advised the London office that "Mr. [William] Robertson, one of the Cape Government's experienced Veterinary Surgeons, left here on the 26th instant with apparatus for making a thorough investigation of the disease."[19] As Orpen later put it,[20] Robertson "brought with him at the greatest speed a complete and bulky equipment for a laboratory with the most up-to-date appliances."

Robertson arrived in Salisbury on or after May 8[21] and completed an interim report by May 21. Robertson began his report[22] by saying that after a careful consideration of the clinical symptoms and post-mortem lesions, he was of the opinion that the disease was not rinderpest but 'what is known as Texas fever in the United States . . . Tick fever in Australia, Redwater in Cape Colony, and Tristeza in the Argentine." He conceded that the disease was unusually severe "but that may be due to the amount of infective ticks infesting the animal . . . as we know . . . all Southern Rhodesia is infested with ticks, I do not think any cordon or barrier can be of any avail . . . and I agree with the Chief Veterinary Surgeon that a quarantine of thirty days be imposed on all herds showing signs of infection." Just as Gray had done, Robertson spoke of typical and atypical cases. For Robertson the presence of fluid in the lungs was the most important feature of the atypical cases: "I have never before seen such a lesion in any case of Redwater . . . whether it is due to the altitude of this plateau or the severity of the disease I am unable to say." As far as parasites in the blood, Robertson rarely found the classic "pyriform stage"; instead he found "strange forms, miniature rods strongly resembling small bacilli." But that did not prove that the disease was not redwater, quite the contrary:

In connection with the above description of the forms of the micro-parasite found in the red corpuscles, Professor Koch, in an official report from Dar-es-Salaam under date of 1897, states: 'With regard to the forms of pyrosoma and the relations of both it and the full grown parasite to mild and severe Texas Fever, I have come to different conclusions from [the] American investigators. I found, namely, in the red blood corpuscles of cases which took a severe form, and rapidly proved fatal, strange forms resembling miniature staves, so that one might take them to be small bacilli. These are frequently curved, and sometimes so strong [strongly curved] that they form rings, and in that case resemble the parasite of tropical malaria. Between such forms and the pear shaped form of the full-grown pyrosoma there are a number of intermediate stages. In the severer cases they are found in extraordinary [sic] large numbers, 80 to 90 per cent of all red corpuscles being invaded. As far as my experience goes, in quite acute cases only the first forms are met with.'

Robertson's sole comment on this passage from Koch was "This bears out my examination and is another proof of the extreme severity of the present outbreak of Redwater." We will hear much more about Koch's studies in Dar-es-Salaam and the errors they contained; Robertson was the first person to refer to them in connection with the new outbreak.

On May 22, the London office cabled:[18] "To Charter, Salisbury. What is the position of cattle disease. Are true nature and remedy known." As a result of Robertson's report, the reply from Salisbury[18] said that Robertson and Gray agreed that the disease was redwater, which had existed in South Africa for many years. Although there had been considerable mortality in Umtali and Salisbury, there had been comparatively little loss in Matabeleland, and the disease would probably drop off after the frosts.

Soon after finishing his report Robertson sent two letters to his chief, Duncan Hutcheon, on June 8 and June 10.[22] On June 8 he again mentioned the presence of bacillary forms "alluded to by Koch in his report upon R. Water in Dar-es-Salaam." Although the typical pear-shaped parasite was often seen in Salisbury, in many cases it could not be found at all. He added that the severity of the outbreak, the mortality, the rapidity of death and the lesions in the lungs had led many lay observers to doubt that this disease was redwater or Texas fever "but I consider that the difference . . . is due to increased severity of infection, not to any mixed disease." On June 10, Robertson wrote "I am having lots of work and lots of vilification as no one, that is of the transport rider class, will believe that the disease is R. Water." He added that he knew that his interim report was very poor "but you can't make bricks without straw & the Gov. here fairly clamoured for my opinion to sort of back up their views."

Gray also wrote an interim report: both his report and Robertson's report were dated May 21 and were in Orpen's hands by May 22.[22] Gray's report began:

Much dissatisfaction has been expressed of late at what the less fully informed public have termed the 'inactivity and apathy of the Government' . . . and many have evinced a desire to lay all blame for the spread of the disease at the door of the Agricultural Department without taking into consideration the fact that the apparent epidemic nature of the disease may be the natural cumulative result of long established infection . . . a statement of the whole case may do much to clear the vision of those (and it is believed that their number is considerable) who have been misled by a mis-representation of the facts.

Gray argued that redwater had infected the fields for many years, so that "given local conditions peculiarly favourable to the multiplication of ticks, we may have an outbreak anywhere . . . hence the futility of attempting to arrest the disease by any cordon . . . [and hence] the abolition of cordons, which are galling and must be ineffective, is advisable and . . . substitution . . . of quarantine is being tried." Gray went on to review the history of the outbreak, again exonerating the Australian cattle and mentioning that severe outbreaks of redwater had occurred in Rhodesia in 1891 and 1897.

As to quarantine, Gray said that Jarvis had tried to impose it in Umtali

but was met with such strenuous opposition . . . that all his efforts to trace cases and isolate affected herds were unavailing . . . [in a report written in December, 1901] Mr. Jarvis says 'all support one another to conceal the disease . . . [the public] openly boast, not only to me, but to the cattle Inspector at Melsetter, that they are "banded together" to conceal the disease, and try as we will we have been so far unsuccessful in tripping them'.

Thus

the attempt to enforce a quarantine was given up and for a time much public satisfaction was manifested [but] when the more susceptible animals had been weeded out and the disease became altered in character by reason of the intensity of the infection, cases of an atypical nature predominating . . . much uneasiness was manifested at what was designated 'the new disease'

"Although compelled by public opinion and absence of public support [to stop enforcing] quarantine measures," the Department had never stopped warning the public not to take clean cattle into infected areas. Nevertheless many people were still moving infected cattle about on clean veld. Finally, Gray said, it had been stated that the Farmers Association of Bulawayo had repeatedly been rebuffed on the frequent occasions when it had demanded that the government seek expert advice. In fact only one such demand had been made, and it resulted in Mr. Robertson being sent for.

On May 22, Orpen wrote a long letter to the Chief Secretary of the B.S.A.C. in Salisbury, H. H. Castens, enclosing both interim reports.[23] Orpen praised the qualifications of Gray and Robertson and said their reports should be published in the next Government Gazette and "simultaneously furnished to the two Salisbury newspapers." The Executive Council agreed on May 26 and, on May 29, ordered the publication of the reports.[23] They appeared in various forms, one of which was an official pamphlet dated June 14, 1902.[24]

What Orpen and Gray did *not* know on May 22, and did not learn until May 26, was that on May 12 the Rhodesian Landowners and Farmers Association had joined with the Chamber of Mines and the Chamber of Commerce in sending a letter to the London office of the B.S.A.C.[25] to demand that Orpen be removed from his position as Minister of Agriculture. The letter stated that the London office was being approached directly because the Administrator had already been asked to replace Surveyor-General Orpen as Minister of Agriculture and had refused to do so. Referring to the epidemic as disastrous, the letter said that

having accepted the dictum of his professional advisers that the disease was 'Red-Water', no action had been taken by the Surveyor-General to prevent its spread, or to ascertain in what way the disease may be cured, and that even when representations were made as to the necessity for stopping the removal of cattle . . . the Surveyor-General stated that it was of no use to [take] any such measures . . . Against this contention, we . . . urge that although the disease has been prevalent for 9 to 12 months past in Mashonaland, [actually 7 months at most; 12 months presumably refers to the Australian cattle] it was only from 2 to 3 weeks ago that any infected cattle were found in Matabeleland, and . . . [they] had travelled on the main road from Salisbury to Gwelo.

The letter accused Orpen of neglect of duty in not prohibiting the movement of cattle across the Shangani river.

It is hardly necessary to point out to the Company that in 1896 there was scarcely a single head of cattle left alive in Southern Rhodesia owing to the ravages of rinderpest. In the six years that have elapsed . . . the country has become stocked with cattle to a degree [which led to the hope that it] would again become one of the great stock-raising territories of South Africa.

But now, "owing to the wilful neglect of the Agricultural Department . . . [the] whole country is to be again denuded of cattle with a great loss of wealth to cattle owners, both white and black, and a great amount of discontent among the native owners." Moreover, the crippling of transport to areas not served by the railway "threatens to temporarily arrest the progress of the country entirely" by making the mining industry unable to afford transport. "The country is under no obligation to maintain in its Government a Minister who has shown himself so incapable of dealing with an epidemic so disastrous as the present one." And, finally, "A copy of this letter has been forwarded to His Honour the Administrator." (The letter was not, in fact, sent to Kotzé, the Acting Administrator, until May 22, and Orpen saw it only on May 26. Since it *was* a letter and not a cable, it did not reach London for some time, although it had arrived there by June 30. The minutes of the London board of the B.S.A.C. show that the letter appeared on the agenda only on July 30, 1902, when Milton was already in London and attending meetings of the B.S.A.C. board.)[26]

A reply was drafted in Salisbury on May 12, but it was sent from London in revised form only on August 16.[27] That reply pointed out that some months before, Ross Townsend had been appointed to relieve Mr. Orpen of the greater part of his duties in connection with the Agricultural Department. Townsend had been unable to serve because of illness but was expected to return before the end of the year. This reply obviously reached the Landowners and Farmers Association too late to have any effect.[28]

Orpen gave the letter of May 12 to Gray on May 26, the same day that he received it. Responding immediately,[29] also on May 26, Gray insisted that the disease had been in existence for over ten years, that it *was* redwater, that Robertson agreed that it was redwater and that

The cordon of whose inefficiency the correspondents complain was instituted temporarily to allay public unrest in Bulawayo, fomented by those who strenuously declined to accept the verdict of the Veterinary Department, that the disease was Redwater. It was only imposed until such time as Mr. Robertson should be able to confirm or contradict the views of the Government Veterinary Staff and was withdrawn when Mr. Robertson declared in their favour.

Gray went on:

While the signatories in the abstract express themselves as being anxious that everything should be done, as they say, 'to arrest the spread of the disease' . . . yet when it comes to be a matter of personal interest . . . the same anxiety is not manifest . . . only a short time ago Mr. Wrey, President of the Rhodesia Chamber of Mines, urged the Veterinary Department . . . to . . . allow cattle amongst which Redwater existed . . . to carry food stuffs to the Beatrice Mine . . . under his management, which was in danger of being shut down . . . at that time he was able . . . to close his eyes to the fact that [this] would . . . spread . . . the infection.

On May 28, 1902 Orpen sent the Chief Secretary of the B.S.A.C. in Salisbury a long and vigorous defence of his actions, followed only three days later by a second, similar letter.[29] The first letter, eighteen pages long, was divided into forty-two numbered paragraphs! Orpen said he had been unfairly attacked as "unfit for any employment whatever"; that the letter of May 12, was "already a fortnight on its way to England" before he saw it; that "His Honour, the Administrator [Milton] had complete confidence in Gray"; that "His Honour and I have acted throughout implicitly on [Gray's] advice"; that Gray is eminently qualified and "has slaved beyond all office hours day and night, in all weather, in town and country." Deserving gratitude, Gray instead has been obliged "for many a night to spend the only hours he has for any natural rest, in defending [himself] against ... bitter and unfounded attacks."

In defence of himself, Orpen said that he had been appointed Surveyor-General to *reform* a department that badly needed it; that he had as "an old practical farmer and member of Parliament [in South Africa]" offered "my gratuitous services to Earl Grey [Administrator in 1896 and 1897] to bring into existence ... an Agricultural Department ... those gratuitous services have remained gratuitous ... [Although] I have had some scientific training" what a Minister requires is "the best professional and scientific specialists he can obtain" – and he had obtained them. After a few paragraphs attacking farmers who think they know more than the experts do, Orpen responded to some of the other complaints made in the letter of May 12 and ended up by suggesting that as a *reformer* of both the Surveyor-General's Office and of the Agricultural Department "I have more than any Head of a Department to say *No*. That is at the bottom of all these baseless representations." (As Surveyor-General, Orpen was required to enforce the most hated of all of the rules of the Chartered Company, a rule that affected the ownership of farms. Having seized so much land from the Africans and having given so much of that land to large landowners, the Chartered Company was not inclined to give a clear title to the small settlers. The small settler could take title to land only if he personally occupied it. As Keppel-Jones says,[30] "there was no question of requiring occupation by the big companies and magnates to whom favours were lavishly distributed." Keppel-Jones adds that even Milton complained that "Jameson has given nearly the whole country away ... there is absolutely no land left which is of any value for ... immigrants ... I think Jameson must have been off his head for some time before the raid." No wonder that Orpen had so often to say *No*.)

In his follow-up letter of May 31, Orpen returned to his charge that he was being attacked by persons whose interests he had been forced to oppose. He said that he was by no means lacking in physical energy (he was 74 years old). "I have worked overtime as I believe no other officer has ever done for six consecutive years . . . The . . . [Veterinary and Agricultural Offices] . . . are 330 yards from my personal office . . . separated by high stairs . . . I walk [to and from] these offices several times a day [but] I do not complain. I require plenty of exercise in order to do plenty of head work." Orpen also complained of shortages of staff and pointed out that Gray had lost his principal aid [O'Neill] and had not been able to replace him, that newly arrived veterinarians require two years to become familiar with the diseases of Southern Africa and that Gray had only recently, with some difficulty, obtained a veterinary surgeon [G. S. Bruce] direct from England.[31]

On June 6, 1902, the Central Farmers Association (of Enkeldoorn, now Chivhu) sent its own letter[32] asking the London office to replace Orpen. The Landowners and Farmers Association returned to the attack on June 14, in a letter to the Chief Secretary of the B.S.A.C. in Salisbury.[33] Having criticized the government for publishing its report in Salisbury but not in the Bulawayo paper, the letter went on to concede that Gray and Robertson were correct in their diagnosis of "an exceptionally severe form of Redwater" and to thank Robertson for his work. But the charges of apathy and inefficiency were renewed. "Mr. Orpen alleges that Mr. Robertson brought with him at great speed a complete and bulky equipment for a laboratory with the most up-to-date appliances. If such a laboratory is needed now, surely it was needed the summer before last and a qualified Bacteriologist." (They were wrong: this is the Australian cattle again. The "summer before last" was not the summer of December 1901–March 1902 but that of December 1900–March 1901, in other words the summer when the Australian cattle were dying of what was in fact redwater. Had a bacteriologist been there then, all he would have found was redwater.) The Association insisted that cordons could have prevented the spread of the disease, and repeated its charge that by "what we can only consider the wilful neglect of the Agricultural Department, it would seem that the whole country may again be denuded of cattle." This letter was sent to the (Salisbury) *Rhodesia Herald* which published almost all of it on June 26.[34]

An early response to the emergency had been to press forward the completion of the railway from Salisbury to Bulawayo. (As van Onselen has pointed out,[35] the disruption of transport had been one of the serious results of rinderpest in South Africa.) Because the Boer War was still in progress, all material for building railroads was held in Port Elizabeth, in the Cape Colony, under the military control of Lord Kitchener. On May 2 the Administrator cabled Kitchener:[36] "In consequence of severe outbreak cattle disease . . . transport difficulties are becoming very great and it becomes of increasing and vital importance in order to keep mining and other industries supplied that railway extension should be pushed forward with all possible speed." The Administrator asked that the supplies for building the railroad be increased from 3,200 tons a month to 5,000 tons. Kitchener replied on May 9: "I have ordered an increase to be made in civil rail permits for Rhodesia Railway material . . . to 4,000 tons per month . . . " The railway south from Salisbury reached Gwelo on June 1 and Bulawayo on December 1, 1902.

In another response to the loss of ox-drawn transport, on July 24 the government of Rhodesia advised the public that "Farmers, Transport Riders and others" could apply for assistance in the purchase of donkeys.[37] An extensive correspondence concerned with efforts to buy donkeys in India or Spain ensued. A delegation actually left London for Spain in early September, with instructions to purchase 1,200 donkeys, armed with a letter of credit of £8,000, but the project was cancelled on September 16 when it was found that it was possible to buy donkeys more cheaply in South Africa.[38]

On July 7 the Chamber of Mines, the Chamber of Commerce and the Landowners Association met in Bulawayo and sent a vituperative telegram to Kotzé[39] referring to the

absolute necessity [to arrange] for two thoroughly qualified experts . . . one from Australia, the other from South America and . . . opening in Bulawayo of a Bacteriological Institute . . . so far as researches have gone at present no tangible result . . . and Robertson may . . . be recalled to Cape Colony leaving country without any expert advice worthy of the name . . . disease is spreading in all directions . . . if no preventive measure be discovered before next wet season all the cattle in the country will be wiped out . . . no expense should be spared . . . we are intentionally keeping this wire from the Press in order to prevent a panic . . . (A marginal note against those words about the press, in the Administrator's copy, reads "very kind.")

The next day the Executive Council met and asked Orpen to refer the letter to Gray and Robertson, which he did. On July 9 Gray replied to Orpen[39] that he could not recommend obtaining experts from Australia and South America since they would have no familiarity with southern African diseases of stock and would be no better qualified than Robertson. Gray said that the disease was very virulent, perhaps because of the passage of the infection through large numbers of highly susceptible cattle and because of the unusually massive infestations with ticks. Inoculation experiments would resume as soon as enough dipping tanks were created. "The advisability of using dips was long ago impressed upon the public ... but persistently disregarded, although it ... might have been thought that the very simplicity of the step would have ensured its possible adoption." As to his research having produced no tangible results, Mr. Robertson had been here only six weeks. Professor Koch had spent 12 months studying rinderpest and the method he had proposed did "not altogether give the results which he predicted." Gray again attacked the Chambers:

the glaring inconsistency of these bodies ... is noticeable in their correspondence. Yesterday they said 'no expense should be spared and only the promptest action can prevail.' Today, July 9, when a rumour has arisen that certain steps are being considered ... to regulate traffic in the Victoria District, which swarms with native cattle [and] to retard the spread of infection by transport riders moving all over ... across native grazing grounds, they wire 'we are informed ... Victoria road ... closed ... if ... not opened at once all Selukwe Mines must close down ... no other source for grain supply' ... Not a word here as to ... promptest action ... Native cattle may die off wholesale – a native rising may be precipitated but the Selukwe Mines must not be deprived ... and no step must be taken to check the disease which clashes with the individual interest of any member of either Association.

A formal reply must have been sent to the Chambers' telegram of July 7, but I have not located it. The suggestion that a bacteriological institute be set up is discussed below.

Kotzé was worried enough to warn Milner, on July 14, that the disease was very virulent and that measures had been taken to prevent cattle being moved outside Rhodesia. Since the boundaries were so extensive, Kotzé advised Milner to prevent cattle entering the Transvaal.[40] As early as June 28 the Agricultural Adviser in

Pretoria had written to enquire about the outbreak; his letter was referred to Orpen who did not reply until July 19. Orpen again said[41] the outbreak was simply one of redwater, and again said that redwater had long been present in Rhodesia and the Cape. He did, however, note that the disease was exceptionally severe, that supposedly immune cattle had died, and that Rhodesia had taken steps to close its borders with the Transvaal and the Protectorate (Bechuanaland). Unfortunately, he said, those regions had not closed the borders from their side, so any animals that did get across from Rhodesia were free to go on their way. Orpen recommended the early burning of grass and the use of dipping as measures to control ticks and he enclosed several pamphlets, among them Gray's report of January, 1902 and the interim reports of Gray and Robertson. In the postscript he added "I enclose a memo on inoculation by the Chief Veterinary Surgeon."

In that memo, also dated July 19, Gray reported[41] that inoculation was not giving satisfactory results but

when the [dipping] tanks are in working order and we can eliminate the factor of tick infection, we will then be better able to decide whether the virulence of the present outbreak is the result of extreme tick infection, whether it arises from the passage of the disease through large numbers of very susceptible animals and is only a temporary phase of the disorder, or whether it is due to climatic influence and is likely to remain . . . I incline to the belief that the present intensity of Redwater here is due to the second cause and will not persist. I advise against inoculation of any description at present until this question has been worked out.

On July 28 Kotzé cabled from Salisbury to the London office:[42] "Re cattle disease erection of dipping tanks at various centres I am advised is absolutely essential I have authorized expenditure as matter extreme urgency this will probably mean with their upkeep £6,000."

Public protest came to a boil in Bulawayo on July 29 when Kotzé met with representatives of the Chamber of Mines, the Landowners and Farmers Association and the Chamber of Commerce. A 20-page-long report (apparently a stenographic transcript) of that meeting was submitted to the Executive Council by Kotzé on August 1.[43] The President of the Chamber of Mines began by saying that "the cattle disease was practically killing off all the cattle in the country, and the people could not see their way two months ahead . . . the mines were face to face with having to close down."

Kotzé expressed his sympathy and said that "I came here with no preconceived notions, but with an open mind to listen to what you, gentlemen, have to say in the interest of the country." The Chairman of the Landowners and Farmers Association said that the first point was to get an expert from Texas or Australia, to study the disease and to do so in Bulawayo. Kotzé replied that he had great confidence in Gray and Robertson whom he had consulted "as a medical man would be consulted in a case of family sickness." They did not recommend that an outside expert be obtained since it was certain that the disease was only a very virulent form of redwater. Moreover, Dr. Hutcheon was leaving Cape Town that night and would arrive in a few days' time. Kotzé added that he was not opposed to getting an expert from Texas or Australia but would like to work in conjunction with the Cape government and would like to consult Dr. Hutcheon [the Chief Veterinarian of the Cape] since he did not wish to seem to cast doubt on Mr. Robertson's ability. Besides it would cost a great deal of money to get an expert, so that he would have to cable to the London board of the Chartered Company for permission to do that.

The speakers repeatedly insisted that the new study be carried out in Bulawayo because of the anxiety of the local people. Kotzé said that as far as an expert is concerned "I have a telegram in my pocket that I would send to the Board . . . but I want to see Dr. Hutcheon first . . . if [he] had no objection the experiments could be carried out in both places [Salisbury and Bulawayo]."

The discussion then turned to the urgent need for importing donkeys; Kotzé agreed but was not sure if the Chartered Company would pay for them. After some further discussion on a "pass system" for the moving of cattle and some discussion about dipping, and about the urgency of the need to complete the railroad and to reduce the freight rates, the meeting adjourned.

As a result of that meeting, on July 30, Kotzé sent an exceptionally urgent cable to the London office, directly from Bulawayo:[44]

Feeling in Matabeleland running so high re cattle disease and want of transport I deemed it necessary to visit Bulawayo Township and, meeting representatives of the various Chambers in conference discussed all points satisfactorily with them and while appreciating the authority to spend £10,000 I feel it absolutely imperative ask for authority £25,000 more to meet pressing necessities and prevent shutting down the mines . . . also requisite that railway company temporarily reduce charges . . . the matter is most urgent and with the necessary funds I will pacify people and tide over all difficulties. Cattle disease is spreading and no means of safe preventative inoculation yet discovered. Please reply as soon as possible to Salisbury.

The reply came the next day, authorizing the expenditure of £25,000; "also if you think it necessary employ another expert for cattle disease."

On July 30, the *Bulawayo Chronicle* reported that Kotzé had accepted the suggestion that an expert be secured "from Australia or Texas," but, as we will see in the next chapter, the Colonial Office's Resident Commissioner in Salisbury, apparently without Kotzé's knowledge, had already asked the Colonial Office to send out an expert from England.

An enlightened and early response of the Chartered Company was its decision to create a bacteriological institute. Had that institute come into being the Chartered Company would have been highly praised: that it did not come into being was no fault of the Company. As early as June 8, 1902, Orpen wrote, apparently to Kotzé, that he had been very impressed by Robertson's qualifications and had learned that Robertson had approached Milner with the suggestion that he be employed as a bacteriologist by the new colonies (the Orange River Colony and the Transvaal).[45] This had given Orpen the idea that a bacteriological institute, headed by Robertson, might be set up in Rhodesia, perhaps supported by part of Mr. Rhodes' bequest. (Rhodes was *always* called *Mr.* Rhodes; in some circles he still is.) Such an institute might investigate "rinderpest, tsetse, Horse-sickness, Gall-sickness, Bush-sickness, Pyaemia, Glanders, etc., etc. These difficulties are even a matter of Imperial and world wide concern." The institute could also produce various vaccines; in fact the institute at Grahamstown actually paid its way by producing such vaccines, although, "what is mainly to be expected are the invaluable results with regard to animal diseases." Orpen said that he had approached Gray, who had not only strongly approved but had obtained a plan and a budget from Robertson. Robertson estimated that it would cost £7,000 to build and equip an institute and about £3,000 a year to operate it, a sum that included a salary for Robertson of £700 a year. Orpen included a resumé of Robertson's qualifications which gave as references Hutcheon, McFadyean and the Chief Medical Officers of the Cape and the Transvaal. The proposal was forwarded to

Milton in London along with a letter saying that Kotzé strongly endorsed it. Robertson was not employed, perhaps because he and Gray had fallen out of favor with the farming and mining communities, but the idea was revived a few months later. I have not located all of the relevant correspondence,[46] but it appears that advice was sought from Cape Town, because A. J. Gregory, the Medical Officer of Health of the Cape Colony, wrote to Milton on December 16, 1902 to introduce "Dr. R. W. Dodgson, who, I am informed, has been invited by the Rhodesian Government to go up to Salisbury in connection with a possibility of entrusting him with Bacteriological Investigation in Rhodesia." Gregory added that

Some time ago I wrote to Mr. Stevens . . . recommending Dr. Dodgson for this work . . . I feel quite confident that Dodgson is a man who will give you value for your money . . . Of course you must not expect . . . results to be turned out like pins from a factory, they may be much or little, be made at once, or only after a long period of research . . . All you can expect is that honest, steady and competent work . . . is put in and, above all humbug and lies are not dealt in. And on all these points I am confident, if you engage Dodgson, you will get what you pay for – a matter which in this Colony, as you are quite aware, we have not so far as Bacteriology is concerned, always been successful in obtaining.[47]

Milton underlined *competent* and placed a line in the margin along the passage beginning "All that you can expect" and ending "humbug and lies are not dealt in." He then wrote on this letter "Write a letter for my signature. I am glad to have secured the services of Dr. D. & feel sure that he will do excellent work for us. W.H.M." On December 24, 1902, Orpen wrote to Milton to say that Gray had formed a high opinion of Dodgson and to enclose Dodgson's estimate of the cost of building the institute, an estimate which, Orpen said, was in accord with that of Robertson. Orpen and Gray suggested that Dodgson be paid £1,200 a year.

Dodgson *was* hired, he did accept, and, before the end of December, 1902 the Salisbury Department of Public Works had drawn detailed plans for a handsome institute, which included a home for the director (with two bedrooms and a sitting room), a five-room laboratory, the main room of which was 18 feet × 30 feet, and a large stable.[48] All these plans, high hopes and enthusiasm came to naught. Dodgson fell ill, and more than a year later, on March 28, 1904, the London office cabled to Milton[49] "Dodgson states illness has been more serious than was thought but if present progress maintained can sail in six weeks. Confidential advise cancel appointment." Milton replied on March 29 "Cancel Dodgson engagement. I have been compelled to make other arrangements for carrying on Dr. Koch's investigations and maintaining Rabies Institute."[50]

A major opportunity was thus lost and Gray and Milton must have been severely disappointed. Fortunately for Dodgson, who was a relative of Lewis Carroll, he recovered and enjoyed a long and successful career in England.[51] But the Bacteriological Institute did not recover. Although Gray, on a visit to London late in 1904, succeeded in recruiting L. E. W. Bevan to head that institute, by the time Bevan arrived in Rhodesia in 1905 whatever facilities had been available had been turned over to the medical department and, much to his resentment, Bevan had to spend the next few years doing practical field work. Bevan quit in disgust in 1908, spent some time at the Pasteur Institute in Paris, and was finally persuaded to return to Rhodesia, having been firmly promised the title of Government Veterinary Bacteriologist; but he did not receive adequate facilities for research until 1922.[52]

In August, 1902 Gray and Robertson published their final joint report, "Report upon Texas Fever or Redwater in Rhodesia",[53] an oversize (8″ × 13″) pamphlet containing about 15,000 words of text, four plates showing photographs of dead cattle, two plates containing eight illustrations of parasites, seventeen large fever charts, a formula for dip and a detailed plan of a dipping tank. Condensed versions of the report, with few or no plates, also appeared in important veterinary journals.[54] This joint report is a document of major importance in the history of East Coast fever. It contains detailed descriptions of the clinical and post-mortem findings in that disease, it contains an excellent description of the parasite that causes East Coast fever, and it contains an early announcement that cattle immune to ordinary redwater are not immune to East Coast fever. Not only was it widely reprinted, at least in somewhat abbreviated form, we know that it was studied by both Koch (see chapter 5) and by Laveran (see chapter 7).

The report continued to argue that the disease was not new. It began with a description of Texas fever and a summary of the work of Smith and Kilborne, and said that "when the data of the present outbreak in Southern Rhodesia are compared with those which occurred in Australia, America and the Argentine, it can be seen that although certain ... symptoms are different in this outbreak, the main train of *symptoms* and *post-mortem* appearances are the same." Gray and Robertson then turned to the history of the disease in Rhodesia. Texas fever had been seen there for at least ten years, which was not surprising since the tick that transmits it (*Rhipicephalus decoloratus*, the blue tick) is widespread throughout the country. Yet one might ask, if that was so, why had the disease not attracted much public attention until then? The answer was to be found in the eventful history of Rhodesia. "First there was war and locusts, then came rinderpest which practically denuded the country of stock, this was followed by a rebellion which at one time threatened to send the settlers after the cattle." With all these distractions, "it is not difficult to see how a disease of this description might be fairly prevalent and yet pass unnoticed by the general public." Outbreaks had unquestionably occurred in 1891 and in 1897, and sporadically ever since, but the disease came to public attention only when it caused the death of the Australian cattle. The present outbreak had begun around November, 1901, initially in Umtali and later in Salisbury. The Umtali outbreak had extended along the roads to Melsetter and Penhalonga. The Umtali stockowners began to claim that a "new disease" had been imported from Australia. In addition, "*Post-mortem* appearances not placed upon record in any literature on the subject of Redwater were also observed." That fact, plus the public agitation, led to the securing of help from the Cape Colony (i.e. Robertson).

In typical redwater, the report went on, two or three days of fever are followed by the appearance of red urine and delirium. In "atypical" redwater, marked fever is not accompanied by other signs or symptoms and the urine is not abnormal. In fact the presence of the disease may be overlooked until the animal suddenly dies from pulmonary effusion, with froth flowing from the nostrils. On *post-mortem* examination, in typical redwater the spleen is much enlarged and the liver is somewhat enlarged. In atypical cases lesions may be seen in the spleen and liver but the lungs are filled with exudate (which was, again, attributed to the effects of anemia and high altitude). In atypical cases the kidney lesions (white infarcts, actually lymphomata) are extremely constant and the lymph nodes are enlarged and hemorrhagic.

The joint report then mentioned Koch's findings in Dar-es-Salaam[55] (as Robertson had done in his interim report) and stated that the "stave" or "bacillary" form of the parasite is almost invariably present. Most strikingly of all, Gray and Robertson reported that "Out of several hundred cases in which the blood was microscopically examined, in twenty cases only was the typical double pyrosoma (alluded to by Smith and Kilborne) met with, and then in conjunction with the bacillary and spherical stages." This suggests that *all* of the several hundred animals thus studied may have been victims of East Coast fever; twenty of them may also have had redwater. But Gray and Robertson had a different explanation. They argued that these "imperfect or miniature forms" of the parasite were seen because the cattle were so susceptible. As a result, the parasite multiplied with such great rapidity that the animal became ill and died before the organisms could attain their full development.

Six pages of the report were devoted to inoculation. They described the methods used to inoculate against Texas fever in New South Wales and in Queensland and even quoted a letter on the subject from W. H. Dalrymple of the Agricultural Experiment Station in Baton Rouge, Louisiana. (Gray had written to Dalrymple for advice; Dalrymple had replied as early as April 3, 1902.)[56] The report noted that experiments on inoculation had begun in Rhodesia as early as January 6, 1902, when three calves had been inoculated by Gray with blood taken from the three Australian cattle that had survived out of the group imported by Rhodes. Other inoculations had been made with glycerinated bile (which Koch had used to immunize against rinderpest). But the results were far from encouraging. Gray and Robertson concluded that the combination of gross tick infestation plus the abnormal virulence of the disease overcame any protection conferred by inoculation. (Baton Rouge was not the only part of the United States to figure in the report, which included detailed plans for a dipping tank "modelled on the plan of those erected at the Santa Gertrude Ranche [sic] Texas", that is, the King Ranch.)[57]

In the summary of their report, Gray and Robertson said,

it is as well to state how in our opinion this epidemic of Redwater differs from that disease as known to us in the Cape Colony and from the description of the workers in other countries in:

1. The severity of the infection and mortality amongst infected herds.
2. The fact that young animals (sucklings) bred and run on infected

veldt contract the disease and die.
3. The fact that one attack ... does not confer any lengthy immunity.
4. The severity of the *post-mortem* lesions.
5. The presence of lung lesions ... and kidney lesions ...
6. The uncertainty of conferring immunity ... [by] inoculation.

But, they concluded, all these differences are to be attributed to the fact that the disease "has developed a virulence which will probably abate at a later date."

How could Gray and Robertson have failed to realize that "atypical" redwater, which they had described so clearly, was a new disease? Presumably because they were influenced by Koch, whose 1898 report of his investigation of 1897 had described the staves, small bacilli and spherical stages as being a form of the parasite of redwater, commonly found in "cases which took a severe form, and rapidly proved fatal." Gray and Robertson found the same parasites that Koch had misidentified, found them, as Koch had done, in cases that took a severe form, and accepted Koch's dictum that the disease was redwater. Koch was, after all, the greatest bacteriologist in the world. Had Gray and Robertson been unaware of Koch's earlier work, they might have realized that "atypical" redwater was a new disease, even though Gray had previously been so certain that it was not.

Small wonder that Gray remarked, in 1908, sourly but accurately, that[58] "further enquiry [in 1897] might have placed him [Koch] in possession of important information which would have made the record of his researches a guide instead of a stumbling block to future investigators."

The joint report by Gray and Robertson had an appendix which reprinted a letter written by Gray to Orpen on July 19, 1902, describing in detail the post-mortem findings on eight head of cattle supposedly immune to redwater that had arrived from Natal on June 16, in charge of Watkins-Pitchford. Two of those cattle died on July 11 and all were dead by July 16. We will hear more about those cattle in chapter 4; to Gray their death meant only that "the present outbreak here is of a more virulent type than is common in Natal, even in the Coast Districts, otherwise some of these animals should have withstood infection." A further appendix, by Duncan Hutcheon, is discussed in chapter 7.

As we will see in the next chapter, a long search for outside expert advice culminated in Robert Koch arriving in Bulawayo in late February, 1903. The knowledge that an outside expert was being sought did not stop the work in Rhodesia and the Transvaal. Gray continued to struggle almost alone in Rhodesia, while maintaining an active correspondence with Robertson, with the Cape entomologist, Charles Lounsbury, with Hutcheon, and with Watkins-Pitchford of Natal.[59] Much of that correspondence reported Gray's growing conviction that dipping did not seem to protect cattle from the disease. That fact led Gray to believe that perhaps the disease was not tick-borne after all; but if it were not tick-borne could it really be redwater?

Gray's doubts made Watkins-Pitchford uneasy. On November 11, 1902 he wrote to Gray, "the conclusion to which you are being forced ... would seem to be bringing us face to face with hitherto unascertained conditions." Even William Robertson was on the defensive when he wrote to Gray on December 11, enclosing some specimens that Theiler had sent him from the Transvaal. Referring to the parasite, Robertson said, "I fancy you will recognize him as a very old friend & what is more important Theiler has submitted such specimens to Laveran who says he can see no reason why this deviation in shape should lead us to doubt it being the real P. Bigeminum. I tell you we are all right on pure R. Water." As we will see in chapter 7, on the very next day, an ox that had been exposed to brown ticks by Lounsbury fell ill in Cape Town. Four days later, Robertson found only the "atypical" rod-shaped parasites in its blood. A few weeks later, Theiler proved that cattle immune to redwater were not immune to the new disease.

Great advances had thus been made before Koch arrived, but the disease continued to spread and the cattle continued to die. Looking back at these events from the vantage point of 1936, the *Cambridge History of the British Empire*[60] said: "Those who settled on the land suffered severe reverses down to 1901 when an outbreak of African Coast Fever among cattle, following upon malaria, the Matabele rebellion, rinderpest and the Boer War, appeared to dispose finally of the idea that Rhodesia could become an agricultural country."

The same idea was put rather more poignantly in the *Rhodesia Advertiser* for July 3, 1902:

Cattle – to eat and trample down the long rank grass; cattle to break the land and carry their transport; cattle to give them the chief item of their daily food . . . Cattle was the secret password which promised success . . . to their children if not themselves . . . for ten years every shilling these farmers made has gone into cattle . . . [and] now . . . the bank into which every shilling is placed, [is] broken.

4

The search for an expert

At the stormy meeting held in Bulawayo on July 29, 1902, Kotzé finally promised that he would take steps to obtain an outside expert. He said that he would act as soon as he had consulted the London office; he also wanted to consult Duncan Hutcheon, who was expected to arrive in Salisbury soon. Kotzé did not know that the matter had already been taken out of his hands. On July 22, alarmed by the death of the Natal cattle, the Resident Commissioner, Marshall Clarke, had urged the High Commissioner, Alfred Milner, to obtain an expert to act on behalf of Rhodesia and the South African colonies and Milner had agreed to do so.

During the search that followed, the Chartered Company often acted without telling Clarke or Milner what it was doing, and Milner often failed to tell the Chartered Company what he had done. For that and other reasons the search repeatedly brought the Chartered Company into conflict with the Colonial Office. On December 19, 1902, the choice finally fell on Robert Koch, who was not necessarily the best candidate. From the point of view of the relations between the center and the periphery of the empire, which are discussed again in chapter 12, the search was such a disaster as to be worth documenting in detail. This chapter offers a case history on how not to search for an expert; the reader who is more interested in science than in its governance may wish to turn to chapter 5.

Alfred Milner

Milner is said to have been brilliant, aloof and gifted at figures; he was also a dedicated supporter of the empire and of British dominance of South Africa. During the Boer War that great phrasemaker, Winston Churchill, managed to provide the titles for *two* later biographies of Milner[1] when he wrote

only at Government House did I find the Man of No Illusions, the anxious but unwearied Proconsul, understanding the faults and virtues of both sides, measuring the balance of rights and wrongs, and determined – more determined than ever, for is it not the only hope for the future of South Africa? to use his knowledge and his power to strengthen the Imperial ties.

During the search for an expert Milner always did the sums correctly and always advised the interested parties what each proposal would cost. During the search, he was not a mere transmitter of messages to and from the Colonial Office but an active player, both as High Commissioner and as Governor of the Transvaal. Nor was Kotzé merely a name to Milner. As we saw in chapter 2, during the events that led to the Boer War Milner was influenced by his conviction that Kruger "was irredeemable and inaccessible to reason," a conclusion that he reached when Kruger dismissed Kotzé as Chief Justice of the Transvaal.

As High Commissioner, Milner exercised whatever powers the Colonial Office had with respect to Rhodesia and the four South African colonies. In addition, he had become civilian administrator of the Transvaal and of the Orange Free State when they were formally annexed during the war and became Governor of those "new colonies" after the end of the war. Thus when Milner consulted two of the four colonies he was technically consulting himself. Milner did always consult the Lieutenant-Governor of the Orange River Colony, but the Lieutenant-Governor always responded promptly and never disagreed with Milner's recommendations. Consulting Rhodesia meant consulting the British South Africa Company.

The Cape Colony played a special role. The Cape hoped to escape the new disease and did remain free from it until 1910. On the other hand it had the best resources to study the outbreak. Its Department of Agriculture was well organized, its veterinary services, headed by Duncan Hutcheon, were efficient, it had a staff of veterinary bacteriologists (of whom William Robertson was one), and its government entomologist, Charles Lounsbury, was already studying ticks sent to him from Rhodesia to see which of them was responsible for transmitting the disease. The Cape thus had its own experts and may well have been reluctant to contribute to the cost of bringing an expert from Europe. In addition, Milner's political relationships with the Cape were strained. Both during and after the Boer War, Milner had considered suspending the constitution of the Cape Colony in order to diminish the Afrikaner influence in its government.

The grim and destructive Boer War had ended with Boer women and children held in concentration camps and Boer prisoners of war held in camps as far away as Ceylon. Some people blamed the war on Milner, but in 1902 he was trying to undo its consequences by resettling the Boers and their families on their farms, by building schools, by restoring the economy of the Transvaal and by trying to establish harmony between the Boers and the English and among the various South African colonies.

Milner and his famous "kindergarten" of bright young men, brought out from England to assist him, were determined to bring the Transvaal up to date in every way, but the new cattle scourge was a major threat to their plans to resettle the Boers on their farms. In addition, Milner had long been interested in the improvement of agriculture by scientific means. He became the civilian Governor of the Transvaal on June 21, 1902 and soon approved plans drawn up by F. B. Smith for the creation of a full-scale and entirely modern Department of Agriculture, complete with its own journal (the *Transvaal Agricultural Journal*), long and detailed annual reports and a veterinary bacteriologist (who was, of course, Arnold Theiler). As a result, Milner not only oversaw the search that brought Robert Koch to Bulawayo, he also created the institutional framework that supported Arnold Theiler's far more useful investigation of East Coast fever.[2]

F. B. Smith

Frank Braybrooke Smith (1864–1950) played a far smaller role in the search for an expert, but a far greater role in the day-to-day involvement of the Transvaal Department of Agriculture with East Coast fever. Smith studied agriculture at Downing College, Cambridge. He joined the staff of the then new South Eastern Agricultural College at Wye in January, 1895, where he was Professor of Agriculture, Director of the College Farm and, later, Vice-Principal. In 1900 he visited the United States and Canada, where he studied the system of agricultural colleges and practical field stations that had done so much to advance agriculture in the United

States. On his return to Great Britain he tried to persuade the Board of Agriculture to use itinerant agricultural instructors to dissemi- nate throughout the farming community the techniques developed by the agricultural colleges and their practical field stations. Although he did not succeed at that time, he did impress Milner, who had been closely involved with the Board of Agriculture.

Early in 1902, before the end of the Boer War, Milner cabled Chamberlain to request the services of an expert to advise on land settlement, the restocking of farms, the introduction of new grasses and crops and the starting of one or two model farms. My summary of Milner's request is based on one of the replies to it since I have not located the cable itself. It is quite possible that Milner may have specifically mentioned Smith as a possible candidate, since Smith's formal application for the post was submitted to the Colonial Office on March 11, 1902, when the Colonial Office had already received letters supporting his candidacy. Having been certified as medically fit (by Patrick Manson), Smith received the appointment on March 27, 1902, and sailed on April 20.

On July 31, 1902, Smith submitted to Milner a "Report on Proposed Agricultural Department." That 25-page-long report recommended the creation of a department of agriculture that would include a veterinary department, a chemical department, a division of soils, a geological survey, a study of irrigation, a meteorological department, a statistical department, an entom- ological department, a botanical department (to deal with botany, plant physiology and pathology, agrostology, seed and plant in- troduction, horticulture and forestry), a publications department (to publish quarterly reports as well as leaflets dealing with practical subjects) and a library. Smith further recommended that the depart- ment conduct a system of agricultural education to convey infor- mation to the farmers by an agricultural journal, by bulletins and leaflets, by encouraging the formation of farmers' clubs or institutes to be addressed by qualified speakers, by giving agricultural shows, by establishing model farms, by organizing "peripatetic instruc- tion" to visit the newly formed settlements, and by arranging experiments on crops and manures in cooperation with farmers.

Smith remarked that his suggestions were "based very largely upon the methods adopted in the United States, which undoubt- edly possesses the best organized, most perfectly equipped, and most practically conducted department of any country in the world." Smith's proposals seem almost audacious, and one might have expected them to be dismissed as impractical and impossibly expensive. The report was presented to the Executive Council on August 13, presumably with Milner's backing; on August 20 that Council voted to create a Department of Agriculture, to appoint Smith as its director, and to provide salaries of £1,200 a year for a chemist, a botanist, a veterinary surgeon/bacteriologist, an irrigation assistant and an entomologist, as well as a salary of £800 a year for a dairy expert. On September 15, 1902, Smith was formally advised of his appointment and was told that he should secure the services of his staff at less than the salaries mentioned if that was possible. On the other hand, "it is His Excellency's wish that should specialists of the high type required be not obtainable at the figures named, you will make your recommendations as to revision in such cases as you think desirable." Smith, backed by Milner's blank check, soon created a system of scientific agriculture in the Transvaal that was the equal of anything in the empire and, from the point of view of scientific resources, superior to that of the Board of Agriculture of Great Britain. I am told by John Garnett of the U.K. Ministry of Agriculture that Smith's influence on Lord Milner and others later led to the introduction of a free, official agricultural advisory service which enabled major advances in the efficiency of British agriculture. Yet he is all but forgotten.[3]

The Natal cattle

Soon after the new disease had appeared in the Transvaal in May, 1902, a single episode of what was feared to be "Rhodesian redwater" occurred in Natal. That episode led the Minister of Agriculture of Natal to ask H. Watkins-Pitchford, who was the Government Bacteriologist and Director of the Veterinary Department of Natal, whether the importing of cattle into Natal from areas in which redwater was enzootic should be banned. Watkins-Pitchford replied on June 2, that[4] "my latest advice both from Cape Town and from Mr. Robertson . . . now at Salisbury is . . . that the disease is the usual 'uncomplicated red-water' . . . of a severe type . . . cattle which have become acclimatized to Rhodesian conditions have succumbed to the disease." Watkins-Pitchford discounted "the existence of an acute or hitherto unrecognized form of Redwater," but he suggested that he go to Rhodesia to enquire into the outbreak and to test the susceptibility of Natal cattle to it. He also recommended that a proclamation should be issued to prohibit the importing of cattle from any country in which redwater was known to exist.

That proclamation was issued on June 4. On June 5, F. R. Moor, Secretary for Native Affairs of Natal, sent a copy of it to Henry McCallum, the Governor of Natal, for his official signature.[5] He also recommended that the Governor warn the High Commissioner against importing cattle from Rhodesia or from Australia. (Milner had already cabled to Australia for advice, on June 2.) Moor's letter of June 5, which was forwarded to Milner, concluded by saying that H. Watkins-Pitchford would "be leaving Natal today for Beira en route for Rhodesia with a view to ascertaining the susceptibility of Natal cattle to the disease, and he is taking with him 8 head of clean Natal cattle free from all disease for the purpose of experiment." Those cattle were presumably immune to redwater, which had long been present in Natal.

On July 19, the Governor of Natal telegraphed to Milner that all eight cattle had died: "Evidently imported type of redwater is of deadly character and will require careful and firm measures to prevent its spreading."[6] On July 21, Milner forwarded that news to Salisbury, Mafeking and Pretoria and to the Colonial Office in London.[7] Watkins-Pitchford had told the Resident Commissioner that he had expected the cattle to die,[8] and for Charles E. Gray, the death of the cattle did "not prove that the disease is not identical with that of Natal, but simply indicates that it is . . . more virulent"; thus there was no need to go to the expense of securing additional experts.[9] But the Resident Commissioner did not agree: whether the disease was a new one or not, if it could kill cattle immune to ordinary redwater, help was needed. On July 22, he sent a telegram to Milner confirming the death of the cattle[8] and adding: "Taking into consideration the difficulties explained in Mr. Robertson's memo on inoculation and the large interests at stake may I suggest that the States in S. Africa be invited to join in obtaining the best qualified expert opinion." Milner replied on July 30:[10] ". . . I agree as to advisability of obtaining best expert opinion. If the Rhodesian Administration desires steps to be taken I am prepared to approach various governments at once with a view to securing their cooperation."

As later events showed, the Chartered Company had the power

to act on its own and the ability to act quickly. Had it initiated the search for an expert and kept it in its own hands, that search might have moved more quickly. But the decision was pre-empted by Clarke and Milner, and their official obligations led to endless consultations with the four South African colonies, with the staff of the Colonial Office, with the Colonial Secretary himself, with the Royal Society, with the Foreign Office and even with the Secretary of State for War.

Was the decision to get an expert in fact taken by Clarke and Milner, acting without Kotzé's knowledge? The Resident Commissioner made his recommendation on July 22. Milner cabled his agreement on July 30, the day after the stormy meeting at which Kotzé placated the local "Chambers" by agreeing to obtain an expert from "Australia or Texas" as soon as he could consult Hutcheon. Had Kotzé known that the Resident Commissioner had urged Milner to get an outside expert as early as July 22, he presumably would have announced that fact instead of saying that he wanted to wait until he could consult Hutcheon.

Moreover, when Clarke had obtained Kotzé's consent, his telegram of August 1 to Milner[10] read:

I am requested by the Acting Administrator [Kotzé] to forward the following message to your Excellency: 'In regard to the Resident Commissioner's telegram of 22nd July and your Excellency's reply of 30th July *communicated to me* [emphasis added] . . . I beg in view of the virulent nature of the . . . disease . . . that the various South African Governments be approached by your Excellency without delay to act together jointly . . . This Administration is prepared to bear its share of the expenditure for the establishment and conducting of a temporary South African experimental station at Bulawayo which is the most suitable spot in addition to what is already being done in that direction here in Salisbury.'

One typed copy of that telegram is actually headed "Copy of telegram despatched to His Excellency the High Commissioner through the Resident Commissioner." Since Kotzé was perfectly capable of sending his own telegrams this suggests that the Resident Commissioner had indeed taken charge. Nearly two weeks passed before Kotzé sent a written confirmation to the Resident Commissioner,[10] on August 12, to say that "this Administration would be much obliged if His Excellency . . . would approach the various Governments . . . as suggested in [his] telegram of the 30th ultimo." That letter makes it seem even less likely that Kotzé had been a party to the original decision. What is certain is that the initial request for outside help was sent to the Colonial Office by Milner, not by Kotzé to the London office of the Chartered Company.

The Chartered Company had acted throughout on the advice of the veterinarians; it seems to have agreed to join in getting an outside expert in part to placate the farmers and miners and in part because Clarke and Milner had already decided that an expert was needed. Whether Clarke had taken any advice I do not know, but he was certainly at odds with the veterinarians, none of whom thought outside advice was needed. It would be interesting to know why Clarke acted against the views of the local experts and the views of the Chartered Company, but the record sheds no light on that question. On July 22 Clarke was right and Kotzé was wrong: outside advice was needed. By July 29, Kotzé had promised the settlers that outside advice would be obtained. But Milner's decision of July 30 took the matter out of Kotze's hands and put it in the hands of a slow-moving and cautious bureaucracy.

During August Milner approached the South African colonies, who were slow to respond. No expert had been invited by August 28, when Kotzé found himself in Bulawayo preparing for another confrontation with a public that was still demanding that action be taken. As a result, on August 28, Kotzé sent a telegram from Bulawayo to the Resident Commissioner in Salisbury[10] saying that if there had not been a reply from Milner "will you . . . ascertain how far matters have progressed as I am pressed here to get further expert assistance. Dr. Hutcheon recommended Professor Macfadyen [*sic*] of Veterinary College London as most suitable and failing him that Macfadyen suggests a competent man." He also said that he assumed the investigation would be conducted in Bulawayo.

On the next day, Friday August 29, Clarke sent Milner a telegram to tell him that Kotzé was anxious to know what progress was being made, that Kotzé assumed that the investigation would be conducted at Bulawayo, and that Kotzé "wishes me to inform you that Dr. Hutcheon of Cape Colony recommends Professor Mac-Fadyian [*sic*] veterinary college London or failing him the man recommended by him for the work."

Duncan Hutcheon had come up from the Cape Colony to take a look at the redwater problem; he spent most of August in Salisbury. I do not know if he had decided by then that an expert was needed.

He may simply have been willing to suggest a name once the decision had been taken.[11] The man he recommended, who actually spelled his name McFadyean, was the leading academic veterinary pathologist and bacteriologist of the United Kingdom.[12]

The first search for an expert

Milner had agreed with the Resident Commissioner on July 30 that an outside expert should be obtained. Nearly five weeks later, on September 1, 1902, he finally cabled to the Colonial Office:[13]

It is proposed that South African States should unite in bringing out first class scientific bacteriologist to investigate redwater which has broken out in Rhodesia and discover if possible means of preventive or protective inoculation ... It is suggested that Professor MacFadyean, Principal of Royal Veterinary College, London, should be asked to come or if he cannot come to recommend someone else. Would you find out and telegraph whether MacFadyean could come or if not whom he recommends. What salary would he ask?

On September 2, The Resident Commissioner advised Kotzé that the request had been forwarded.[14] He added "it can be settled later where investigation should take place. What are the appliances like at Bulawayo. There is a very well equipped laboratory at Pretoria." There was indeed a very well equipped laboratory at Pretoria: Arnold Theiler's laboratory. Had the outside expert, who eventually turned out to be Robert Koch, gone to Pretoria, the entire character of his investigation of East Coast fever might have been different. For Kotzé, however, it was crucial that the investigation be conducted in Bulawayo. The state of the economy and the effects of East Coast fever had led to public meetings being held to demand that the Colonial Office abrogate the charter of the British South Africa Company. The Bulawayo Landowners and Farmers Association had held a special meeting on August 29 and voted to oppose such demands, but one reason they had done so was that Kotzé had promised them that an expert would soon arrive to investigate the cattle disease and would carry out his studies *in Bulawayo*. The situation must have been tense: the *Bulawayo Chronicle* of August 30 reports the presence at the meeting not only of Kotzé but of Hutcheon, Gray, Gray's assistant (C. R. Edmonds) and Robertson.

Hence Kotzé's angry reply on September 2:[14] ". . . I must point out that I made it a condition . . . that the investigation or experiments were to be conducted here in Bulawayo." He asked Clarke to remind Milner of this since ". . . the matter is of the utmost and immediate importance. I must ask for a speedy assurance that it is definitely understood the experimental station is to be here at Bulawayo where the disease exists."

Milner replied to Clarke on September 3,[14] that while he did not suppose there would be any objection to the investigation being conducted at Bulawayo, it was important that the work not be delayed in any way, and since it had been suggested that full laboratory facilities might not be available there, the expert might wish to begin his work elsewhere. "If scientific appliances are immediately available, there will be no difficulties as to stationing expert at Bulawayo. Please explain that to Administrator."

On September 6 Clarke sent the gist of Milner's reply on to Kotzé and again asked what scientific appliances were available in Bulawayo. There were none, of course, but on September 9, Kotzé telegraphed directly to Milner[14] to say that although he had been told that the "place of experiment may stand over for the moment," experts, including Hutcheon, had advised him that Bulawayo would be the most suitable place "as the disease is prevalent here." More than that, "I have authorized the purchase of the buildings at Hillside Camp Bulawayo as an inoculation station and as we have as yet no laboratory there I will be obliged if your Excellency would let me know who is coming out as expert. He should bring out all necessary equipment and appliances for a suitable laboratory." Kotzé won the argument: all experts who were later approached were asked to bring out their own "appliances," and Koch did work at Hillside Camp, which was a disused army barracks in Bulawayo.[15]

As Dwork has pointed out,[16] the Colonial Office minutes relating to Milner's request that McFadyean be approached "indicate a cautious response." The file that was opened on September 2 began with the comment "Mr. Graham. I presume we should communicate substance to Prof. MacFadyean and ask whether he would be disposed to undertake the work." Graham replied: "I think we [should] first find out something, privately, about this Professor. It is my experience that such proposals are sometimes made, quite wildly, on hearsay evidence." On September 5, we find "Make private inquiry at the Agricultural Department – about Professor MacFadyean." The next minute reads: "I have seen the Private Secretary there who says that he is at the very top of his profession and would do well if he would accept." A letter was finally sent to McFadyean on September 10, explaining the situation and asking him if he would undertake the investigation.

McFadyean replied the next day that his duties at the College made it impossible for him to accept.[17] He advised the Colonial Office to approach either German Sims Woodhead,[18] or Auguste Sheridan Delépine.[19] Before the Colonial Office wrote to Woodhead and Delépine, it had heard from Milner again. In early September, Kotzé was still being bombarded by complaints from the farmers and the miners to whom he had promised some kind of action as long ago as July 30, and he lost patience. On September 13 he complained to Milner, who responded on the same day that he had sent another telegram to the Colonial Office:[20]

has answer yet been obtained from MacFadyean. Most important to lose no time … could expert who comes out bring with him necessary laboratory equipment. It is proposed to conduct investigations at Bulawayo where disease is most virulent and there is no laboratory there at present. Would bringing out of equipment involve any delay and what would be approximate cost.

The letters that were sent to Woodhead and Delépine, on September 18,[21] did stipulate that laboratory equipment would have to be brought out, which the letter to McFadyean had not done. In a preliminary reply[21] of September 19, Delépine said he would explore the possibility of being granted leave by his University, but he added that he could not claim to have any special knowledge of redwater. On September 21, he wrote that he and the Principal of Owens College had agreed that he could not leave the college for any length of time.[21] Woodhead was also a distinguished medical bacteriologist who had had no experience with redwater or with cattle diseases other than tuberculosis. He also declined. Neither McFadyean, Delépine or Woodhead suggested David Bruce;[22] two months later Bruce would be the instant choice of the Royal Society. Why his name did not come up earlier I do not know. Having declined, Woodhead kept the search alive by looking for a possible expert on his own. On October 3, he wrote[23] that "two of the men to whom I have written cannot get away … A third has wired for more information and I am to see him in Cambridge on Monday

... I have also made a rough calculation of the cost of apparatus ... about £1,200 or £1,300 would be required." Woodhead's "third man" was T. S. P. Strangeways.[24] Woodhead recommended him very highly in a letter to the Colonial Office, dated October 14, and added that Strangeways could get away for eight or ten months.[25] (At this point the Colonial Office was receiving the name of the third choice of one of McFadyean's two candidates.) Strangeways was never offered the position, since the Chartered Company had decided in favor of Koch before Strangeways' name was put to them.

Why did McFadyean not recommend a veterinary bacteriologist? McFadyean's biographer, Iain Pattison, has told me[26] that he is not surprised that McFadyean declined "because he had so much on hand at that time, particularly the human/bovine tuberculosis experiments stimulated by his disagreement with Koch." Pattison adds that

Very few veterinarians in Britain at that time had the research experience needed to investigate East Coast fever. Two possible candidates were otherwise engaged – Albert Mettam had recently been appointed Principal of the new veterinary school in Dublin, and Stewart Stockman[27] was in the Army in South Africa ... Britain was far behind continental countries in veterinary research; a government enquiry in 1922 revealed only five full-time veterinary research workers in the whole of the United Kingdom.

The political situation in Rhodesia

While the McFadyean phase of the search for an expert dragged on, a three-way struggle over the political and economic future of Rhodesia was in full swing. As analyzed by Keppel-Jones,[28] the struggle involved the Chartered Company, the settlers and the Colonial Office. Vacancies had occurred on the London board of the Chartered Company because of the deaths of Rhodes and Sidney Shippard. As a result, three new directors were elected in July, 1902: Alfred Beit (who had been forced to resign after the Jameson raid), Jameson himself, and Rhodes' banker, Sir Lewis Michell. And, in September 1902, those new directors actually visited Rhodesia, to inspect the estate, as Keppel-Jones puts it. A session of the Legislative Council was due in November. Public meetings were held in both August and September to debate whether the Colonial Office should be asked to abolish the Chartered Company by revoking its charter and "the three visiting directors ... were besieged by deputations, with grievances, requests and demands." Among those demands was the creation of a separate Department of Agriculture, which of course meant the removal of Orpen from his post as Minister of Agriculture. The Directors agreed to this; although an independent Division of Agriculture was not created until July 23, 1903, Orpen's successor, E. Ross Townsend, had long before taken over the duties of the Minister of Agriculture. They also agreed to other demands but "far outweighing all these concessions, the directors promised a reform in the constitution." That reform, which did not take effect until March 6, 1903, provided for a significant increase of settler representation on the Legislative Council. Although this reform appeared to give the settlers more power, Keppel-Jones suggests that it was really intended to give the settlers plus the Chartered Company more freedom from Colonial Office oversight: "the Company men, after chafing in silence under the imperial yoke, seized on the idea of a more popular legislature as a means of casting off the yoke." An important part of the proposed reform "was that the High Commissioner should have power to amend the constitution ... when asked to do so by the Legislative Council." Thus the Company, the settlers, the Resident Commissioner and the High Commissioner could make an agreement without interference from the Colonial Office.

The "reform" of 1903 was to lead to more and more local control of the affairs of Rhodesia. Twenty years later the Chartered Company withdrew entirely, and the colony was granted full local "responsible government" (still subject, however, to Colonial Office oversight). Keppel-Jones suggests that the proposed "reform" of 1903 was a sort of unilateral declaration of independence, a precursor of the actual unilateral declaration that occurred in 1965.

Milner and Chamberlain agreed to this reform only because of the position into which the Chartered Company maneuvered them, and even then they retained the Colonial Office power to veto further amendments of the constitution. Keppel-Jones cites a confidential dispatch from Milner to Chamberlain as saying that if the Colonial Office did not agree, the Chartered Company would say "We are prepared to give the people a greater voice in the management of this country, but, as you see, the Colonial Office has refused to allow it." Keppel-Jones adds that the Chartered Company had decided that "on balance, the Company did better by calling the people to its support in opposition to ... Downing Street than by counting on Downing Street to help it to defy the people" and suggests that "the most important decision had been taken along the road to an independent Rhodesia under white domination." And that is why Keppel-Jones chose the year 1902 as "a natural terminal date" for his book *Rhodes and Rhodesia: The White Conquest of Zimbabwe 1884–1902*.

Thus 1902, which was the year of East Coast fever and the year of the search for an expert to study East Coast fever, was also a year in which the settlers, the Chartered Company and the Colonial Office were at odds over many crucial issues. The effects of East Coast fever on farming, ox-drawn transport and mining threw fuel on the fires of the political and economic struggles.

The first request for Koch

Milner had cabled the Colonial Office on September 1, and again, even more urgently, on September 13.[29] The Colonial Office did not reply until October 1. On October 3, Milner forwarded the news to Kotzé:[30] "MacFadyean declines and also two persons recommended by him ... he is making further enquiries and pressing matter as much as possible." On October 8 the Colonial Office sent Milner the tentative budget that Woodhead had drawn up, along with a hint that the recommendation of an expert was imminent;[31] Milner forwarded that news to Kotzé on October 9.[32]

More than ten weeks had passed since the events of July 29 and July 30, and the beginning of the rainy season was only three weeks away. Ticks and tick-borne diseases would start to flourish soon. If an expert came out immediately, he might be able to do something to arrest the upsurge of disease that was expected to occur between November and the following March. If an expert began work only in March, 1903, he would be able to do relatively little until October, 1903. In spite of repeated warnings, that is exactly what happened.

Not only was there no reply from the Colonial Office, there was a new factor at work in Salisbury. As we will see in more detail in chapter 7, Gray had decided that the outbreak might, after all, be the result of either a new disease or of redwater plus a new disease. And he (and perhaps Hutcheon) had told the officials of the Chartered Company that Robert Koch had investigated a similar outbreak in East Africa in 1898. Less than three months after the events of late July, the veterinarians, the farmers and the Chartered Company agreed that an outside expert was needed, and that he should be Robert Koch. But the Colonial Office was still waiting for Woodhead to tell it whether Strangeways was available.

As a result, presumably on Gray's advice, on October 11 Kotzé sent Milner another telegram:[33]

... next to Professor MacFadyean there does not appear to be in England any really first class scientific bacteriologist suitable for our purpose and I much fear that unless we obtain a master mind time and money will be wasted. I ... beg that a cable be sent ... cancelling any selection to be made in England and that Professor Koch be approached [it may be] that after all cattle outbreak is due to a mixed infection of redwater and some hitherto unknown unclassified disease. Koch in German East Africa so I am informed experienced a similar difficulty ... necessary money [will be] advanced by this Administration ... the cost and expense to be afterwards adjusted between the various South African Governments.

On October 11 Milner telegraphed the Colonial Office:[34] "Please defer final selection till you hear further from me." Undeterred, the Colonial Office cabled its recommendation of Strangeways to Milner on October 15.[34] On October 12 Milner asked the governments of the Cape Colony, Natal and the Orange River Colony to approve securing the services of Koch.[35] The Orange River Colony agreed on October 13 and Natal on October 16, but the Cape Colony, invariably slow to reply, did not agree until October 22. Milner then cabled the Colonial Office, on October 23:[36]

... Rhodesian Government have suggested that Professor Koch be approached if possible. Unsatisfactory results of dipping in Rhodesia ... indicate possibly a mixed infection of redwater and some disease hitherto unknown and Koch is said to have experienced similar difficulty in German East Africa ... Cape, Natal and Orange River concur ... Could you ascertain whether Professor Koch would come and what his terms would be.

Unfortunately Milner did not tell Kotzé that his request for Koch's services had been forwarded to the Colonial Office, nor did the Colonial Office keep Milner informed of subsequent developments. Kotzé's request of October 11 received a reply only on November 12.

Joseph Chamberlain intervenes

Milner's telegram of October 23 led the Colonial Office to open a new file and to send a letter requesting that the Foreign Office approach the German government to see if Koch's services were available. That request had to be withdrawn when the matter came to the attention of Joseph Chamberlain. Sometime on October 27, Chamberlain scribbled an angry and all but illegible letter that was to delay the choice for another eight weeks.

Ask F.O. [Foreign Office] to delay this [until] we have communicated with R.S. [Royal Society].

It seems to me scandalous that we should have in the U.K. no one competent for this work & be obliged to ask German assistance.

What I would first ascertain [is] whether Prof. Koch is really the only possible scientist – and if R. Soc. has another candidate I would suggest to Rhodesian Gvt. that Bacteriology is not entirely 'made in Germany'.

Then if they still want Koch they may ask him themselves.

There was national[?] irritation when he was sent to the Cape about Cattle Plague [rinderpest] & I believe his prescription was a failure. J.C. 27/10.[37]

The Royal Society

Kotzé had asked Milner to obtain Koch's services on October 11, Chamberlain scribbled his angry note[38] on October 27, and on Monday November 3, Gilbert Grindle paid a visit to the Royal Society, where he left a message. On November 4, the members of the Malaria Committee were summoned by telegram[39] to a special meeting to be held on Wednesday November 5. John Burdon Sanderson and Clifford Allbutt were unable to attend. Those who did attend formed an impressive group: Lord Lister, Prof. Bradford, Lt.-Col. David Bruce, Sir Michael Foster, Sir John Kirk, Professor Ray Lankester, Dr. Patrick Manson and Charles Sherrington (I will discuss the Malaria Committee, its members and its connection to Chamberlain in chapter 6).

The Malaria Committee recommended that[39] David Bruce "be entrusted with this investigation having ascertained that ... [he] would be willing to undertake the investigation if certain difficulties connected with his membership of the Army Medical Advisory

Board could be overcome. Sir Michael Foster undertook to personally communicate this decision of the Committee to the Colonial Office authorities." The Malaria Committee clearly took the matter very seriously and wanted its case for Bruce to be made as strongly as possible. As soon as the committee had met, the Assistant Secretary of the Royal Society, Robert Harrison, wrote to Gilbert Grindle of the Colonial Office[39] that Sir Michael Foster "would like to communicate personally . . . the views taken by the Royal Society Committee . . . and will therefore call at the Colonial Office tomorrow morning [Thursday] about 12 o'clock when he hopes to have the pleasure of finding you there."

Ray Lankester felt strongly enough to send a note to the Colonial Office from the Arts Club, where he presumably went as soon as the meeting had adjourned. Lankester said that he was writing unofficially and was doing so because it was important that the Colonial Office know "something about the remarkable qualifications of Colonel Bruce . . . there is . . . no possibility of doubt that he is the man whom you would wish to employ – as being really capable and one whose performance and reputation can be preferred to those of Dr. Koch."[40]

The Colonial Office could act quickly, at least when Chamberlain was present. On Thursday November 6, Chamberlain received a persuasive hand-written report[37] advising him that

Sir Michael Foster has seen me this morning . . . [the Royal Society] can fully recommend one – but only one – Englishman, for they say that this is a particular branch of pathology that is not much taken up here in as much as it doesn't pay.

That man is Lt. Col. David Bruce, F.R.S. He conducted an enquiry into the Nagana (Tsetse fly) disease in Zululand and the Society are greatly pleased with the results (You may recollect that the Natal Govt. were very angry because Sir W. Butler took him off the investigation when Enteric broke out among the troops in Newcastle in 1898–9).

The difficulty is that he is a member of the permanent Advisory Board of the W.O. [War Office] on the R.A.M.C. [Royal Army Medical Corps], and that while he would like to go out to S.A. for the investigation he would not do so if it meant resigning from his position on the Board. The Board would not like him to go, but Sir Michael Foster says that they would grudgingly acquiesce in his being lent if you would use your influence with Mr. Brodrick [Secretary of State for War] to press them to do so.

Failing him, the Royal Soc. can only suggest that Professor Koch be approached.

The matter is urgent, as the [Advisory] Board meets at 5 p.m. today, and not again for a fortnight.

If you agree as to Colonel Bruce, would you speak to Mr. Brodrick on the subject, & ask that he be lent (without having to resign his position), provided that the S.A. Colonies agree to ask for his services?

In that case we should telegraph to Lord Milner, explain matters, pointing out that in the opinion of the Royal Soc. it is not necessary to go to Germany, asking if the S.A. Colonies would accept the recommendation of Bruce & asking what terms they would offer? (An assistant would be wanted).

Chamberlain must have approached the War Office at once, because a hand-written note[37] was sent on Friday November 7:

Dear Monk Bretton.

Mr. Chamberlain was anxious to have the services of Lt. Col. Bruce, R.A.M.C. placed at his disposal – that matter is arranged, but I conclude the usual official correspondence will emanate from you.

[signed] J. Stanley Williams[?].

Quick work indeed: the Royal Society was approached on Monday and summoned the Malaria Committee on Tuesday, the Malaria Committee met on Wednesday, Michael Foster visited the Colonial Office Thursday at noon, and the War Office made Bruce's services available later the same day!

On November 11 Chamberlain telegraphed Milner:[41]

Your telegram 23 October. Before acting on suggestion that Professor Koch should be engaged I thought it desirable to refer matter to the Royal Society. A committee of that body unanimously recommended Lieutenant Colonel Bruce F.R.S. who discovered the cause of tsetse fly disease as well as that of Malta fever and whose merit is universally recognized both at home and abroad. There is no one in their opinion who has so special an aptitude for the kind of investigation required. The Secretary of State for War is prepared to place his services at the disposal of the governments interested.

This excellent advice reached Milner too late: the Chartered Company, frustrated by the delay, had committed itself to getting Koch before Bruce was suggested as an alternative.

The Chartered Company acts on its own

The disease continued to spread, the cattle continued to die, the public became increasingly angry and the Chartered Company's officials in Salisbury received no reply to their request that Koch's help be secured. As a result, on October 28, the day after Chamberlain wrote his note, the Chartered Company decided to act on its own. Since this decision caused further delays and conflict I had wondered whether it was taken for some arbitrary or discreditable motive. Letters that have survived only in the National Archives of Zimbabwe show that the Chartered Company acted as it did out of understandable impatience.[42]

Kotzé had proposed Koch to Milner on October 11. Milner forwarded that request to Chamberlain on October 23, but he did not tell Kotzé that he had done so. As a result of that omission, the officials of the Chartered Company in Salisbury were under the impression that nothing had been done. (As a matter of fact the search had been stopped, by Chamberlain's objections to Koch, but even Milner did not know that. If either Milner or the Chartered Company had known that *something* was being done it might have been helpful. As it was, Chamberlain's recommendation of Bruce on November 11 was the first real reply to the request initiated by the Chartered Company on October 11.)

On October 23, Gray wrote to Milton's Chief Secretary (H. H. Castens) and referred to "Procuring an expert of European reputation." Milton, who had been on leave in London, presumably had asked to be brought up to date, since someone wrote a note in the margin of Gray's letter that read "What is the position in this respect?" Castens responded, also by hand, in a note dated October 27:

... Lord Milner has been instrumental in getting the Cape Natal and the Transvaal to agree to share the expenses of getting a good expert out from home & Professor MacFadyean was approached but was unable to come. Mr. Kotzé then thought of suggesting to Lord Milner that Professor Koch should come out but whether he did so or not just prior to his Honour's arrival I am unable to say as Mr. Kotzé was communicating directly with Lord Milner.

Orpen had been as busy as Chamberlain on October 27. On October 28 he wrote to Milton to say that on the previous evening he had finally had a chance to discuss the procuring of an expert with Gray, who had told him that if McFadyean could not come "then Koch should if possible be obtained . . . he has already partially investigated similar disease at Dar-es-Salaam. If Koch cannot be obtained then he would advise Professor Nocard be obtained if possible." Orpen added that since the disease was spreading in Swaziland, Natal and the Transvaal, the High Commissioner and the other colonies might agree to sending a cable to Europe "to secure the services of an expert of European reputation."[43]

Orpen's letter was minuted by Milton on the day that he received it: "The Atty Gen'l for personal expression of views W.H.M. 28/10." Kotzé replied immediately and incisively:[42]

I think we have already lost much valuable time. It is three months ago since the High Commissioner was first approached by this Administration. The matter has always been represented to the High Commissioner as of urgent and pressing importance, and I am of opinion that we are now quite justified in sending a final telegram to His Excellency. I would draw attention to the telegrams that have passed in connection with this matter, particularly to the telegram sent some three weeks ago [on October 11] by the Acting Administrator to the High Commissioner requesting that negotiations be broken off with Professor McFadyean and urging that Dr. Koch be approached without delay. *To that telegram no reply has been received* [emphasis added]. What is required is not merely a scientific and skilled bacteriologist, that we have had in Mr. Robertson and possess in Dr. Loir from the Pasteur Institute at present in Bulawayo,[44] but a master mind, and Dr. Koch seems peculiarly suited for the object in view. He was successful in South Africa with Rinderpest; has had experience of the red-water disease in German East Africa . . . and is besides at the top of his profession as a Scientist. Failing Dr. Koch we should as formerly suggested by Dr. Hutcheon and now by the Surveyor General obtain the services of Professor Nocard. It was promised the Joint Chambers at Bulawayo that the experimenting and inoculating station would be at Bulawayo, and the buildings at Hillside Camp . . . have been purchased for the purpose.

On October 30, Milton wrote on Kotzé's letter: "[Private Secretary] to draft [telegram] stating that as no definite reply has been received in view of the importance of the matter to this territory if not to S.A. I propose asking the Directors to engage Koch's services exclusively for this Government." On the same day, Milton put that draft before the Executive Council; it included the words "I recommend with advice of Council immediate engagement either Koch or Nocard to come direct to Bulawayo and investigate exclusively on our behalf."

Milton then sent a telegram to Milner, also on October 30:[45]

. . . this Administration does not consider that it will be of any advantage to obtain the services of any but the recognized Heads of the profession . . . in view of the importance of the matter to this Territory and the urgent necessity that action should no longer be delayed, I propose asking my Directors by telegraph to engage the services of Dr. Koch or Dr. Nocard for this Administration.

Milner's rather cool reply, also dated October 30, said:[46] " ...
Secretary of State was asked ... on 23rd October to engage services
of Dr. Koch ... It might therefore be advisable for your Directors
to ascertain from Colonial Office whether offer has already been
made to him." Milton telegraphed to the Cape on October 31, to
tell Stevens that the Colonial Office had already been asked to
approach Koch and that "It might therefore be advisable for Board
to ascertain from Colonial Office whether offer has already been
made to him. Not withstanding this I think our cable should be
sent." The telegram that was finally sent to London, via the Cape
Town office on October 31, 1902,[47] read:

> ... as such serious delay is occurring in securing united action with regard
> to obtaining advice of expert(s) to enquire into cattle disease and as the
> matter is of most pressing importance I do recommend with advice of
> Council immediate engagement either Koch or? Nocard to come direct to
> Bulawayo and investigate exclusively on our behalf. Koch is preferred as
> having previously knowledge of redwater though exact nature of disease
> is still doubtful ... High Commissioner cabled Colonial Office on 23rd
> October to engage Koch ... you should enquire whether any offer has
> been made to him.

Koch or Bruce: Act I

As of early November, 1902, Milner had asked the Colonial Office
(on October 23) to secure the services of Koch on behalf of the
South African colonies and Rhodesia, whereas Milton, who had
not been advised of that, had urged his London board (on October
31) to secure Koch's services solely for Rhodesia. By then there had
been two more failures of communication. When Chamberlain had
intervened on October 27, no one had advised Milner that he had
done so. For all Milner knew, the Colonial Office was moving
ahead, on his recommendation, to get Koch. Nor did the Chartered
Company know that Chamberlain was opposed to the employment of Koch. It might have learned that if the London board had
discussed its plan to hire Koch with the Colonial Office, but it had
not told the Colonial Office anything about that plan.

Milner presumably learned of Chamberlain's opposition to Koch
only when he received Chamberlain's telegram of November 11. In
that telegram, Chamberlain made it very plain that he had intervened personally ("I thought it desirable to refer matter to the
Royal Society") and that he endorsed the Royal Society's rec-

ommendation. Milner could hardly ignore a recommendation personally endorsed by Chamberlain. Nor was the Chartered Company in a position to ignore such a recommendation: to ignore the staff of the Colonial Office was one thing, to defy Chamberlain himself in a direct way was quite another matter. The possibility of employing Bruce thus had to be explored.

On November 12, Milner telegraphed to the governments of Natal and of the Cape and Orange River Colonies and to Milton:

Secretary of State . . . has consulted Royal Society and the Committee of that Body unanimously recommended that investigation be entrusted to Bruce who discovered cause of Tsetse fly disease and also of Malta fever and who has a wide reputation both at home and abroad. Bruce's services are available. I am inclined to think it would be well to accept this opinion and ask Bruce to come out at once. Do you agree?

The Orange River Colony agreed the next day and Natal agreed on November 14, but no reply was received from the Cape or from Milton, so Milner telegraphed them again on November 18 asking for a reply.[48]

Milton's delay in replying resulted from further consultation. The Chartered Company had a (presumably illegal) source of information in the Colonial Office since on November 11, *the day before Milner had cabled him*, Milton received a cable from the London office of the Chartered Company:[49]

PRIVATE. Referring to your telegram of the 31st October. Colonial Office object to employing German if Englishman available but they will approach Koch if South African Governments insist. Colonial Office are telegraphing High Commissioner asking if Surgeon Major Bruce will be acceptable to South African Governments. If Bruce approved and starts at once do you want Koch still exclusively for Rhodesia. Whoever goes out for joint Governments will visit Rhodesia first without a doubt.

Milner's telegram to Milton was not sent from Johannesburg until 6.20 p.m., November 12 and reached Milton on November 13, by which time Milton *had already asked Orpen to consult Hutcheon*. Orpen did that on November 13

. . . Royal Society . . . unanimously recommended that investigation should be entrusted not to Koch but Surgeon Major Bruce who is prepared to start at once and would doubtless come first to Rhodesia. Gray is of opinion that Koch is preferable to Bruce do you concur with him.

Hutcheon replied from Kimberley on the morning of November 14:[49]

... my preference for Koch is because he has already given considerable study to this same problem as it occurs in German East Africa and is therefore in a better position to take the matter up than anyone else. Surgeon Major Bruce did some excellent work in connection with tsetse fly disease previous to that however he was not known as a bacteriologist of any note. I would certainly prefer that Koch should be trusted with this investigation without in any way disparaging Bruce.

Hutcheon's reply was misplaced for two or three days: according to a minute of November 17,[49] it "got mixed up, i.e. attached itself to a report of Dr. Moore's." Milton met with Orpen and Kotzé on November 18 and then, on November 19, replied to Milner:[48]

... we are still strongly of opinion that if possible Dr. Koch should be secured ... especially in view of his intimate acquaintance with the nature of the disease acquired in German East Africa. My Board of Directors are willing to endeavour to obtain his services exclusively for this country should other South African Colonies decide otherwise.

On November 20, the Governor of the Cape Colony advised Milner:[48] "re Bruce, Ministers will shortly send formal reply; meanwhile, I hear that they will suggest that Dr. Koch be applied for."

A little arm-twisting was applied by the Minister of Agriculture of the Cape Colony, who cabled to the Principal Under-Secretary of Natal on November 19:[48] "Our veterinary service [Hutcheon] favours ... Koch in preference to Bruce. Do you concur?" The Governor of Natal put the matter to his Minister of Agriculture and received a revealing reply on November 21:[48] "I concur ... no doubt Koch is the better man but, in view of the recommendation of the Royal Society and the tenour of the Secretary of State's telegram I thought it better ... to fall in with his suggestion." On November 21, the government of Natal actually suggested[48] that *both* Koch and Bruce be employed! The question was also put to F. B. Smith, who wrote an interesting note which was received by the Colonial Secretary in Pretoria on November 21:[50]

It is rather a difficult question to decide. Bruce is I believe a thoroughly good man but of course he has had neither the opportunities or experience of Koch, so on the whole I should incline for the latter. Nocard of Paris has I believe conducted more research on redwater than any other man, & he is also a most able scientist & quite at the top of the tree.

On November 21, nearly a month after he had originally asked that the Colonial Office get Koch, Milner sent a telegram to Chamberlain:[50]

Administrator Southern Rhodesia still asks that Koch may be sent for and states that British South Africa Company would try to get Koch in any case ... I have just heard from Governor Cape of Good Hope that his Ministers also wish Koch to be tried. In these circumstances I think the best thing to do is to ascertain at once by cable whether Koch will come and if he refuses to arrange with Bruce. Will you do this it is important that there should be no further delay getting a man out.

Milner had thus accepted and acted on the Chartered Company's decision, but, once again, he did not tell Milton that he had done so.

The Chartered Company invites Koch

Only one day later, November 22, not knowing that Milner had finally asked the Colonial Office to approach Koch rather than Bruce, and to do so on behalf of Rhodesia and the colonies, the London board of the Chartered Company did what Milton had urged it to do on October 31, and wrote directly to Koch. Nor did it tell the Colonial Office that it had done so. The letter to Koch[51] described the problem and went on: "I am to ask you whether in the event of its being decided to send out an expert, you would be willing and ready to undertake the work in question, and if so for what remuneration?"

Koch accepted only two days later, but his conditions were that he be paid £6,000 for one year's services and that he have two assistants, each to be paid £1,000. Those fees, plus other expenses outlined by Koch came to a total of about £10,000.[52] Koch ended his letter with the comment that he could not reduce his personal fee "as I lose during the period ... my existing pay and also other revenue."

The Chartered Company, which had so boldly decided to hire Koch on its own behalf, backed away the minute it learned how much that would cost. The London office cabled to Milton on November 26:[53] "... Koch available states his expenses will exceed £10,000. We hesitate accept such heavy expenditure unless you can arrange with Viscount Milner. Reply by telegram." The responsibility had thus been put on Milton, as a private letter[54] on November 28 to Milton from the London board shows:[55] "We did not know if you realized what an enormous expense the engagement of Koch will entail, we therefore thought it better to let you know the figure before finally settling it ... the decision must come from you." The cable of November 26 was minuted: "Show to Mr. Orpen. Urgent does sum asked by Koch include assistants laboratory equipment and all other expenses."

Milton was in a very awkward position. On the one hand he did not know that Milner had already requested the Colonial Office to invite Koch rather than Bruce. On the other hand, he now had to tell Milner that the Chartered Company had bypassed the Colonial Office, and, having received Koch's agreement, felt that his services were too expensive. Even worse, from the point of view of the Chartered Company, referring the search back to the Colonial Office was bound to, and did, reopen the question of getting Bruce. But Milton had no choice: on November 28, he sent a long telegram to Milner[56] that included the words: "Dr. Koch is willing to come here ... the expense will probably not be less than £10,000." After giving the details of Koch's terms, Milton went on "I feel some hesitation in accepting his offer solely on behalf of this Government and before deciding beg to enquire whether any of the other South African Governments are prepared to contribute."

Milner sent another cool reply:[57] "As other South African governments ... [concur] in getting Dr. Koch if possible I think you may assume that they will bear a share of expense. I had already telegraphed to Secretary of State on 21st November to secure Koch if he would come and if not to send Bruce. I presume your present information comes from your London Board." Following this up with another telegram, sent the same day, Milner added "presume you will arrange through your London Office for supply to Dr. Koch of appliances referred to in the last part of your telegram of September 9." Perhaps alarmed by the coolness of Milner's replies, Milton cabled to the London Office on December 1:[58] "... High Commissioner ... telegraphed Colonial Office on 21st November asking on behalf of South African government(s) that Koch might be obtained you should see Colonial Office and leave them to arrange terms. MILTON." The London office did no such thing, although it did approach Nocard, presumably to see if his services would be cheaper than those of Koch. Nocard declined to serve and suggested Maurice Nicolle as a possible alternative.[59] Nicolle was never approached.

The Colonial Office approaches Koch

Chamberlain was no longer actively involved in the search: he was about to leave for South Africa and he sailed on November 25. Koch had been invited by the Chartered Company on November 22 and had replied on November 24, but the Colonial Office did not know that. On November 27, three days after Koch had replied to the Chartered Company and six days after Milner had asked it to approach Koch, the Colonial Office asked the Foreign Office[60] to "ascertain whether Professor Koch would be inclined to undertake the proposed investigation." On November 28, the Foreign Office sent a telegram to George W. Buchanan, Chargé d'Affaires in Berlin:[61]

Unsatisfactory result of dipping cattle in Rhodesia for supposed Redwater Fever possibly indicates mixed infection of red-water and some unknown disease. Koch alleged to have had same difficulty in German Territory – Ascertain whether he would undertake investigation at Bulawayo and if so on what terms and what would be approximate cost of requisite laboratory equipment and how soon it could be shipped to S. Africa.

On November 29, Buchanan replied that Dr. von Muhlberg had offered to procure Dr. Koch's address and had also offered to place the memorandum in Koch's hands.[62] On December 1 Buchanan advised the Foreign Office by telegram that he had learned from Dr. von Muhlberg that Koch had already sent his terms to the British South Africa Company.[63] That telegram, which reached the Colonial Office on December 3, began ". . . I have to report that Doctor Koch has telegraphed his acceptance to the British South Africa Company on the following conditions." This produced a Colonial Office minute[63] estimating the cost of a year's study at £10,000. On the same day, December 3, the Colonial Office received the same information from Milner in a telegram sent on December 1:[64]

Administrator of Southern Rhodesia telegraphs that he has ascertained that Koch will come. I presume this is through London Board of British South Africa Company. I had already heard that they proposed to invite him and suggested that they should communicate with you on subject as you were approaching him. Will you make arrangements with them and let me know result.

The receipt of these telegrams by the Colonial Office produced a marvelous minute:[64] "I think we ought to tell the B.S.A.C. how the matter stands or there may be a muddle."

Muddle may or may not be the right word to describe the situation. On November 21, Milner had asked the Colonial Office to approach Koch. Working through the Foreign Office, it did not receive Koch's terms until December 3. Starting a day later, on November 22, by December 3 the Chartered Company had approached Koch, received his terms, thought them high, ascertained that the Cape found them high, and, as we will see below, offered to pay two-fifths of the cost of Koch's services in order to lessen the cost to the other colonies.

Koch or Bruce: Act II

The Chartered Company still wanted Koch but it was no longer willing to employ him on its own because his services were too expensive. And even though Hutcheon had persuaded both Milton and the Cape that Koch was to be preferred to Bruce, the Cape Colony now declined to share in such a costly venture. The Chartered Company then came up with the notion of drawing the rest of the colonies back into the arrangement by paying more than its share. An undated note (December 1?) from Kotzé to Milton[65] says that Castens had suggested paying two-fifths of Koch's expenses, and that "I would even suggest that we pay the *half* . . . I feel very strongly that the Military Surgeon [thus did Kotzé describe David Bruce] will not be a success and then *that* expense will not merely be thrown away but much valuable time lost. It will really in the end prove cheaper for us if we even pay half . . . that will fetch the other S.A. Governments." On December 2, Milton cabled to the London office:[66] "Cape Colony thinks Koch's charges excessive and will not contribute we still desire him and suggest we pay two fifths of cost."

On December 3 the Colonial Office received two telegrams advising it that Koch was available and what his services would cost, one from the Foreign Office and one sent by Milner on December 1. On the same day it received yet another telegram, sent by Milner on December 2:[67]

Administrator Southern Rhodesia states that Cape now inclined to think Koch's charges excessive . . . Rhodesian Government . . . still strongly in favour of getting Koch . . . prepared to find two fifths of sum required leaving £6,000 to be divided among other Colonies. Would this be much in excess of their share of what would be paid to Bruce . . . if so I think Bruce should be sent otherwise Koch.

On December 3, the Colonial Office appears to have sent a letter to the B.S.A.C. asking that a representative call to discuss the matter. I have not located that letter, but it must have been strongly worded, because, on December 4, the Joint Manager of the B.S.A.C., Wilson Fox, appeared at the Colonial Office for what must have been a fairly unfriendly interview with Mr. Fred Graham, the Assistant Under-Secretary for South African Affairs. As a result, on December 5, J. F. Jones, Joint Manager and Secretary of the B.S.A.C., sent a letter to the Colonial Office that mentioned that interview and, for the first time, provided the Colonial Office with a copy of its letter to Koch of November 22,[68] a copy of Koch's reply of November 24, and copies of other "private" letters. Jones wrote further that "I am also to confirm . . . that in the event of the engagement of Professor Koch, Rhodesia will be prepared to contribute two-fifths of the expense . . . Rhodesia will not be prepared to make this contribution . . . to secure the services of some expert other than Professor Koch . . . it is most important . . . [that] steps [be] taken before the end of the rainy season." On the same day, the London office cabled Milton:[69] "Colonial Office has received from Koch same terms as were offered us they are finding out now cost of sending Bruce before deciding. We have intimated that Rhodesia will not contribute two-fifths of expense of Bruce [intimated indeed!]"

By December 5 the Colonial Office had received Koch's terms *four times*, once from Milner and once from the Foreign Office on December 3, and once from the Chartered Company and once again from the Foreign Office on December 5.[70] And Milner had put to it a specific question and a specific recommendation:[71] "Would [£6,000 divided among the colonies] be much in excess of their share of what would be paid to Bruce . . . if so I think Bruce should be sent." But the Colonial Office had not asked Bruce for his terms, although it had known since November 7 that he was willing to accept the assignment. Presumably no one had thought that the cost of an expert study might become important because no one had expected Koch's services to be so expensive. The Colonial Office therefore sent Bruce a letter that contained a statement of the problem, a request for an estimate of costs, and a query as to whether Bruce was willing to undertake the investigation. That letter was sent on the same day (December 5) that Bruce wrote to Sir Montagu Ommanney:[72]

Dear Sir, It dawned upon me a few minutes ago that perhaps you expected a letter from me as the result of our talk on Wednesday last [December 3]. I on the other hand was waiting for a letter from you. As it can at any rate do no harm, I send the information you asked for.

I may say that delay at present in regard to this work is bad. This is the time to be hard at work.

The disease will probably die out more or less from May to October, viz, in the cold months.

Yours most sincerely,
David Bruce

Bruce asked that he be paid only his annual army salary, which was less than £900. His wife would serve as an unpaid assistant and a second assistant would receive perhaps £100 a year. Other expenses would include those for travel, per diem living expenses, and equipment.

The Colonial Office did the sums[72] and concluded that Koch wanted £10,555 whereas Bruce wanted £2,880. Bruce then confused the issue by writing, on December 6[73] that he would need "large numbers of cattle . . . herd boys, cattlemen and at least one veterinary surgeon . . . If possible Vet. Surgeon Theiler [!] . . . in regard to the total cost . . . I should put it down at not less than £10,000." But the Colonial Office correctly noted that "The incidental cost . . . is a fixed quantity: it is only the personal renumeration that can make a difference between Koch and Bruce." The minute continued: "shall we tell H.C. [High Commissioner] by telegraph about Theiler? G.G." The reply was: "We may as well wait." The B.S.A.C. was notified of Bruce's terms on December 6, as was Milner. In Chamberlain's absence, the Earl of Onslow sent a cable to Milner:

Bruce's terms work out from £6,000 to £7,000 less per annum than Koch's for self and assistance which he will bring with him. Those terms include apparatus he would take with him but he stipulates in addition that he shall have use of local laboratory, materials and appliances be supplied with experimental animals and have services of an experienced local Veterinary Surgeon. Bruce has been careful to impress upon me that no comparison can be instituted fairly between their terms in view of Koch's unique position in the profession. It is for the local Governments to consider whether it is worth paying additional sum demanded in order to secure

confidence due to weight attaching to Koch's name. British South Africa
Company decline to contribute two-fifths if any one other than Koch is
employed.

On December 8, Milner sent identical telegrams to the colonies.
His telegram began by quoting Onslow's cable in its entirety,[74] thus
letting the colonies know that Koch's services would cost much
more than those of Bruce. He went on:

Governments of Cape Natal and Rhodesia have all expressed preference in
favour of Koch if he can be secured but his terms which work out at least
£10,000 for a year's work for himself and two assistants are thought high.
Please inform me by telegraph: whether in the circumstances your
Government advocates employment of Koch. Secondly whether it will be
prepared to share expenses involved. Thirdly, Whether in event of other
Governments not agreeing to share extra expense of Koch your Government agrees to employment of Bruce. It is understood that in the event of
Koch being employed Rhodesia is willing to bear two fifths of whole
expense, but if anyone else is employed it will bear only an equal share
with other governments.

Milton replied the next day:[75]

first: This Government advocates employment of Koch. Second – It will
be prepared to bear two-fifths of the cost. Third – It is not disposed to
contribute towards cost of employment of Bruce . . . this administration is
not now so much concerned in the matter as other South African Governments are. The disease has gone through this country and any steps
recommended by Koch will not affect what is past, whereas Colonies who
have not yet suffered will have the full benefit of Koch's advice as to
preventive and curative measures . . . this administration is fully satisfied
with services of Mr. Robertson [and do] not consider it of any advantage
to obtain further advice other than that of the acknowledged leader in this
branch of science, who has, moreover special acquaintance with this
disease.

Milton advised the London office of his reply to Milner on the same
day.[76] Milner immediately (i.e. still on December 9) telegraphed to
the other colonies[76] that Rhodesia would pay nothing towards the
cost of Bruce if Koch was not employed. "The alternative is therefore either to send for Koch or to drop the enquiry unless the other
Governments wish to go on with it apart from Rhodesia in employing Bruce. What is the view of your Government?" On December
11, Natal recommended employing Koch. On December 11, the
Orange River Colony replied that it would contribute to the costs
of either Koch *or* Bruce.

The Cape Colony sent an interesting reply on December 13.[75]

Someone (who?) had advised the Cape Colony that the Orange River Colony favoured Koch, when in fact, that colony was willing to go with either Koch *or* Bruce. The reply from the Cape Colony said that *since* Rhodesia was willing to pay two-fifths *and since all the other colonies wanted Koch*, Ministers "on re-consideration . . . now disposed to support . . . Koch." One wonders what might have happened if the Cape Colony had not been misinformed and had known that the Orange River Colony was willing to get Bruce?

Milner had approached the South African colonies six times. Apart from Rhodesia, every colony had, at some point, either preferred to or agreed to hire Bruce. Had Milner made a seventh approach and advised the South African colonies that the Orange River Colony was willing to get Bruce, that the Cape Colony had agreed to Koch only after reluctant reconsideration and that, even without a contribution from Rhodesia, it would cost the South African colonies about £700 each to bring out Bruce whereas it would cost them about £1,500 each if they were to divide three-fifths of Koch's charges, the balance might well have tipped in favor of Bruce. Perhaps Milner wanted to get the matter settled; perhaps he had decided that it would be better to get Koch; perhaps he wanted to keep Rhodesia in the consortium. Milton's threat to contribute nothing and do without any expert was presumably only a bluff designed to force the selection of Koch. It came only six days after his offer to pay two-fifths of the cost and public pressure to get an expert had certainly not abated. Bluff or not, it worked. On December 16, Milner cabled the Colonial Office:[77] "Cape, Natal and Orange River Colony now agree to employment of Koch . . . I presume you or London Board of British South Africa Company will now make agreement with him." On the next day Milton sent a message to the London board[78] that ended "you should see Colonial Office and arrange with them for early departure Koch."

William Robertson had surmised as much. Five days earlier, on December 11, he sent Gray a sparsely punctuated letter that ended with the words:[79] "I think Koch will come out £10,000 seems a tidy sum to pay for him & his assistants, but I suppose the best costs money personally I should like another shot in at the Rhodesian Texas fever".

Koch

On December 17 we find several minutes referring to Milner's cable.[77] "Sir M. Ommanney, send copy to F.O. ask that it may be ascertained when Prof. Koch will start? And inform B.S.A.C. and Col. Bruce? G.G. 17/12." "In the circumstances I should be inclined to let B.S.A.C. go on with the arrangements – cf Mr. Chamberlain's minute ... and inform Col. Bruce and R. Soc. privately." The reply read "Yes – tying them down to their offer of a contribution of 2/5th – and leaving them to settle with the different colonies what each is to contribute." Lord Onslow had the last word: "I much prefer that B.S.A.C. should do the work."

On December 18 the Colonial Office sent the Chartered Company a letter[80] that ended "it is understood that the offer of the Directors ... to contribute two-fifths of the expense from Rhodesian funds holds good and that they will take the necessary steps to engage Professor Koch's services." Chamberlain had had one modest success: "if they still want Koch they may ask him themselves."

On December 19 the Chartered Company cabled Koch[80] to accept his terms of November 24 and said that a confirming letter would be sent (as it was, on December 20).[81] On the same day that the confirming letter was sent Koch cabled "Can start twelfth January." On December 22[80] the Chartered Company duly notified the Colonial Office that it would indeed contribute two-fifths of the cost, adding that "Professor Koch ... will sail for South Africa on the 12th of January."

On December 19, Sir Montagu Ommanney sent Bruce a gracious private letter[82] telling him that the B.S.A.C. had chosen Koch:

the matter was, of course, entirely one for their decision and I can only say that if their choice had fallen upon you, we should have felt sure that their interests in this important question could not have been in better hands. I want to thank you for the talk we had together the other day and must express my regret for having imposed upon you a good deal of fruitless trouble. Believe me, yours very truly.

The Colonial Office also told the Royal Society what had happened. On December 20 Michael Foster replied:[82] "Bruce will not be disappointed since he expected that they would want Dr. Koch. We must try and raise an Englishman with Koch's virtues without his – – – –." (One would indeed like to know exactly what Foster had in mind when he wrote "– – – –.") Bruce may have "expected that they would want Dr. Koch," but he had some reservations about the decision. He wrote a letter that has since been destroyed; a clue to its contents is found in the register of letters received by the Colonial Office:[83] "24 Dec. 1902. [Bruce] asks letter reporting selection of Prof. Koch ... Thinks result will be interesting as his previous work has been principally among the bacteria."

Thirteen possible experts had been suggested or considered between July and December: McFadyean, Delépine, Woodhead, two unknown persons whom Woodhead had approached, Strangeways, "a man from South America," "a man from Australia," "a man from Texas," Nocard, Nicolle, Bruce and Koch. Bruce had asked for the assistance of Arnold Theiler and it seems unlikely that he would have *prevented* Theiler from carrying out the work that Theiler already had in progress, work that was so successful that the disease would eventually be called bovine theileriosis and its causal parasite *Theileria parva*. If Bruce had left in mid-November he would have reached Africa just when Lounsbury was about to identify the brown tick as the vector of East Coast fever and just as Theiler was about to complete his proof that animals immune to redwater are not immune to East Coast fever. But that work went ahead anyway, and since Bruce was not chosen, he was free to accept the next recommendation of the Royal Society and go to Uganda. While Koch was in Bulawayo, Bruce was in Uganda, establishing the fact that human sleeping sickness is transmitted by the tsetse fly and the fact that it is caused by a parasite very similar to the parasite that he had earlier shown to be the cause of tsetse fly disease of cattle.[84]

Why was Bruce's name not suggested long before November 6, 1902? He had already studied Malta fever in both man and animals and he had already discovered the cause of the tsetse-fly disease of cattle. In late July the Chartered Company had asked for McFadyean or for someone McFadyean might recommend. Perhaps Bruce was *not* famous: his work on human sleeping sickness and eponyms like brucellosis, *Brucella* and *Trypanosoma brucei* lay in the future. Perhaps his name simply did not occur to McFadyean. Then again, if Bruce had been suggested by McFadyean in early September, the War Office might not have made his services available – it did so only at the strong urging of Chamberlain, who acted on the unqualified recommendation of the Royal Society. And neither Chamberlain nor the Royal Society had been drawn into the matter in September.

Nor did Chamberlain's telegram to Milner really convey the intensity of the Royal Society's support for Bruce. Milner in turn advised the South African colonies only that "Bruce had discovered the cause of Tsetse fly disease and also of Malta fever and . . . has a wide reputation." Besides that Milton requested Hutcheon's advice on the basis of the secret cable from his London office which told him nothing at all about Bruce's qualifications. Hutcheon in turn knew nothing of Chamberlain's strong recommendation, of Lankester's letter, of Foster's visit to the Colonial Office: Milton told him only that "Royal Society . . . recommends Surgeon Major Bruce." A good deal of lobbying and good advice had gone to waste.

Hutcheon was the key to the whole affair. He was the best known veterinarian in the whole of southern Africa, and the only person to whom Kotzé or Milton could reasonably have turned for advice. The first expert from outside Rhodesia was William Robertson, sent from the Cape by Hutcheon. When it was decided to obtain an expert from England, Hutcheon recommended McFadyean. When McFadyean declined and could not produce another candidate, Hutcheon recommended that either Koch or Nocard be approached. Finally, when Bruce was proposed as an alternative to Koch, Milton sought Hutcheon's advice, and Hutcheon recommended Koch. The only part of the story that is not explained by the role of Hutcheon is the equivocal nature of the Cape Colony's replies to Milton, but that may have resulted simply from the fact that the Cape government was reluctant to spend so much money to get Koch no matter how strongly Hutcheon supported him. Nor can one suggest any bias on Hutcheon's part. He knew as well as anyone could have that Koch's work on rinderpest had not been an unqualified success but he also knew that Bruce had never studied redwater whereas both Koch and Nocard had done so.

It is easy to think of various unworthy motives or unconvincing reasons for the choice of Koch. Koch was "famous," he was a "master mind," he had had "experience with rinderpest," his name would "reassure the public." (The latter would not have been a wholly "unworthy" motive, considering the level of public anxiety.) But the Chartered Company insisted on Koch because he was repeatedly recommended by Hutcheon and by Gray, who recommended him for none of those reasons. Hutcheon and Gray recommended Koch because they knew that the lethal form of redwater that Koch had studied in German East Africa resembled the disease that had broken out in Rhodesia. They were even more right than they knew: although he did not know it himself, the disease that Koch had studied in East Africa was actually East Coast fever.

5

Robert Koch in Bulawayo

As soon as he received written acceptance of his terms, Koch wrote to the London office of the B.S.A.C., on December 22, 1902 to suggest that he should travel to Bulawayo not by the fast mail ship from London to Cape Town, but via a slower route, along the east coast of Africa to Beira.[1] He recommended that he take that route because the disease had apparently broken out in Beira and spread from there. Moreover, "I could institute researches into the occurrence of this or similar diseases at the different stopping places at which the steamer may touch." He added "I shall be glad if you will send me the report on Texas Fever or Redwater in Rhodesia by Mr. Gray and Mr. Robertson and any other reports upon diseases affecting human beings and cattle." Koch thus asked, explicitly, for a copy of the final joint report in which Gray and Robertson had given a detailed picture of clinical and post-mortem findings, had carefully re-described the "juvenile form" of the parasite and had noted that the juvenile form had been seen in hundreds of cases, only twenty of which also showed the typical pear-shaped parasite. That report, discussed in chapter 3, was published as a pamphlet in August, 1902, and had been reprinted in the November issue of the *Agricultural Journal of the Cape of Good Hope*. Whether Koch had seen one of those versions or had merely seen a reference to the report is not clear, but he obviously had heard of it. On December 24 the B.S.A.C. sent him that report,[2] along with Gray's report of January, 1902, the "interim" reports by Gray and Robertson of late May, 1902, and Gray's annual report to the Agricultural Department for the year ending March 31, 1902, which was still unpublished.

Before we follow Koch to Bulawayo we must review the work he had done in Dar-es-Salaam in 1897 and 1898, when he had studied what he thought was a "virulent form" of Texas fever and had observed and described unusual forms of the parasite in lethal cases.[3] In an official report in the form of a letter dated November 15, 1897,[4] Koch said that although many cattle in the East African region die of surra [trypanosomiasis], "a far greater percentage [die from] a disease which . . . is so similar to a certain cattle pest known in the United States as Texas fever . . . that I have no hesitation, despite certain variations in character, in saying that the cattle pest that prevails here is Texas fever." Koch added that he had confirmed both the clinical and post-mortem findings that are characteristic of Texas fever. The blood was very watery and the serum had a distinctly yellow color. The organs had a typical icteric (i.e. jaundiced or yellow) color. The spleen and liver were greatly enlarged and the urine was bloody although "strange to say, this important symptom had been locally overlooked." But, Koch remarked,

the greatest interest centred, of course, in the microscopic examination of the blood, in which as is well known, Th. Smith and F. L. Kilborne[5] have discovered a parasite, which they regard as the cause of Texas fever.

This parasite is found in the red blood corpuscles, and is, when fully developed, of a pear-shaped form. As a rule two of these parasites are lying next to each other in a red blood corpuscle, on account of which this particular micro-organism has received the name of *Pyrosoma bigeminum*.

The discoverer of the *Pyrosoma* states that the parasite has, in its earliest stage, forms which look like very fine points or at most assume the size of micrococci. These are said to be found exclusively in mild cases of Texas fever, but then in large numbers, so that 5 to 50 percent of the red blood corpuscles are infected with them. In acute cases of Texas fever the only parasite found is said to be the pear-shaped form.

In a certain number of the animals examined by me I could trace the developed *Pyrosoma bigeminum*. It answered the description of it given by Smith and Kilborne so perfectly that no room for doubt was left regarding the identity of the parasite here found with that discovered in American cattle.

Only with regard to the earlier forms [*Jugendformen*] of the *Pyrosoma* and the relations of both it and the full-grown parasite to mild and severe Texas fever, have I come to different conclusions from the American investigators. I found, namely, particularly in the red blood corpuscles of cases which took a severe form and rapidly proved fatal, strange forms resembling miniature staves, so that one might take them to be bacilli. These are frequently slightly curved, and sometimes so [strongly curved] that they form rings and in that case look very much like the parasite of tropical malaria. Frequently these little staves are slightly thicker in the centre. They then clearly show a double outline and assume the form of a willow leaf. Between such forms and the pear-shaped form of the full-grown *Pyrosoma* there are a number of intermediate stages, and I have in consequence formed the conviction that the parasites I found are the real first forms [*eigentliche Jugendformen*, i.e. 'true juvenile forms'] of the *Pyrosoma*.

Koch added that he could not, for the present, decide whether the differences between his findings and those of the American investigators were the result of the time of year, the climate, the race of cattle or, perhaps, of the experimental method.

Koch thus saw two kinds of parasite, one large and pear-shaped, and one much smaller and "stave-like." And he followed Smith and Kilborne in regarding the smaller parasites as being the juvenile form of the larger parasites. Smith and Kilborne had associated the small parasites with a mild form of Texas fever and the large pear-shaped parasites with a severe form of Texas fever. Only on that point did Koch say that he differed with Smith and Kilborne, since he found the small parasites in severe cases of the disease and the large parasites in less severe cases.

Having described the post-mortem findings and the parasites, Koch noted that he found areas where "Texas fever" was endemic. In those areas, the cattle were more or less immune and seemed to suffer little from the disease (that state of affairs can, in fact, be found in both East Coast fever and Texas fever). On the other hand, when non-immune cattle were brought into an area where the disease was endemic, the disease broke out among them. Cattle brought to the coast from inland soon fell ill. This suggested to Koch that the disease was endemic on the coast and that cattle brought from inland to Dar-es-Salaam or other parts of the coast contracted it there.

Koch therefore devised an ingenious experiment which unfortunately yielded extremely misleading results. Rather than bring more cattle from the mountains to the coast, or bring cattle from the coast to the mountains, he decided to bring ticks from the infected coastal area to the mountains to see whether those ticks would infect healthy cattle in the mountains. "At Dar-es-Salaam . . . ticks were taken from animals belonging to an infected herd but which had a healthy appearance . . . [and] from a calf suffering from Texas fever (the blood of this calf contained a very large number of Texas fever parasites, but only the early forms of them; it died the next day)."

The ticks began to lay eggs even before Koch left Dar-es-Salaam but larvae developed from the eggs during the journey to the mountains, which took two weeks. In the mountains, Koch placed the larvae on healthy cattle. If the larval forms had descended from ticks originally removed from healthy cattle on the coast, the animals on which they were placed in the mountains remained healthy. But if the larval forms had descended from ticks removed from the diseased animal on the coast, the animals on which they were placed in the mountains were found, at the end of twenty-two days, to have many parasites in their red blood cells. Those parasites were pear-shaped, the illness was mild, and the cattle recovered. Yet the larval forms had grown from the eggs of ticks removed from an animal whose red blood cells showed what we now know to be the parasite of East Coast fever and, indeed, from an animal that had died the very next day.

How can this be explained? Rather simply, in fact. The eggs that Koch used must have been eggs of the species of tick that can transmit Texas fever, the blue tick. And, in that species of tick, as Smith and Kilborne showed in 1893, the parasite is transmitted from the tick to its eggs and thus to its larval descendants. The ticks must have fed on an animal infected with both East Coast fever and Texas fever. The larvae of those ticks could and did cause Texas fever when they were allowed to feed on a healthy animal in the mountains because the parasite had been transmitted from tick to egg to larva.

East Coast fever is transmitted by a different tick, and its parasite is *not* passed forward via the egg. (That was not discovered until 1903, by Lounsbury and by Theiler.) If Koch had taken "East Coast fever ticks", i.e. brown ticks, from infected cattle, and allowed them to lay eggs, the parasite would not have appeared in the eggs of those ticks, and the resulting larvae could not have infected healthy cattle with East Coast fever (or with Texas fever). Koch had thus transmitted *ordinary Texas fever* by larvae that had hatched from infected eggs, whereas what he had hoped to do was reproduce, in the mountains, the "severe form" of the disease and the "juvenile forms" of the parasite that he had seen on the coast.

Once he had succeeded in infecting cattle, Koch made further studies in the mountains. Knowing that Texas fever (redwater) can be transmitted by injecting a healthy animal with blood taken from an infected one, Koch took blood from one of the animals that had developed Texas fever after being exposed to the larval form of the tick and injected it into four healthy animals. They rapidly came down with Texas fever, complete with pear-shaped parasites, but of course, no juvenile forms; although they became very ill, they all recovered.

Koch then did a *third* test. He injected blood from infected animals into six more animals. Two of those animals were healthy and previously untested and two were the cattle that had remained healthy after being tested with the larval descendants of the eggs of ticks taken from healthy animals back on the coast. All four of those animals became ill. The remaining two animals were those that had recovered after a mild attack of Texas fever, induced by the larval forms of ticks originally taken from infected animals on the coast. When those two cattle, which had recovered from Texas fever, were injected with infected blood they remained completely healthy: they were immune as the result of the earlier mild attack. But Koch seems to have thought that he had induced immunity to the "severe form," and that seems to be why, when he realized in 1903 that the "severe form" was East Coast fever, he thought that he could induce immunity to East Coast fever by the inoculation of blood.

Koch was an exceptionally clever investigator and he realized that there were two gaps in his evidence. He knew that, in his experiments in the mountains, he had *not* reproduced the severe and usually fatal form of the disease that he had seen in non-immune animals brought to the coast, and he knew that he had not reproduced the small "juvenile forms" of the parasite. He thought that the difference in climate between the mountains and the coast might explain that, but he was well aware what the crucial experiment would be, and he did that experiment. He took six immunized animals down from the mountains to the coast at Dar-es-Salaam to see if they were immune to the naturally occurring form of the disease *and* to see what would happen if he injected them with blood containing the juvenile form of the parasite. Injection of blood does not readily transmit East Coast fever, but, since the animals were not immune to East Coast fever, they should have died soon after they were brought to the coast and exposed to ticks infected with the East Coast fever parasite. In a sense Koch had, partly by accident, devised exactly the right series of experiments. By using larvae that could transmit only Texas fever he had produced animals immune to that disease. If those immunized animals, after having been brought to the coast, had fallen ill and died, with their blood full of "juvenile forms," Koch would surely have realized that he was dealing with two separate diseases.

But the final experiment was not completed before Koch had to leave Dar-es-Salaam. He states clearly in his letter of February 14, 1898, that he had brought the cattle to an area where they surely were exposed to East Coast fever. If they had died, he certainly would have said so, having raised the question so explicitly. They must have contracted East Coast fever, but they presumably did so only after Koch had left. East Coast fever has a latency period of up to two weeks; in Lounsbury's first experiment (see chapter 7), the parasites appeared in the blood nineteen days after the animal was bitten by the tick. Koch's last letter from Dar-es-Salaam is dated March 6; the cattle should have shown signs of serious illness a day or two later! As Gray said in 1908:[6]

Koch's observations appear to have gone no further at this time, or if they did they were not considered of sufficient interest to place on record . . . if the projected experiment had been carried out [it was begun, but it was not completed] . . . he might have found out that the disease which he produced in the . . . mountains was not the rapidly fatal form . . . which killed off animals so quickly at the coast, and further inquiry might have placed him in possession of important information which would have made the record of his researches a guide instead of a stumbling-block to future investigators.

What does this mean? It means that Koch had seen a new disease and an old one and had lumped the diseases and their causal parasites into a single disease and a single causal parasite. He had described only the typical post-mortem findings of genuine Texas fever. As to clinical findings, he noted only that "Texas fever" sometimes assumed a lethal form. He saw the parasite that causes East Coast fever and said it was a juvenile form of the parasite that causes Texas fever. And, from the misleading results of his ingenious experiments with ticks, he concluded both that he had transmitted the disease and that he had evoked immunity to it. His report certainly influenced Gray and Robertson in their conclusion that the virulence of the disease, and their finding of small parasites, did not mean that the disease was other than Texas fever (redwater), since Koch had already shown that Texas fever could appear in a "severe form" and that its causal parasite could appear as a "juvenile form."

As we will see, in 1903 Koch came close to implying that he had discovered "Rhodesian Redwater," i.e. East Coast fever, *and* its causal parasite as long ago as 1897. He had, of course, seen both the disease and the parasite, but he certainly had not "discovered" East Coast fever in 1897 and 1898. Why did he imply, and perhaps believe, that he had done so? Presumably because as soon as he heard of "Rhodesian Redwater" he recalled and began to re-evaluate his experiences of 1897 and 1898. Why else would he have suggested travelling to Bulawayo not via the fast and comfortable mail ship from London to Cape Town but by a far more tedious route along the east coast?[7] On the other hand, during that long and tedious journey he had the results of Gray and Robertson in hand. And he surely studied the reports of those results during his two-month-long voyage to Beira. In their reports Gray and Robertson had skillfully and accurately described both the clinical and the post-mortem differences between "typical" and "atypical" redwater. They had also described the prevalence of the parasite that Koch had previously regarded as being only the "juvenile form" of the parasite that causes redwater. And they cited Watkins-Pitchford's evidence that eight Natal cattle immune to ordinary redwater were not immune to the new disease.

Koch arrived in Beira on February 18, 1903, having made "investigations and enquiries . . . along the East African coast [at seven places, including Mombasa and Dar-es-Salaam]." Rhodesia had been waiting for his arrival for a very long time. A cable to Milton from the Cape Town office,[8] dated February 6, 1903 reads:

following from Sir Lewis Mitchell begins Koch lands Beira 18th Feby. Major M. Heany states that Redwater is rapidly gaining ground in Matabeleland cattle having died on the town commonage Bulawayo he thinks that public opinion will be strong against the delay incurred by adoption of Beira route this is now unavoidable that route was probably wisely selected to trace the disease from its source but I suggest that one of Koch's assistants should proceed to Bulawayo sharp which would give great satisfaction.

Koch and his party were met at Beira by Gray; two days later they were in Umtali. Little could be done in Umtali because "the disease had spent itself and only a very few head of cattle were left." The same condition was found at Salisbury and the group went on to Bulawayo where the army barracks at Hillside Camp awaited them, still undergoing renovation. Because of the delays in securing his services and because he had taken a time-consuming route,

Koch reached Bulawayo close to the end of the rainy season. As we will see, he was never able to evoke cases of the disease by the use of ticks. And because the disease and the ticks died down between April and September, he found it difficult to test animals to see if he had immunized them. The only way he could do that was by exposing them to the infected fields and the fields were not to become infective again for some months. (Ticks and East Coast fever die down so much between July and October that farmers in Zimbabwe are legally entitled to dip cattle less frequently during those months.)

The young veterinarian, G. Stanley Bruce, who had joined the Rhodesian veterinary service in July, 1902, seems to have struck up an acquaintance with David Bruce before leaving England. On March 5, 1903 he sent a fairly shrewd summary of the situation to David Bruce:[9]

I have now been some time in Rhodesia and thought a few lines on the cattle disease would interest you. Dr. Koch and his two assistants arrived last week, having come up from Beira. They have gone on to Bulawayo. The disease is worst at that place just now . . . I am sending you a report which some time ago was published by Mr. Gray . . . & Mr. Robertson . . . which gives a good description of symptoms, P.M. [post-mortem] & microscopical examinations . . . so far none of their suggested methods of inoculation have been successful . . . Dipping did not further the success of inoculation . . . in my opinion ticks get on to cattle in the larval stage and infect at that time . . . You will notice reading P.M. [post-mortem] notes the frequency of lung complications . . . only in a few cases is haemoglobinuria present . . . The greatest death rate has been amongst transport cattle & on farms adjoining transport roads. In most cases where no transport has been no Redwater has broken out . . . Rabies broke out about 5 months ago . . . [in addition to muzzling] 40,000 dogs have been destroyed in Matabeleland alone.

On March 26, 1902, less than a month after his arrival in Bulawayo, Koch submitted his first or "Interim" report.[10] That report is a marvel of style, content and lucidity. Koch noted that while waiting for the stables to be rebuilt so that "healthy animals can be kept without danger of infection" . . . "we have lost no opportunity of studying the disease by observing its course in sick animals, by making post mortems and by examining the various organs therefrom . . . [an] extraordinarily high mortality characterizes this disease. In Umtali, of 4,000 head of cattle, scarcely 200 survive."

"The symptoms of the disease and the post mortem appearance

... correspond to those given in the most excellent report of Messrs. Gray and Robertson." It had been supposed that the Rhodesian disease was identical with Texas fever but "important differences appear." In Texas fever, as Koch pointed out, large pear-shaped twin parasites are found in the red blood cells, a great number of red blood cells perish, much of their coloring matter is liberated to discolor the blood serum and to cause hemoglobinuria or red water. And, of course, a marked anemia is seen. In "Rhodesian Fever," as studied by Koch up to the time of his first report, the parasites were smaller and of a different shape, there was not the same destruction of red cells, hemoglobinuria was rarely seen and no remarkable anemia developed.

Moreover, in "Rhodesian Fever" one finds lesions not seen in Texas fever. These are found in the kidney, lungs and liver, and in the swollen and bloody lymph glands. And, "we find in all these . . . parts that the organisms are unusually abundant and there we have observed a peculiar form which up to now has not been described, a form which leads to the conclusion that here an increase of parasites takes place." (These "peculiar forms" are the "macroschizont" form of the parasite. Known as Koch's blue bodies,[11] their presence provides an important means of diagnosing the disease and they had not been described by Gray and Robertson. In the light of later insights into the effect of the parasite of causing multiplication of lymphoid cells, Koch's conclusion "that here an increase of parasites takes place" was truly remarkable.)

Koch went on to argue that one must distinguish between Texas fever (redwater) and "Rhodesian Fever" because "the causal parasites, the symptoms to which they give rise, and the pathological changes in the organs, are different." He went on to say that:

bearing out my opinion that the Rhodesian Fever is a specific disease, I may instance another fact considered of considerable importance at the present day in the classification of infective [*sic*] diseases, and this is that it has been proved through direct experiments by Gray, Robertson, Pitchford and Theiler, that cattle from Natal and the Transvaal which are, as we know, immune against Texas Fever as existing in Natal and the Transvaal, and even cattle from Texas itself will catch the Rhodesian Fever and die of it. Were the two diseases of exactly the same character, a complete or at least a certain degree of immunity should have been manifested, but this is not so; therefore they cannot be considered identical, nor is the view that Rhodesian Fever is merely a more than usually virulent form of Texas Fever a tenable one.

The importance of this passage will become entirely clear in chapter 7. At this point, I will only argue that Koch's reference to the fact that "Rhodesian fever" can kill even cattle brought from Texas proves that he was aware of the results of experiments that Theiler had begun in August 1902 and brought to a successful conclusion in early 1903. Those experiments had shown that cattle imported from regions where all cattle were immune to Texas fever (redwater) *and* cattle artificially immunized against "ordinary" redwater died soon after being exposed to the "new disease." Koch's correct and influential assertion was not based primarily on evidence that he had obtained himself. While Theiler held back, Koch strode forward, to a conclusion that, even if it was not fully tested, was correct: "Rhodesian Redwater" was not Texas fever.

Koch went on, in his interim report, to discuss the Australian cattle, which he assumed had caught the disease at Beira and had carried it to Umtali. But how, he asked, could those cattle have become infected? They had been healthy in New South Wales, where no such disease existed, they had remained healthy on the long sea voyage and there was no apparent disease in Beira. At this point there is a major break in Koch's logic, because there were many serious diseases in Beira to which the local cattle were resistant but to which the Australian cattle were wholly non-immune, including, of course, ordinary redwater. Koch ignored the possibility that the Australian cattle might have died of other diseases to which they had no immunity in favor of suggesting that the Australian cattle had contracted the "Rhodesian Fever" in Beira that is, to say, on the *coast*.

Koch's use of that argument almost suffices to prove that he arrived in Rhodesia all but convinced that the disease that he had come to investigate was the same disease that he had seen in 1897, namely a disease that is endemic along the coast but normally absent inland. And, indeed, he went on to say:

The problem would be well nigh insoluble if there was not one piece of evidence in our possession which I became cognizant of some years back, namely that the same disease exists on the East African coast, as has now broken out in Rhodesia . . . the [symptoms] of this disease are the same as those of Rhodesian Fever and in the blood of these infected animals which I have many times examined, I have always found the same small blood parasites which I have again seen at Umtali, Salisbury and Bulawayo.

All that he needed to confirm his conclusion was the additional, still unpublished, evidence that he must have learned from Gray. That was the evidence provided by Theiler that cattle unquestionably immune to redwater (Texas fever) were fully susceptible to the "new disease." (That evidence is considered in detail in chapter 7.)

Having announced that the disease was a new one, Koch went on to argue that the disease had long been endemic on the coast at Beira and that it had been brought to Rhodesia by the Australian cattle that had contracted it while at Beira. He also argued that it must be endemic on the coast at Delagoa Bay in southern Mozambique, from where it had recently invaded the Transvaal. The disease had thus "conformed to a natural law . . . it has been brought inland from the infected coast districts as it has previously been in many other instances and [therefore should be called] 'African Coast Fever' [rather than] 'Rhodesian Fever'."

We must pause to recall that, although the disease was new to Rhodesia, it almost certainly was not brought in by the Australian cattle. Moreover, it seems most unlikely that it had for a long time been prevalent on the coast at Delagoa Bay in Portuguese East Africa (Mozambique). Not only was there constant trade between Beira and Umtali, but the two towns had been connected by railway since February 1898, and that railway certainly carried cattle. The disease *had* long existed in Tanganyika and it is almost beyond doubt that it was brought to Beira and Umtali late in 1901 by cattle imported from Dar-es-Salaam. Moreover, the low veld of the Transvaal is very close to Delagoa Bay and is not as thoroughly separated from the coast by mountains as Umtali is. The Transvaal could hardly have remained free from East Coast fever if that disease had for a long time been endemic in southern Mozambique. Why had the disease not appeared sooner? Because Dar-es-Salaam is a long way from Beira, at that time at least a week by sea, and to ship cattle from Dar-es-Salaam to Beira presumably had become economically feasible only because of the need to restock after rinderpest had been brought under control. But Koch, like so many others, was misled by the death of the Australian cattle, deaths which, in any case, fit so neatly with his preconceived notion that the disease was "coastal."

As to the identification of the tick responsible for transmitting the disease, on March 27 Koch wrote to his colleague Wilhelm Dönitz[12] that he had gathered very important material at each stop along the coastal route, including specimens of ticks. As a result, Koch said, he had already acquired a complete and exact knowledge of all of the species of ticks that occur both along the coast and in Rhodesia. This seems like a rash claim, the more so because he announced in his interim report that as a result of the collections of ticks that he had made along the coast and in Rhodesia he had established that the blue tick (*Rhipicephalus decoloratus*, as he called it) was responsible for transmitting the disease. He was completely wrong, but he never realized that and left Rhodesia still convinced that the blue tick was the carrier. The blue tick is the tick that transmits Texas fever in southern Africa but, since it cannot transmit East Coast fever, all of the results of many later experiments in which Koch used ticks to transmit East Coast fever must be viewed with skepticism. The matter goes far deeper. All of the work that Koch did in Rhodesia was hampered by his inability to induce East Coast fever at will. He expected to induce the disease by injecting blood: that procedure will transmit Texas fever but not East Coast fever. And, because he did not identify the brown tick as the transmitter of the disease, he could not induce the disease by the use of ticks. Having announced that the new disease was *not* Texas fever and that the parasite that causes it is *not* a form of the parasite that causes Texas fever, Koch spent the next year trying to transmit the new disease either by the blue tick, which transmits Texas fever but does not transmit East Coast fever, or by the inoculation of blood, which also transmits Texas fever but not East Coast fever. (Why Koch did not welcome the fact that the disease was not carried by the blue tick as further evidence that the disease was a new one I have no idea.)

It is exactly at this point that we can see the most serious consequence of the demand by the British South Africa Company that Koch work in Bulawayo. Had Koch worked in Pretoria he would surely have been in regular communication with Arnold Theiler and, through Theiler, with Lounsbury. And he could hardly have overlooked their evidence, described in detail in chapter 7, that the new disease was not transmitted by the blue tick but by the brown tick. And so the public meetings in Bulawayo that demanded abrogation of the B.S.A.C.'s charter helped to shape the direction of Koch's research.

Having expressed some doubts about whether cattle can develop a lasting immunity to Rhodesian fever, Koch went on to say that he had some hopes in that direction because of his previous experience at Dar-es-Salaam. (He was right in the sense that he had seen herds along the coast that were more or less immune to a disease that swiftly struck down animals brought to the coast, and that disease was almost certainly East Coast fever. In regions where East Coast fever is endemic, calves became ill from it. Many die, but those that survive do become immune.) Koch pointed out that a major problem would arise from relying on naturally acquired immunity, because such immunity would develop only in the 10 to 20 per cent of animals who survived an initial attack of the disease. That would be a very long and very costly way to acquire large immune herds. On the other hand, since it hardly seemed possible to eradicate the ticks, much effort would have to be directed at finding a way to induce immunity. "It is my intention to do my utmost to obtain a suitable stock vaccine as soon as possible. I will experiment simultaneously in many different lines in order to save time, and for the purpose many healthy cattle will be required."

Gray was about to write his report for the year ending March 31, 1903.[13] In that report, he said that Dr. Koch had concluded that a new disease is present, which "he proposes shall be called 'African Coast Fever' . . . This conclusion, while it negatives the view that our local disease is ordinary Redwater which has undergone intensification . . . does not necessitate any change in . . . policy . . . as ticks alone are responsible for dissemination . . . the steps necessary to check the spread of virulent Redwater apply equally to 'African Coast Fever'." Gray went on to list the results of forty-two attempts that he had made to induce immunity by inoculation of blood. Since the results had not been encouraging he reiterated the need for dipping, which had, however, remained very unpopular among farmers and the transport riders. The disease was not abating in virulence and about 90% of the cattle had died in various townships. It is, Gray said, to be hoped that Drs. Koch, Kleine and Neufeld will find a means "to cope with this slowly spreading [disease: crossed out] scourge."

As of the end of March, 1903, Koch had thus correctly surmised, largely on the basis of evidence that had been obtained by other investigators, that the disease was a new one, given it a name, identified the wrong tick as its carrier, made the remarkable observation that the parasite multiplies in lymphoid tissue and begun a year-long search for a method of immunization. As a result of that year-long search he did develop a technique that he believed induced immunity to East Coast fever but both his method for producing immunity and his evidence that it did produce immunity were to be shown to be baseless.

Koch's interim report reached the Colonial Office on May 9, 1903, where it was duly minuted:[14] "Prof. Koch finds that the Rhodesian disease is similar to one indigenous for generations on the German East African Coast but differs from Texas Fever . . . the disease is spread by ticks and protection by inoculation is the goal." Copies of the interim report were sent to the Foreign Office, the Royal Society and Professor McFadyean.

On April 2, 1903, the Administrator of Rhodesia (Milton) cabled to High Commissioner Milner:[15]

Important preliminary report by Dr. Koch. Your Government should know at once that he thinks that disease, although allied to Texas Fever . . . is a distinctly different disorder, the causal parasites, the symptoms and the pathological changes . . . being different . . . He advises that Ports on East Coast used for introduction of cattle . . . [be examined for signs of African Coast Fever] and those so infected should be closed against cattle . . . He advises that we cannot at present reckon upon lasting immunity but he is convinced that such a thing exists.

What are we to make of the fact that Koch had said in his interim report that he had some years ago been cognizant of this disease on the East African Coast, since it is clear that he had been cognizant of no such thing? In his report of 1898 he said that the cattle he had studied in 1897 and 1898 showed the classic post-mortem findings of redwater and that the unusual parasite was only a juvenile form of the redwater parasite. It was Gray and Robertson who described the clinical picture and the pathological changes that distinguish "typical" redwater from "atypical" redwater. It was Gray and Robertson who reported finding the unusual form of the parasite in the blood of *all* of the several hundred cattle they had studied, the typical form also being present in only twenty of those cattle. Moreover, the joint report by Gray and Robertson gave full details of the death of the cattle that Watkins-Pitchford had brought from Natal, deaths that proved that animals immune to redwater quickly died of the new disease. And all of that information was in the reports that Koch had with him during the two-month-long voyage to Beira.

As his interim report shows, soon after he arrived in Rhodesia, Koch learned, presumably from Gray, that Theiler had produced further proof that cattle immune to redwater were not immune to the new disease.[16] With the clinical and post-mortem observations of Gray and Robertson in hand, and with the proof that cattle immune to Texas fever were susceptible to "Rhodesian Redwater" in hand, it is not surprising that it took Koch only three weeks in Bulawayo to announce that the disease was indeed a new one, which should be called African Coast fever. Koch certainly deserves great credit for that insight, one that Gray and Robertson had failed to make. But Gray and Robertson were held back from the insight, at least in part, because they had relied on Koch's assertions of 1898 that the disease that he had seen in 1897 and 1898 was Texas fever and that the unusual parasite that he had seen was only a juvenile form of the parasite that caused Texas fever. I wonder how Gray felt when Koch said something like: "Yes, of course, this is the disease that I saw some years ago in German East Africa and described in 1898"?

In a letter to Dönitz[17] of March 27, 1903, Koch said "the disease itself . . . is, as I had suspected from the beginning, the same that prevails on the German East African Coast." This indeed suggests that as soon as Koch had been advised by the British South Africa Company that a "virulent" form of redwater had appeared in Rhodesia he suspected that he might have seen the same disease in 1897 and 1898 (although without having realized at that time that it was a new disease). This interpretation of the events leads to a story in which everything falls into place: with a view to testing his hypothesis, Koch travelled to Rhodesia along the east coast of Africa, looking for parasites like those he had seen in 1897 and 1898. While *en route* he studied the report by Gray and Robertson, whose observations fit in with that hypothesis. But, with appropriate caution, he waited until he could see for himself, and announced his conclusion only after he had seen many sick cattle, done many post-mortem studies and examined many slides of the blood and other tissues. Even with this reconstruction of the events, one cannot argue that Koch gave Gray and Robertson full credit for their careful re-description of the parasites and for their description of the different clinical findings in "typical" and "atypical" redwater. That may be a small matter since Koch was generous in praising their post-mortem findings. But we have yet fully to deal with Koch's assertion that he had been "cognizant" of the disease in 1898. Had Koch been more candid in 1903 he might have said that in 1897 and 1898 he had thought and said that the disease he saw in

German East Africa was Texas fever. Koch might have added that it was only after he had been asked to investigate "Rhodesian Red-water" that he had realized that the disease he had seen in 1897 and 1898 might not have been Texas fever after all. (Stanley Portal Hyatt actually said[18] that "the great German scientist himself told me that he knew all about the matter before he came out, that he had known all about it for the past seven years, and had long ago given the authorities warning." The statement that Koch claimed to have warned the authorities must be taken with more than one grain of salt, since it reflects Hyatt's hatred of the Chartered Company.)

Questions of candor aside, Koch was not much given to self-effacement. Had he known that he had discovered both a new disease and its cause in 1897 and 1898 he surely would have said so at the time. But Koch's candor is not of much importance compared to a more interesting question, which concerns the consequences of the fact that he had both *made* those findings *and* misinterpreted them. Consider what *might* have happened as well as what did happen. (1) If Koch had interpreted his findings of 1897 and 1898 correctly, the lethal nature of East Coast fever and the microscopic appearance of its causal parasite would have become known when he published in 1898. As a result, the importing of cattle from Tanganyika might have been prohibited well before 1902. And even if such importing had not been prohibited, any outbreak of East Coast fever in Rhodesia might have been diagnosed very quickly and its spread might have been prevented. (In other words, as Gray said in 1908, Koch's report of 1898 would have been a guide instead of a stumbling block to future investigators.) (2) If Koch had not made his studies of 1897 and 1898 at all, his misinterpretation of those studies would not have been published in 1898 and thus would not have provided the stumbling block that helped Gray and Robertson to become convinced that they were dealing only with a virulent form of redwater. Without that stumbling block, they might well have realized that they were dealing with a new disease. (3) On the other hand, if Koch had never made that study, he would not have been in a position, in late 1902, to begin to re-evaluate his findings and to realize that the new "Rhodesian Fever" was probably the same disease that he had seen in 1897. (4) Finally, if Koch had not made those studies in 1897 and 1898, he might well never have been invited to Rhodesia. The pressure to invite Koch rather than some other expert came from Hutcheon and Gray, who argued that Koch was the man to get because Koch had already studied a similar "virulent" form of redwater! And if Koch had not been invited to Rhodesia the credit for announcing that East Coast fever was a new disease might eventually have gone to Gray or to Arnold Theiler.

In his interim report, Koch may have been disingenuous in implying that he had recognized the disease in 1897 and ungenerous in not praising the careful studies Gray and Robertson had made of the symptoms of East Coast fever and of the parasite. But that seems rather unimportant compared to the realization that so much of what happened between October, 1901 and March, 1903 flowed exactly and all but inevitably from two facts, namely the fact that Koch *had* studied the disease in 1897 and 1898 *and* the fact that he had misinterpreted his findings.

The interim report was just that – a report published before the real work had begun. Koch had been brought out to Rhodesia in the hope and expectation that he would find some way to prevent the disease by immunization and he obviously expected to do just that. Where was he working and under what conditions?

In 1903 Bulawayo was the largest city of colonial Rhodesia. Today it is the second largest city of independent Zimbabwe. Relaxed and friendly, it has wide streets, blessedly few tall buildings, a beautiful park and botanical garden, and Zimbabwe's finest historical museum (all in all, a city well worth a visit). On April 2, 1903, Koch wrote to his friend Gustav Theodor Fritsch:[19]

I do not know if your [visit] to South Africa included this region . . . If so you would be amazed at the changes that have occurred. Cities grow like mushrooms . . . where ten years ago only an African village stood . . . now Bulawayo stands . . . looking like a European, or even more like an American city, with a railway station, a large hotel, electric lights, a few magnificent buildings and many houses and cottages, built, by and large, of sheet metal. Even my experimental station, which, to be sure, lies outside the city, consists of a number of tin boxes [In the German original, "Tinboxes" is in English]. In many respects it is, however a great pity that the European culture so unmercifully sweeps away all that had earlier made the country so interesting. On the railway journey I have seen very few . . . native villages, even in regions where traces of their remains showed that they had once been. Where earlier one could everywhere see countless herds of wild animals, not a trace remains. Men and animals who had earlier dwelt on the land have drawn back from the Europeans. I still, however, hope to have the opportunity to learn more about the yet untouched parts of the country in which there is no digging for gold.

In 1932, Kleine, who was one of Koch's two assistants in 1903,[20] looked back at his experiences. Here is a condensed and freely translated version of his reminiscences:[21]

I had the good luck to accompany Robert Koch [on two of his journeys to Africa]. The first time [was in] 1903/1904 . . . a few years after rinderpest had died out . . . South Africa again became the home of the death of cattle. Thousands of cattle fell to 'Rhodesian Red Water.' In December, 1902 both English and German newspapers announced that Koch's help had been sought. At that time Koch had only two assistants in his private laboratory, Neufeld and myself. One morning I mentioned the rumor and begged Koch to take either me or Dr. Neufeld with him to Africa. Koch replied 'You can both come . . . but I must first be summoned myself.'

The next morning a cable arrived from the Chartered Company, which ruled Rhodesia. In a few days everything was arranged by telegram . . . and in January Robert Koch, his wife, Dr. Neufeld and I left Naples . . . *en route* along the coast to Beira . . . where we were met by the Chief Veterinary Surgeon of Rhodesia . . . After a many-day-long journey by rail, we reached Bulawayo.

Founded by Cecil Rhodes, Bulawayo at that time consisted of a few streets, on which were the town hall, the court, the banks, a club, and a few large businesses and shops . . . We lived in the Grand Hotel. During the second half of the year that we were there I came to know many of the English colonists. The real goal that they longed to reach was the coal, gold and copper that had been discovered to the north and could be reached by the new Zambezi bridge. Together with the German General Consul we visited the nearby Matopos hills where Cecil Rhodes had found his last and wildly romantic resting place.

Our daily work was strictly regulated. A brief 7 o'clock breakfast was followed by a 25 minute journey to our experimental station, Hillside Camp. It consisted of a few houses where the three English veterinarians who had been brought together by Koch resided, a large barracks, with three rooms, and a number of stables. The barracks served as a laboratory, stables housed the experimental animals . . . Before our arrival the veterinarians had prepared all the necessary blood smears. We stained them and began the microscopic studies while Koch and the Chief Veterinary Surgeon visited all of the cattle stalls. Long hours were devoted to the autopsy of the fallen animals. Koch stood attentively at each dissection, not fatigued by the intense African sun . . . After a brief midday rest at the hotel we returned to the laboratory. When the sun set, our work ended. So it went every day but Sunday.

We sometimes saw, in the blood of sick animals, the parasite of Texas Fever, but Koch soon noted that these parasites signalled only a secondary infection. Little staves and rings within the red cells are the true cause of an entirely new and unknown disease . . . anatomical findings pointed the same way. One found lymphomas in the kidneys, the lung and the liver . . . the lymph glands were swollen and hemorrhagic. Koch recalled that he had seen these small parasites in his earlier study on the east African coast and gave the illness, which the transport of cattle had brought inland from the coast, the name 'African Coast Fever.' The brilliance of Koch in discovering this new disease can only be appreciated by those who have studied the tangle of mixed infection in the tropics.

A preventive injection against coast fever was not achieved and remains out of reach. We hope that a chemotherapy may be found. Up to now the disease is combatted by destruction of its carrier, the tick, through dipping cattle in tanks filled with water, sodium arsenite, petroleum and green soap.

The interim report appeared on March 26. Having spent two more months under the burning southern African sun, Koch submitted his second report, dated May 28, 1903.[22] In it he said that he could only indicate the direction in which his research might proceed. He said that the study of African Coast fever is necessarily slow if compared to the study of rinderpest, because African Coast fever has a longer incubation period and, when transmitted by ticks, has an even longer incubation period.

Animals that previously suffered from redwater might again show symptoms of it if attacked by African Coast fever. That might explain the occasional presence of large pear-shaped organisms in the blood and the occasional occurrence of hemoglobinuria.

[In ninety-one sick animals] in every instance we have found the small parasites of African Coast Fever, but only in ten cases have we found these parasites in conjunction with the larger pyriform organisms, and in six of the latter cases we have observed blood-coloured urine. These observations bear out the view ... that ... animals [immune] to ordinary Redwater ... again developed this disease [after being attacked by African Coast fever].

Koch went on to say that he had expected to be able to produce African Coast fever "without difficulty by subcutaneous inoculation with blood taken from sick animals, an easy matter in ordinary Texas Fever." But such inoculations did not produce the disease. Since the question was of such great importance, he tried the effects of larger doses, of using warm fresh blood, of injecting subcutaneously, or into a vein, or into the peritoneal cavity. In some cases a mixture of blood, spleen and lymphatic glands was injected; in others, a large volume of virulent blood was injected. But the disease was never induced. "In our many experiments we found no evidence that the direct inoculation of healthy animals will cause African Coast Fever . . . This remarkable fact separates African Coast Fever still further from Texas Fever."

In spite of this, Koch persuaded himself that he was on the trail of a procedure that might immunize cattle against "African Coast Fever." Although the initial injection did not cause the disease, a second injection sometimes caused a mild attack of fever "characterized by the appearance of the usual small parasite in the blood." Whether such a mild attack produces any immunity "I cannot say at present. That question cannot be answered until we can reproduce the disease artificially . . . perhaps through the medium of the tick . . . and tick experiments are tedious and take up much time."

Meanwhile, Koch said, he was at work on a curative serum. He proposed to obtain what we would now call a "hyperimmune" serum by injecting animals with increasingly large doses of "virulent" blood. As to immunity acquired by animals that survive an attack, Koch said that the situation was not clear. Many animals whose blood contained the small parasites had since been attacked by "African Coast Fever" and had died.

On April 24, G. Stanley Bruce had sent David Bruce a second letter, in which he summarized Koch's interim report. He wrote again on August 14,[23] expressing a wistful hope that he might be allowed to work with Koch:

Dear Dr. Bruce,

I was very pleased to receive your letter [of May 2, 1903] and to hear that you were tackling this most peculiar disease, Sleeping Sickness. Do you still think that a Trypanosoma is probably the cause? Koch is still in Bulawayo along with my chief Mr. Gray, and I am still based in Salisbury but Mr. Gray has promised to endeavour to let me have a month or two with Koch if he can possibly manage it. Koch is working hard at the Rhodesian Cattle Disease and is certainly making progress although slowly. He says that it is the most interesting disease that he has yet worked at. I sent you copies of his [first and second] Reports. You will observe a marked difference between them. In the majority of cases there is a mixed infection [of] ordinary R.W. combined with African Coast Fever, the latter indicated by the small bacillary like parasites pointed out in Gray and Robertson's Report a copy of which was sent you. It is quite possible that he may obtain a curative anti-toxin or immunizing serum but he has a very difficult task. It is also probable that he will bring forward a new theory as to immunity . . . Through Mr. Gray I informed Koch of your discovery in sleeping sickness.

I quite agree with you that there is plenty of scope for Research here and when the Government have got a new laboratory built some of the unknown causes of disease ought to be found out . . . Kind regards, I am yours truly, G. Stanley Bruce. P.S. I shall continue to let you hear when anything new crops up. G.S.B.

There is indeed a marked difference in tone between the first report and the second report, which was dated May 28. Nearly four months passed before Koch submitted his third report, on September 25.[24] From that report we learn that Koch had continued to inject healthy animals with blood from sick animals and from animals that he thought had recovered from the disease, but lacked a means to test the possibility that he had induced immunity because he had no way of exposing possibly immune animals to a virulent attack. Passage of the organism through a series of healthy animals did not increase its virulence, and attempts to induce a full-scale attack by ticks had failed. (Koch had been raising ticks for that purpose but never produced a virulent attack, because he used the wrong kind of tick.) From this point on, we hear more and more often about the presence of "small" parasites in the blood of animals that had supposedly been infected with East Coast fever by inoculation, recovered and become immune. Since East Coast fever cannot be transmitted by a single injection of infected blood or even by a series of such injections, and cannot be transmitted by the blue tick, Arnold Theiler later argued that those "small" parasites were forms of the parasite that causes Texas fever; still later he showed that they were a relatively harmless parasite that is related to the parasite that does cause East Coast fever. Even in his second report, Koch had noted that he had studied a group of twenty-nine animals taken from the Bulawayo commonage whose blood showed a few "small" parasites, and that thirteen of those cattle had already died of East Coast fever. Koch nevertheless argued that "the presence of such small parasites can be taken . . . as a proof that the cattle came from areas where African Coast Fever infection exists."

The third report, dated September 25, 1903, reported work done during the winter, when the ticks and the disease tend to subside. At that point Koch had returned to the method that he had used in 1897 and 1898, i.e., he was trying to transmit the disease by using ticks bred from eggs. He hatched large numbers of tick eggs, but when the young ticks so hatched were placed upon healthy animals "we failed to reproduce a characteristic attack." Koch might have concluded either that he was breeding the wrong kind of tick or that the ticks he was breeding did not carry the infection forward via their eggs. Instead, he decided to create a more "natural" means of infection by filling a field with young ticks that he had raised. The field thus sown with newly hatched young ticks was not, however, a clean field, since cases of East Coast fever had occurred there. In Koch's words, the field *was* clean because "only occasional cases had occurred"; the fact that any cases at all had appeared actually shows that the field already contained brown ticks.[25] Koch also noted that he was working in the cold, dry season when both the ticks and the disease almost vanish.

As spring approached, the field became infective and many cases of East Coast fever appeared in animals that grazed in that field. But, of course, the approach of spring caused both the blue tick and the brown tick to flourish. Whatever this proved as to which tick was the carrier (and it proved nothing), it did provide Koch with an infected field, in which he could place cattle to see whether or not he had successfully immunized them against East Coast fever. Healthy cattle turned out into that infected field rapidly became ill, which meant that possibly immune cattle could be similarly challenged. Eight animals that had been "immunized" by a series of injections of blood were exposed to the infected field; all but three died. As Koch said, "A remnant of three out of eight is small," but he thought that if the animals had had a larger number of protective injections more of them might have been immune. "At present it is impossible to say definitely how long immunity will last . . . how many injections should be made . . . what space of time between the inoculations is best . . . or what class of recovered animals are most suitable for inoculation from."

Koch then reported on his experiences with a serum that he hoped would be "curative." Animals were injected three or four times, at two- to three-week intervals, with doses of blood as large as two liters, always with blood containing many parasites. When serum from such animals was injected into sick animals, there was a striking decline in the number of parasites in the sick animals. Unfortunately all animals treated in that way died of massive hemolysis (destruction of the red cells) before they could recover from East Coast fever. Moreover some of these animals seemed to develop true redwater, to which they had previously been immune. All in all, treatment with this serum seemed unpromising: the injection of as little as 50 cc of such serum could cause fatal hemolysis.

That being so, Koch asked: what should be done? Ideally one would stamp out the disease by rigorous quarantining, but that would require "absolute control of all cattle and of all movements of stock." Since the country was largely unfenced and the African-owned cattle were widely dispersed there was no hope of stamping out the disease in that way. Thus, although he would have preferred to devote more time to the study of his method for producing immunity, Koch recommended that it be used as widely as possible, since that seemed to be the only way to combat the disease. The rainy season was approaching, the disease would soon recur on a large scale, and his method would have to be tried since nothing else was available. He closed his third report with "do it yourself" instructions on how to inoculate cattle, directed at farmers who could not obtain the assistance of a veterinarian. But he added "too much must not be expected of the method, nor must good results be looked for ... in herds in which the disease has gained a thorough foot hold."

On December 23, 1903, the Farmers and Landowners Association once again attacked the government, claiming not only that inoculation was of no value but that it was actually killing cattle. This produced the usual referral of the matter to Gray and a long reply in which Gray called attention to Koch's warning in his third report that four to six inoculations are needed to give any protection.[26] Thus, Gray said, if cattle acquire East Coast fever after having been inoculated only once or twice, that proves nothing. There is no risk of conveying East Coast fever by inoculation, Gray said, but if newly imported cattle are inoculated they may contract other blood-borne diseases to which they are not immune, including redwater itself. Gray added that no disastrous results had as yet followed the inoculation of over 3,000 head of cattle in the Victoria district.

It is far too early in the day to assert that the method is either brilliantly satisfactory or otherwise. Time alone is going to show how it is going to turn out ... Dr. Koch does not claim that the ... inoculation ... will protect every animal ... he rather hopes that when the disease appears in an inoculated herd, recoveries will be the rule, instead of being the exception.

Koch wrote his fourth and last report on February 29, 1904. Before doing that he attended a conference on cattle disease that was held on December 3–5, 1903, in Bloemfontein, in the Orange River

Colony.[27] Hutcheon and Gray were there, as was Watkins-Pitch-ford, who had taken the eight Natal cattle to Rhodesia, where they had all died. And a new team was there, Arnold Theiler and his associate, Stewart Stockman. Theiler and Stockman had been working on East Coast fever in the Transvaal for many months.

On the second day of the conference, Koch was invited to open a session on East Coast fever (which was, at the conference, still called African Coast fever) and to state his views. Koch said that the disease was a specific new disease, new, that was, for that country. It was not Rinderpest and it was not Texas fever. It was caused by a specific parasite. The disease was a new one for that country but it was not a new one for science. Koch said: "We have known this disease for seven years . . . I saw it seven years ago in German East Africa and I am sure the Rhodesian [disease] is exactly the same; with the same parasite and the same characteristic symptoms . . . that I found in German East Africa." It was prevalent on the east coast of Africa and was spread inland when cattle were moved inland from the coast. It was not infectious, i.e. it was not transmit-ted directly from one animal to another, but only by ticks. If healthy cattle were placed together with cattle affected with East Coast fever, they would remain healthy as long as there were no ticks present to transmit the disease.

Koch went on to say that animals that had recovered from East Coast fever still had the parasites in their blood, so they became carriers. Ticks that feed on them could infect other cattle. (The question of whether immune carriers of East Coast fever exist was to be debated for many years.) He had developed a method of immunization that should be used in any region where there was a danger of the disease appearing. Quarantine would "involve con-siderable expense and the disease would come after all." Texas fever "went through the whole of South Africa and the country became immune. In the same way South Africa will become immune [to East Coast fever] in a certain time. But we can make it so in a very short time in an artificial way, with a very small loss of cattle."

Although the audience treated Koch with great deference, he was roundly attacked. Theiler insisted that the disease was carried not by the blue tick but by the brown tick; moreover the disease had not been long prevalent at Delagoa Bay but had been brought there within the past two years. The delegate from Portuguese East Africa (Mozambique), Dr. Amalal Leal, said the disease had not been long endemic there but had been brought in recently from the German East Africa coast or from Zanzibar, first to Beira and afterwards to Lourenço Marques (Maputo). A delegate from Natal, S. B. Woollatt, said that cattle had for years been taken from the coastal districts of Natal into the Transvaal without causing outbreaks of East Coast fever. In short, no one who spoke to that point agreed with Koch's claim that the disease had long been endemic along the east coast of *southern* Africa, i.e. Africa south of Tanganyika.

As to the spread of the disease, Theiler said that Koch's prediction that it would spread throughout all of South Africa was wrong. If it was carried by the brown tick, it could spread only in the regions where the brown tick flourished. As to immunizing by inoculation with blood, that procedure was likely to transmit other serious blood-borne diseases of cattle. The time had not arrived to start inoculation in the Transvaal and, he said, they did not intend to do anything in the Transvaal until they obtained more experience, apart from isolating outbreaks and strongly recommending fencing. Stockman pointed out that if Koch was correct in saying that recovered animals became carriers, inoculation would introduce another permanent plague in the country, since all cattle already there would have to be inoculated, as would all imported cattle. Dipping, fencing and quarantine seemed like a better approach (Koch agreed, but pointed out that dipping, fencing and quarantine could not succeed in countries that had a large population of African-owned cattle). Only Gray and Koch defended inoculation. As to the "small" parasite, Theiler said that he and Stockman had seen it in ordinary redwater, that it might even be a previously unknown species of parasite, and that it certainly had nothing to do with East Coast fever.

In the afternoon session of December 4, Watkins-Pitchford launched a savage attack on Koch: "Was the early Dar-es-Salaam disease referred to by Professor Koch identical in all respects with the existing Rhodesian disease?" The learned Professor had stated during the course of his remarks that the differential features of the two diseases microscopically were 'very easily recognized.' Writing from Dar-es-Salaam some six or seven years ago he stated that the disease existent there was Texas fever. Might he ask if this term was intended to suggest the existence of a hematozoal disease simply, the term "Texas fever" being used rather in a generic than an exact sense? . . . He might say that the differential points upon which the Professor justly laid such stress were fully recognized [when] the disease first came under observation by himself and others. If the microscopical differences were now "very easily recognized" he presumed that they could hardly have been so obvious at . . . Dar-es-Salaam. He was anxious to avoid any controversy but thought it probable that Professor Koch had good reason for the alteration of his opinion and therefore he was asking him . . . was the Dar-es-Salaam outbreak identical with the present disease?

Alas, the conference reporter condensed most of Koch's reply by saying that "Dr. Koch explained the matter fully." Fortunately the reporter added that Koch had remarked that at the time he had made his report [in 1898] it had not been so easy to distinguish between the two diseases as now and an error made at that date was excusable. He had made the mistake of thinking that the small-sized parasites were the young of the pear-shaped ones.

Theiler defended Koch, saying that when specimens had been sent to Laveran and Nocard, both of them had declared the disease to be Texas fever. The rest of the session was devoted to a discussion of official recommendations favoring fencing, the control of movements of cattle and the quarantining of infected fields. The possibility of recommending inoculation was not even mentioned. At the end of the session, Duncan Hutcheon "moved a vote of thanks to Dr. Koch for his kindness in addressing them and the manner in which he had submitted to their criticisms that day . . . The vote of thanks was passed unanimously amid applause."

Koch returned to Bulawayo in time to celebrate his sixtieth birthday on December 11, 1903, amidst a shower of congratulatory telegrams and resolutions. A *Festschrift* was published in Germany and a committee in Berlin agreed that on Koch's return from Bulawayo a marble bust of him would be dedicated at his institute.

Koch wrote to his daughter on December 14, 1903. In that letter, which I summarize in free translation, Koch thanked his daughter for her good wishes and said that he felt reasonably well, but had begun to detect a few symptoms of heart trouble and shortness of breath and could no longer climb high hills. He told her that he had recently spent a few weeks in the Victoria district which is full of hills and wonderfully shaped granite rocks [the famous "Castle Kopjes" that are so distinctive a part of the beautiful landscape of Zimbabwe]. "At the foot of such hills are the astonishing Zimbabwe ruins, which we were able to visit ... But it was not only these ruins that made an unforgettable impression but the landscape, the inhabitants and the vegetation – all carrying a distinctively African character." Nor, he added, did lions fail to appear![28]

Koch and Gray inoculated a very large number of cattle in the Victoria district, as Koch's fourth report[29] of February 29, 1904 reveals. Five "immune" cattle in whose blood "the ring forms of the parasite were present" were brought from Bulawayo to provide the blood necessary for the inoculations. On an average, 300 head of cattle were inoculated every day, although on several occasions over 500 were inoculated in one day. The rains had begun, which meant that the danger period for a resurgence of the disease was at hand. It had already begun to spread, so "that instead of having to inoculate a thousand head ... over four thousand had to be dealt with" [the goal was to inoculate all animals in infected herds and all animals in the vicinity of such herds]. The study continued for many months, although Koch did not remain in the Victoria district the whole time.

After analyzing the preliminary results, Koch said "I do not contend ... that the results of our field experiments prove that the method so far has afforded a high degree of protection ... Sufficient time has not elapsed for this to be apparent. Our work only shows that the establishment of artificial immunity is a much more gradual process than I at first hoped it would be." But, he added, "I feel certain that in the course of the next few months proofs of increased immunity in the infected herds will be forthcoming."

There is little more to tell. By January, 1904, Neufeld had decided that the studies had progressed to the point that he could leave and return to Berlin to continue work that he found more congenial, namely serological studies related to tuberculosis.[30] Koch had originally agreed to work for one year, travel time being included in that year. In September, he had proposed to extend his term to 18 months and the B.S.A.C. and the South African colonies agreed,[31] committing themselves to a further expenditure. (The authorities in the Transvaal were strongly opposed to extending Koch's services, being by then completely out of sympathy with him. The Commissioner of Lands wrote "As far as this Colony is concerned I think Professor Koch's services should terminate with his present agreement. We should in the meantime pursue our investigation vigorously under Dr. Theiler." C. H. Rodwell, the Acting Imperial Secretary, was more blunt:

I venture to suggest that Dr. Koch should be invited to stay on till March and be provided, free of charge, with all necessaries in the way of equipment and animals for experiments but that any further remuneration should take the form of a lump sum, to be handed to him only in the event of his finally solving one or both of the two problems of redwater and horse sickness. I do not suppose for a minute that he will accept such an offer, but . . . it seems a waste of money to go on paying him.

On November 9, 1904, writing in connection with proposed further investigations of horse sickness, F. B. Smith said "Perhaps you may recollect that when the proposition for keeping on Dr. Koch came before us we strongly advised against it and though our advice was not accepted, events proved its soundness."[31]

African horse sickness, which Koch had begun to investigate in July, 1902, is a serious viral disease of horses. (The prevalence of horse sickness was one reason why oxen were so widely used.) He published two reports on horse sickness. I have not looked into that work, but the historical part of the chapter on horse sickness in Henning's textbook[32] does not mention Koch. According to Henning, the fact that the disease is caused by a virus had been shown by John McFadyean in 1900 and confirmed by both Arnold Theiler and Edmund Nocard in 1901, and much of the later work on the subject was done by Theiler. (An attenuated virus capable of giving immunity was developed in the 1930s, using a method developed in studies of yellow fever by Arnold Theiler's son, Max Theiler.) Henning's historical summaries are excellent and detailed, and he cites neither of Koch's reports on horse sickness. Gray himself eventually reported that Koch's method for immunizing against horse sickness had not been a success.[33]

The *Bulawayo Observer* for April 2, 1904 reported that a garden party had been given on Monday, March 28 to bid farewell to Professor and Mrs. Koch, "who leave Rhodesia this week . . . The Doctor speaks in high terms of the treatment he has received in Rhodesia and says he likes the country well . . . We trust the results of the Professor's labours amongst us may prove as successful and beneficial to the country as he himself anticipates." (A splendid photograph of the guests at the garden party has been preserved in the National Archives of Zimbabwe.)[34] Koch sailed home via the same route he had taken on the way to Rhodesia. He reached Dar-es-Salaam on April 12 and Naples on May 10, 1904.

The British South Africa Company kept meticulous financial records. On April 5, 1905, it sent an audited account of the cost of Koch's studies to the South African colonies. The audit, which had been certified on February 18, 1905, was supported by hundreds of vouchers covering such expenses as a ton of hay (four pounds), two packets of soap (two shillings and four pence) and the dispatch of some blood smears (one shilling). The various South African governments were no doubt pleased to learn that they had advanced a little too much, and were entitled to divide up a surplus of some 268 pounds.[35] The entire undertaking had cost £22,981/2/8, at a time when, according to Baedeker,[36] a room in the most expensive hotel in London could be had for ten shillings a night. In 1898, the starting salary for a "boy copyist" in the Colonial Office was four pence an hour, and, in 1888, soon after his well-known services to the King of Bohemia, Sherlock Holmes was of the opinion that an annual income of £100 received from an investment of £2,500 was a large sum and that "a single lady can get on very nicely upon an [annual] income of about £60."[37] It is all but impossible to translate such costs into modern terms, but £23,000 in 1904 in some ways had the purchasing power of perhaps £800,000 in 1989.[38]

It remained for Gray to pick up the pieces. The next Intercolonial Veterinary Conference was held in Cape Town on May 25–31, 1904.[39] The first order of business was East Coast fever. Gray was asked to report and he did so: "The work of inoculation in the Victoria district had been continued until the time prescribed by Dr. Koch," which was the end of April, 1904.

Dr. Koch's system of inoculation had certainly done no harm, but the amount of good it had done was problematic . . . The fact was, that the inoculated animals seemed to show no more resistance to the disease than did those that were not inoculated . . . Taking matters all round, the experiments with inoculation had been rather disappointing.

On top of that, Theiler announced that the ring-shaped parasites, whose presence Koch had taken to mean that he was dealing with an animal that had recovered from East Coast fever, had nothing to do with that disease. He had said as much at Bloemfontein but at that time he thought they might be a new kind of parasite. But since then he had found that they were a regular feature of animals that had been injected with blood taken from animals suffering from ordinary redwater. He concluded that "the rings on which Dr. Koch bases his immunity have nothing to do with East Coast Fever, and if such immunity is really brought about, which does not seem to be the case, then it must be in another way." I will discuss Theiler and his work in chapters 7 and 10; at this conference, held in May, 1904, he was able to present convincing evidence that the disease was transferred from one animal to another by the brown tick and not by the blue tick and to cast grave doubts on the theoretical basis for Koch's method of producing immunity.

On July 11, 1904, Gray wrote an official report about the usefulness of inoculation.[40] In it, he said

I regret to say that while Dr. Koch's prediction that herds infected at the time when inoculation was begun would not be benefited thereby has been fulfilled, neither have those herds been protected which were clean at the time when we started, nor has the percentage mortality in such herds been diminished when the disease appeared. I cannot conscientiously recommend the public to depend on such means of inoculation.

When this report reached London it produced a qualm at the Colonial Office:[41] "I presume that the fact that Mr. Gray casts some doubt on the value of Dr. Koch's process is no reason why we should not distribute it as usual? It is a matter of general scientific and practical interest." The minute in reply read "No, We clearly should do so." Copies were duly forwarded to the Foreign Office, the Board of Agriculture and the Royal Society, and to McFadyean.

Gray's report was published twice in 1904,[40] once in Rhodesia and once in England, thus letting the whole world know that Gray could not

conscientiously recommend the public to depend on such a method of inoculation [and that] the failure of Dr. Koch's method leaves us at present with no other weapons to combat the progress of the disease other than those which previous experience has dictated, those are the suspension of movement of cattle so far as is possible, fencing, systematic dipping or spraying (which must, however, be kept up for at least two years before any benefit will be apparent) and the exclusion of all cattle from infected areas for at least 15 months, in order to give the veld time to become clean again.

More than a year after writing my comments on Koch's lack of candor I came across a similar but far more polemical analysis that was actually published in the *Natal Witness* on July 17, 1903, i.e. some six weeks after the appearance of Koch's second report. That article, headed "The Inconsistency of Dr. Koch," was written by a prominent Natal farmer, G. D. Alexander.[42]

Alexander began by comparing the scientist to

a man in an uninhabited country, without a compass, or other means of 'laying his course,' trying to reach a certain point unknown to him. He starts on his journey and proceeds until he is stopped by some sign that shows him beyond doubt that he is on the wrong track, and, retracing his footsteps, he puts up a notice board for the benefit of future travellers, with the sign 'This is not the road. I have tried it and found it a cul de sac.'

But

a scientist however, must be extremely careful that he has explored a path, and not just taken a look round before he puts up any sign; otherwise he not only fails himself, but causes disaster to many other searchers. I maintain that Dr. Koch has put up a misleading signboard, and has thoroughly misled other workers in the field, and, further, he has not had the grace to say: 'I was wrong in my conclusions, and I regret having misled fellow scientists.' Dr. Koch is a scientist of European celebrity, and has done, no doubt, a great deal of scientific work of value: but it is not the first time that he has made an assertion on a scientific subject of the greatest importance, which on further investigation, has been proved to be wrong. In fact, if the eminent scientist is not careful, one will almost be entitled to say it is becoming a habit.

Alexander then quoted at length from Koch's 1898 report and commented that

it is to be noted that in 1897 Dr. Koch 'has no hesitation in saying' and 'that no room for doubt was left' that the disease on the East Coast of Africa was Texas fever (South African red-water), and that he 'formed the conviction' that the small stave-like forms . . . were the 'real first forms' of the pyrosoma (the parasite which is regarded as the cause of Texas fever).

Alexander went on to quote some 500 words from Koch's interim report (which he incorrectly referred to as the report of May 23, 1903), in which most of the same facts are taken as evidence that the disease is a new one. After commenting that this should convince the reader that Dr. Koch had misled fellow scientists, Alexander rather devastatingly cited brief passages from the 1898 report and the report of March 26 (again incorrectly cited as May 23). In the 1898 report Koch had spoken of coming across severe cases of Texas fever at Mohesa, the terminus of the Usambara railway. Those cattle had been taken from Kilimanjaro to Tanga, "where naturally they had been exposed to the infection of Texas fever," but by mistake had then been sent inland to Mohesa. But in his report of March, 1903, Koch says that six years ago, at Tanga, he had seen an outbreak of "exactly the same character as the present Rhodesian one," an outbreak in a herd "which was brought into the infected area at Tanga . . . became infected there [and] carried the disease . . . to Mohesa in the interior." And, Koch added,

As we know that in the pyrosomal diseases, whereto the Rhodesian fever belongs, ticks play a most important part as agent for the dissemination of infection, I have occupied myself thoroughly with this side of the question. For this I have had special facilities, [since] in my earlier work on the pyrosomal disease at Dar-es-Salaam, which I have identified with Rhodesian fever, I produced it with infected ticks in the far-distant Usambara Mountains, and so proved that the ticks are also the intermediary agents in this disease.

Thus, Alexander says,

Dr. Koch has made one thing very evident, and that is, if Rhodesian fever is the same as the cattle fever on the East Coast, then his conclusions on the former investigation, made by him on the East Coast were wrong, and have been the cause of misleading other scientists who had not the opportunity of making the investigation, and who took Dr. Koch's dictum as being that of a careful and distinguished scientist.

There are some scientists who, on making a discovery, test the correctness of it, attack it from every point, and if it still stands, test it again, and when they finally divulge it, it is worthy of credence.

There are others who evidently arrive at a conclusion, and who do not change their coats in the rush to the newspaper office to gain publicity, in the fear that someone may get in front of them.

Now the result of Dr. Koch's inconsistency is that he has given faulty information and has, therefore, led other scientists astray. Mr. Gray, Mr. Robertson, and Mr. Pitchford had only to satisfy themselves that [the] Rhodesian disease was the same as the West [*sic*] African disease, then, according to Dr. Koch, [the] Rhodesian disease was the same as redwater.

In concluding his article, Alexander attacked not only Koch but those who employed him:

Having arrived at this conclusion [in 1898], and published it to the world, Dr. Koch is sent for at the great expense, and he finds that the West [*sic*] African disease is the same as the Rhodesian disease, but that the Rhodesian disease is not redwater, and the world says, 'wonderful man, Dr. Koch, what would we do without him. Look at that Rhodesian disease, all the other investigators were astray until Koch took it in hand.' Great is the name of Koch, Selah. The world does not know, or overlooks . . . the misleading signboard.

Alexander then commented that there was a time when British

singers had to adopt foreign names in order to receive applause and suggested that "Herr Pitchforditsha, Signor Graysini and Monsieur Robertsoni" might have done better than Pitchford, Gray and Robertson, who received a bare living wage while

when any investigation is needed the powers that be wire at once for some continental scientist, and give enormous sums and a blank check for expenses ... I have drawn attention to the inconsistencies of Dr. Koch because 'fair play is bonnie play,' and I consider Dr. Koch has not given his fellow scientists fair play. His desire to annex all credit, whether belonging to him or not, is very apparent.

Alexander closed with a number of remarks about the unappreciated virtues of Watkins-Pitchford, who had been denied recognition: "that recognition will, I suppose, as in the case of most able men who are deficient of trumpet manipulation, come after he has left us." Watkins-Pitchford may well have had a hand in Alexander's article, expecially since he had repeatedly announced, during 1902, that the new outbreak was only one of redwater. In doing so he relied on Robertson, and on Koch's report of 1898. On June 6, 1902, he said that the ability of redwater "to assume a virulent form ... [seems] to be giving trouble in Rhodesia." On July 18, 1902, he said that "there is no cause for anxiety concerning the spread of the disease in this country [Natal]." On August 1, 1902, he said, in italics, "*The disease is, without doubt, the disease known in Natal as redwater*" and added that "I do not consider any apprehension need be entertained as to its spread in Natal." And on November 21, 1902, he said: "that Professor Koch, in his East Africa investigation was dealing with the same disease now threatening us, there is little doubt in my mind" and he quoted Koch's remarks about "the miniature staves" as evidence that the disease was only a form of redwater. He thus had some reason to feel aggrieved at having relied so heavily on Koch's 1898 report.[43]

Alexander's article, in part calmly reasonable and in part almost a tirade, was reprinted a few months later in the *Veterinary Record*[44] with some, but by no means all, of the rude bits left out, but, as far as I can see, it drew no comment or response, either in the *Natal Witness* or in the *Veterinary Record*. Whether Koch or his assistants ever saw it I do not know.

Many years later, L. E. W. Bevan[45] wrote that

Koch cost the country some £60,000 [it was only £23,000] but conferred no material benefit upon it except that he left behind him a little travelling

Zeiss microscope which Mr. Gray promptly appropriated. He subsequently handed it over to me and I used it for many years. Attached to my saddle I used to take it with me on my journeys. Together we must have travelled tens of thousands of miles.

In 1908 Gray wrote a historical review of East Coast fever.[46] In it he said:

Dr. Koch spent over a year in Rhodesia, and as I was privileged to assist him ... I am in a position to testify to the energy with which he devoted himself to his work, and although he did not achieve success, he certainly deserved it. Unfortunately, however, Dr. Koch departed from our midst ... leaving us with a long record of negative experiments, an erroneous assumption regarding the identity of the tick by which the disease is carried, and the repetition of a conviction expressed in a previous report that it was possible to immunize animals against East Coast Fever, if they were inoculated with the blood of animals which had recovered from the disease.

6

Joseph Chamberlain

In late October, 1902, Joseph Chamberlain tried and failed to prevent Robert Koch from being employed to investigate East Coast fever in Rhodesia. If that brief episode were all that Chamberlain had to do with science or the empire at the turn of the century, he would hardly deserve even this short chapter. But he was involved in the study of rinderpest, he was involved in Rhodesian and South African policies, he was involved in the Jameson raid, which influenced so many later events, and he and Milner were involved in the events that led to the Boer War, in the war itself, and in the reconstruction that followed it. And in him and in his career, an interest in science and a belief in empire were united as they seldom have been in one person before or since.

Who was Joseph Chamberlain, apart from being the father of Neville Chamberlain? Why, in 1902, was he so bitterly opposed to the Chartered Company's proposal to employ a *German* bacteriologist? Why did he express his opposition to the employment of Koch by using a phrase associated with trade and manufacturing: "made in Germany?" And why, on October 27, 1902, was he certain that if an English alternative to Koch existed, that alternative could be identified by the Royal Society?

The brief answers to those questions are that Joseph Chamberlain was, in 1902, Colonial Secretary, as he had been since 1895. He had presided over the growing conflict between German and English colonial ambitions in Africa and had presided over the approach, onset, conduct and conclusion of the Boer War, a war in which the Germans were strongly pro-Boer. Before and during the war he relied heavily on Alfred Milner and, after it ended, he gave Milner every possible support in his efforts to repair the ravages of the war, support that included the expenditure of large sums for a new, scientifically oriented Department of Agriculture in the Transvaal, a department based on the plans of an English agricultural expert, F. B. Smith.

As Colonial Secretary, Chamberlain had reason to distrust the British South Africa Company. He had even more reason to distrust German colonial ambitions in southern Africa. His hopes for an alliance with Germany had collapsed only weeks before the proposal to hire Koch came to his attention. Having made his fortune as a manufacturer he was deeply concerned with the threat to British manufacturing of the rising competition from the United States and Germany. In late 1902 he was wholly committed to his battle to restore the supremacy of British manufacturing by instituting tariff reforms that would favor trade between Great Britain and the empire and he was losing that battle. As to medicine and science, he began his political career as a reformer in the field of public health. And as to the Malaria Committee of the Royal Society, he knew that it existed because it had been created at his request.

Chamberlain was born in London in 1836.[1] He did not grow up in anything like Dickensian poverty, since his father was a comfortably well-to-do small businessman in the leather trade. The child of Unitarian dissenters, he was born neither into the aristocracy nor into the upper class. Nor did he attend a university or an influential public school (he did, however, attend the remarkable University College School).[2] He went to work in his father's office in 1852 and was soon thereafter sent to Birmingham to join his cousin Joseph Nettlefold in a company that was owned by Chamberlain's father and Nettlefold's father, whose wives were sisters. The firm that Chamberlain joined had been engaged in the hand manufacture of old-style flat-ended wood screws (which we would now call bolts). Assisted by an investment by Chamberlain's father, the new firm acquired, from the United States, the patents and machinery needed to manufacture the recently invented self-tapping wood screw. The firm of Nettlefold and Chamberlain was so successful that Joseph Chamberlain became rich enough to retire at the age of thirty-eight. From that time on he devoted himself to politics and to becoming the most colorful and controversial figure on the British political scene.

Chamberlain became rich in Birmingham. He entered politics in Birmingham. Many years later he helped to create the University of Birmingham, of which he said in 1905[3] that "it's *raison d'être* was to teach, as it had never been taught before, science, and also to proceed in the work of scientific research." As reform mayor of Birmingham, he led and won the battles for municipal ownership of the gas–light system and the water works, created a system of pure water and safe disposal of sewage, and fought for and obtained better public housing. On October 12, 1874[4] he said:

I am a Radical Reformer because I would reform and remove ignorance, poverty, intemperance, and crime from their very roots . . . intemperance itself is only an effect produced by causes that lie deeper still . . . these causes, in the first place, are the gross ignorance of the masses and, in the second place, the horrible, shameful homes in which many of the poor are forced to live . . . I do not think we will ever secure success until we follow [the example of] . . . the United States, the people of Switzerland, and Sweden . . . and set up a general system of free schools . . . How can we tell a man to be good and decent and moral when we find him living in a place that is not fit for a beast to live in, much less a human being? . . . we attempt to apply remedies to diseases that ought never to exist in the social state at all . . . We must endeavour to get all the houses made fit for people to live in, and then we must induce the occupants to keep the places clean. I count it a first duty that people shall communicate with the sanitary officers when they find nuisances existing on premises; and, remember, the Corporation will always be ready to exercise the powers they possess in removing any cause that interferes with the health of the inhabitants.

Early in 1875, Chamberlain, while still Mayor of Birmingham, gained national attention by calling together a conference of mayors and other public officials "to create a public opinion on the sanitation of large towns." In addressing that conference[5] he spoke with characteristic vividness of a 'ghastly total of 100,000 persons annually done to death by our stupidity and negligence – annually murdered by the neglect of proper sanitary regulations."

Chamberlain entered Parliament in 1876, but he did not stop giving vivid and provocative speeches. When he was a member of the Cabinet, in 1885, he gave a speech in Birmingham in which he said ancient communal rights had passed away:[6]

some of them have been sold; some of them have been given away by people who had no right to dispose of them; some have been lost through apathy and ignorance; some have been destroyed by fraud; and some have been acquired by violence. Private ownership had taken the place of these communal rights and . . . it might be . . . impossible to reverse it. But then I ask what ransom will property pay for the security which it enjoys? . . . property has obligations as well as rights. I think in the future we shall hear a great deal more about the obligations of property, and we shall not hear quite so much about its rights.

The word "ransom" caused Chamberlain so much trouble that he replaced it by "insurance" in later speeches in which he advocated free education, stronger local government, decent public housing in the cities, land for agricultural laborers, *and* a graduated income tax:[7] "We are told that this country is the paradise of the rich; it should be our task to see that it does not become the purgatory of the poor."

Did he mean what he said or was he only a self-serving demagogue? One of his biographers, Denis Judd, in *Radical Joe*, offers three views of Chamberlain.[8] To his detractors he was

a political manipulator, supervisor of the Birmingham party machine and of a local spoils system . . . an unprincipled *nouveau riche* capitalist, mouthing Radical slogans in order to win the popular support that would enable him to get his tainted provincial hands on the highest offices of state; an ally of 'money-bags' imperialism . . . an atheist, a republican . . . a slick opportunist . . . a man who helped break up the Liberal party . . . and who twenty years later smashed the Unionist alliance.

To his admirers he was

a dedicated reformer . . . impelled by a burning desire to root out social inequality and economic distress . . . a municipal activist who pushed aside the forces of reaction and self-interest and made a bid to establish Birmingham as a beacon of progress and enlightenment.

According to "a more realistic view" (presumably Judd's own view), Chamberlain's career was that

of a man of obscure, though not uncomfortable origins, who, possessing quite remarkable powers of persuasion and analysis, set out to make his country a better place to live in. Lacking the advantages of high birth and assured preferment, Chamberlain was obliged to fight his way to the top through the exercise of his demagogic and organizational abilities. He remained a radical throughout his life; a political radical at the outset of his career, a fiscal and economic radical at the end of it. Even as a municipal reformer and the proposer of the doctrine of 'ransom,' however, he was no social revolutionary: his tactics were Fabian, his objectives essentially ameliorative.

When the young Winston Churchill first entered Parliament,[9] Chamberlain was, for him "incomparably the most live, sparkling, insurgent, compulsive figure in British affairs . . . 'Joe' was the one who made the weather. He was the man the masses knew."

Marked to become Prime Minister, which he never became,

Chamberlain was President of the Board of Trade in the Gladstone cabinet of 1880–5 and Colonial Secretary, under Salisbury and Balfour, from June 5, 1895 to September 18, 1903. Although he turned from a radical reformer into a full-blown supporter of the empire, he never lost his interest in matters related to medicine and public health. That interest was noted both by the *Dictionary of National Biography* and by one of his biographers, Amery, who said:[10] "In none of his many sided activities did Chamberlain discharge ... the statesman's function more successfully than in the field of Tropical Medicine. Indeed, when the final account comes to be drawn, it may well be judged that he did here, his greatest service to humanity." According to Amery, Chamberlain was instrumental in supporting the Colonial Nursing Association, which was founded in 1896; in persuading the Royal Society to back the work of David Bruce by founding a Tsetse Fly Committee; in having Patrick Manson appointed Medical Advisor to the Colonial Office; in persuading the committee of the Seamen's Hospital Society to extend their facilities to include and create what was to become the London School of Tropical Medicine, raising both private and government funds for that purpose; in persuading the Royal Society to create a Malaria Committee; and, after the Malaria and Tsetse Fly Committees had been merged into a Tropical Diseases Committee, in persuading various branches of the government to contribute to a Tropical Disease Research Fund. But Chamberlain might have done none of those things had he been driven from office as the result of the Jameson raid.

The Jameson raid

The Jameson raid, mentioned in chapter 2, had nothing but disastrous results. For Winston Churchill, in 1930,[11] it was "an event which seems to me, when I look back over my map of life to be a fountain of ill." Soon after Jameson and his raiders were captured, the Kaiser suggested that Germany would have intervened on the behalf of the Afrikaners had it been asked to do so, a suggestion that poisoned British–German relations for years, and inflamed the feelings that culminated in the First World War.[12] And as Churchill said in 1930,[11] "The Emperor, for his part, seeing himself completely powerless in the face of British sea power, turned his mind to the construction of a German Fleet." Chamberlain, accused of

complicity in the raid, had to defend himself during a public enquiry. The fact that he was blackmailed during that enquiry by
Rhodes and the Chartered Company certainly deepened his distrust
of the Chartered Company.

The Jameson raid of 1895 may seem to have only a tenuous
connection with East Coast fever in 1902, but, apart from its effect
on Chamberlain's view of the British South Africa Company, it led
to the creation of the post of Resident Commissioner in Rhodesia,
responsible to the Colonial Office, and it was a later Resident
Commissioner who began the search for an outside expert. The
Jameson raid led to the High Commissioner for South Africa (Sir
Hercules Robinson, later Lord Rosmead) being replaced by Alfred
Milner and to Earl Grey replacing Jameson as Administrator. The
raid led to the Colonial Office enlarging its authority over Rho-
desia. It led the Chartered Company to bring Milton from South
Africa to reform the handling of native affairs; by December 1898
Milton was, in effect, Administrator of all of Rhodesia. The
government of Rhodesia, and its relationship to the High Com-
missioner and the Colonial Office, were restructured as the result of
the Jameson raid: it was that restructured government, headed by
Milton and subject to Milner's oversight, that was to deal with East
Coast fever. The raid even affected Arnold Theiler, who was in
Johannesburg and, as a new citizen of the Transvaal, was prepared
to take up arms against the raiders if need be.[13]

The withdrawal of the Chartered Company's police and soldiers
from Rhodesia, and the exposure of their vulnerability, was one of
the causes of the 1896 uprising, rinderpest having been another
cause. The fear that a new cattle plague would lead to new African
unrest was never absent in 1902, as we shall see in chapter 9. The
Jameson raid led to the Boer War, which was the direct cause of the
economic depression in Rhodesia in 1902 that made the effects of
East Coast fever seem like the final blow to the viability of the
country. Finally, as the direct result of the Jameson raid and of the
Boer War, division and distrust between the English and the Afrikaner settlers in Rhodesia was intensified: a frequent charge made
by the veterinary officials was that it was the Dutch farmers who
were particularly prone to violate quarantine and dipping regulations. (Both Arnold Theiler and Stewart Stockman made the
same change against the South African farmers, singling out the
Boers.) As for Chamberlain, had he been driven from office, the

recommendation of Koch would have been approved without objection and Koch's services secured sooner than they were! But Chamberlain's career did survive the raid, and with it, his activities in the area of tropical medicine and his support of Milner.

Chamberlain, Lister and Manson

There is much to suggest, but little to prove, that Chamberlain had a long working relationship with Lister, perhaps beginning with Chamberlain's interest in the sanitary conditions of cities. Chamberlain was elected to the Royal Society, in 1882, under a provision that allowed members of the Privy Council to be elected by a special ballot that was not put to the membership at large but only to the Royal Society's Council for its automatic approval. But only a few members of the very large Privy Council were elected to the Royal Society in that way: only twenty-two during the period 1880–95. Such candidates must, by and large, have been selected for election because they were seen as being sympathetic to the goals of the Society or were seen as being potentially useful to the Society. Lister was entitled to sign those special ballots but he rarely took the trouble to do so. Of the fourteen special ballots for members of the Privy Council that appear in the Certificate Book from 1875 to 1880, Lister signed none, and he signed very few in the period 1881–95. But he did sign the ballot for Chamberlain in 1882.[14] This is admittedly a very indirect argument but, as we will see, when Joseph Chamberlain was Colonial Secretary and Lister was President of the Royal Society, Chamberlain often sought the advice of the Royal Society. In his Presidential Address of 1899[15] Lister mentioned Chamberlain's "enlightened action regarding malaria and allied disorders." And, in 1903, Lister, aged seventy-six, having had a stroke and being in poor physical health and with no expectation (or need) of personal gain or advantage, nevertheless wrote:[16] "I propose to run up to London on Thursday to attend the reception of Chamberlain at the Guild Hall, and the lunch to him at the Mansion House on Friday." This certainly suggests a close relationship between Lister and Chamberlain, as does the fact that Lister received three major honors from governments of which Chamberlain was a member.[17] Lister was made a baronet in 1883, when Chamberlain was the President of the Board of Trade, a baron in 1897, when Chamberlain was Colonial Secretary, and, in

1902, while Chamberlain was still Colonial Secretary, Lister became one of the original members of the Order of Merit. The possibility that Lister and Chamberlain worked closely together on matters of public health, and did so over a long period, might well repay further investigation.

Chamberlain unquestionably had a close working relationship with a major figure in the field of tropical medicine, Patrick Manson. In 1897, Chamberlain intervened (at Lister's behest) to have Manson appointed as Medical Advisor to the Colonial Office,[18] and on July 22, 1902 he asked the Royal Society to appoint Manson to the Malaria Committee.[19] Moreover, as Manson's biographers remark, "Chamberlain strongly supported Manson in the founding of the London School of Tropical Medicine and helped raise funds for it, both from government and private sources." Peter Alter comments that[20] "The London School of Tropical Medicine was also . . . financed from a mixture of sources, funds in this case coming from private endowments and the Colonial Office. This Office, which had supported the work of the school and that of its sister institute in Liverpool, especially during Joseph Chamberlain's period of office, granted the School an annual subsidy." Similarly, "the Sleeping Sickness Bureau and the African Entomological Research Committee, which studied the transmission of tropical diseases by insects, were almost totally funded by the Colonial Office's budget." Alter adds that Chamberlain served as Deputy President of Lockyer's British Science Guild and that he was one of a large group of Members of Parliament who signed a petition calling for more support for the National Physical Laboratory. Overall, Alter concludes that "of the politicians, Joseph Chamberlain provided the most active institutional and financial aid for science."

Chamberlain and Kew

According to a little-known eulogy of Chamberlain, The Royal Botanic Gardens at Kew "owed to him, as to no other of our time, stimulus, encouragement and support." Not only did Chamberlain personally help Kew financially, he induced his friends to do so. In 1894 he played an important role in securing government funds to complete the Temperate House which had remained unfinished since 1863. Finally, the eulogy points out that Chamberlain often turned to Kew for expert advice on agriculture in the colonies and, in 1902, arranged for the Director of Kew (W. T. Thiselton-Dyer) to be given the official position of "Botanical Adviser to the Secretary of State for the Colonies." On August 2, 1898, Chamberlain told the House of Commons: "I do not think it too much to say that at the present time there are several of our important Colonies which owe whatever prosperity they possess to the knowledge and experience of, and the assistance given by, the authorities at Kew Gardens."

Chamberlain's connection with Kew and with Thiselton-Dyer was thus by no means simply that of a rich patron who loved flowers and was famous for wearing an orchid in his lapel. Kew had for some decades been active in collecting new species from all parts of the empire, but it was Thiselton-Dyer who began the period of modern botanical research at Kew. Moreover, as Worboys points out, Chamberlain sought out and accepted the then comparatively unimportant post of Colonial Secretary because he "hoped to use the post to initiate a new phase of imperialism, perhaps leading to the creation of an imperial economic community, if not political union" and that he regarded the colonies as an "estate" that needed development guided by the results of applied science, especially scientific agriculture as represented by Kew.[21]

Chamberlain and the Royal Society

Chamberlain approached the Royal Society twice in 1896. On July 1, perhaps after consultation with Lister, conceivably even at Lister's instigation, he asked the Society for its advice and assistance in the tsetse fly problem. As a result the Tsetse Fly Committee was formed, made up of the Society's President (Lister), its Secretary (Michael Foster), Sir John Kirk, Professor E. Ray Lankester, Mr. Salvin and John Burdon Sanderson, with Dr. Kanthack and Mr. W. F. H. Blandford as "accessory" members.[22] That committee was reappointed, with some changes in membership, every year until December 11, 1902, when it was merged with the Malaria Committee; by then the two committees had almost identical membership. The Tsetse Fly Committee became the principal supporter, promoter and recommender of Bruce and his work on the tsetse fly and on trypanosomal parasites.

On September 5, 1896, Chamberlain again approached the Royal

Society, to ask for advice on rinderpest.[23] An *ad hoc* committee was appointed, again including Kirk, Burdon Sanderson and Ray Lankester, as well as Emmanuel Klein and Kanthack. That committee recommended that Kanthack and his assistant, Dr. Stevenson, be sent to South Africa as soon as possible, but on November 20 the Colonial Office replied that the Cape of Good Hope had declined to accept that proposal. Chamberlain ended up having to ask the German government for the services of Robert Koch![24]

The forming of a Malaria Committee seems to have been Chamberlain's idea, but he may have been put up to it by Manson, who involved himself in the committee because of his support of Ronald Ross.[25] On June 6, 1898, Manson wrote to Ross that he had seen Chamberlain the week before and that Chamberlain "wants investigations made on the African fevers, and . . . is willing to make a grant." But Manson told Chamberlain that important work was in progress in India and suggested waiting for a week or two to get Lister's opinion of that work. Meanwhile, as Manson wrote to Ross, "I got Lister to come to my house, and had some six or seven microscopes with your preparations for him to study. He expressed himself convinced . . . I shall see or write to Chamberlain and tell him this is his opportunity . . . I shall ask him to communicate with Lister [for an opinion on Ross's work]." Finally, on July 8, Manson wrote to Ross: "things are going well on this side. Mr. Chamberlain has written to Lord Lister . . . that he wants something done on the malaria line . . . Lister called on me yesterday and I posted him again on the mosquito business, so that he might be ready for the [Malaria] Committee meeting of the Royal Society yesterday afternoon."

On July 5, Chamberlain had written to Lister to ask the Royal Society to form a committee to confer with the Colonial Office regarding researches into malaria in Africa and to offer financial support for such studies. Presumably forewarned, Lister replied at once, on July 7, that the Society had agreed[26] and had appointed such a committee, to consist of the officers of the Society plus J. N. Langley, E. Ray Lankester and John Burdon Sanderson. As to the officers, Lister was President and Michael Foster was Secretary. (The Treasurer, Sir John Evans, who was an archeologist and numismatist, did not join the committee.) The committee, whose membership overlapped with that of the Tsetse Fly Committee, held its first meeting on July 13, with Lister, Foster, Langley,

Lankester and Burdon Sanderson present. They immediately resolved to ask the Colonial Secretary for a copy of Ross's report on
malaria and they voted to add Sir John Kirk to the committee.

The early members of the committee were an interesting group.
Lister was, of course, famous as the inventor of antiseptic surgery;
Michael Foster was the Professor of Physiology at Cambridge and a
very skillful medical politician. J. N. Langley was a physiologist
who had made fundamental studies of the sympathetic nervous
system, while Ray Lankester was an eminent zoologist. John
Burdon Sanderson's early interest in public health had led him to
study bacteriology and pathology;[27] a search for even more basic
mechanisms led him to become an eminent electrophysiologist. In
1895 he was Regius Professor of Medicine at Oxford, still keenly
interested in bacteriology and pathology. Burdon Sanderson,
Langley and Michael Foster had long been colleagues in the field of
physiology.[27]

Ample information about Lister, Foster, Lankester, Langley and
Burdon Sanderson is available in the *Dictionary of Scientific Biography*. Since the most interesting and colorful member of the Tsetse
Fly Committee and the Malaria Committee did not find his way
into that work, I will say more about him. Sir John Kirk was an
obvious choice for both committees, being a physician, a naturalist
and, above all, an old Africa hand. On his first visit to Africa he
accompanied David Livingstone, serving as physician and naturalist on the second Zambezi expedition from 1858 to 1863. Forced
to return to London because of illness, he soon went to Zanzibar,
where he spent 21 years as physician, political agent and finally
Consul-General and gained enough influence over the Sultan to
become the "virtual ruler" of Zanzibar. (Old-movie buffs may
recall Kirk, in *Stanley and Livingstone* as the consul who was so
hostile to Stanley and to Stanley's search for Livingstone. The
portrayal is probably accurate: there was certainly no love lost
between Stanley and Kirk.)

Kirk checkmated German attempts to take over Zanzibar, played
a key role in the struggle between England and Germany for
colonies in East Africa, obtained from the Sultan the concessions
that led to the creation of British East Africa (Kenya and Uganda)
and fought the slave trade. During all of his many years in Africa he
studied its flora and fauna, discovered many new species of plants
and animals and wrote important articles about them. He was

responsible for a definitive botanical survey of Zanzibar and arranged for exchanges between his private botanical garden in Zanzibar and Kew Gardens, as well as with Natal, Mauritius, India, Ceylon and Malaya. He had been as natural a choice for the Tsetse Fly Committee in 1896 as he was in 1898 for the Malaria Committee. (He may well have been the only member of the original Tsetse Fly Committee to have actually been bitten by tsetse flies, as he assuredly was during his five years on the Zambezi with Livingstone.) He seems well worth a biography, both as a scientist and as a figure in imperial history.[28]

On July 22, Chamberlain suggested that two persons be added to the Malaria Committee to act as representatives of the Colonial Office to that committee, a civil servant, C. P. Lucas and, of course, Patrick Manson.[19] Manson tried, but failed, to take the Malaria Committee by storm. The committee had its own ideas about who, if anyone, should be sent to India to study Ross's work and Manson finally had to settle for a representative of the Colonial Office being added to the party chosen by the Royal Society; he also had to get Chamberlain to propose that he and Lucas be added to the group that would oversee the investigation of Ross's work. A long correspondence between the Royal Society and the Colonial Office reveals ample evidence of friction between Manson and the Malaria Committee, and reveals serious reservations about how Ross's findings should be investigated. But Manson's battle on behalf of Ross is another story, mentioned here only because it was wrapped up in the founding of the Malaria Committee and because it shows, once more, how often Chamberlain became directly and personally involved in matters affecting public health.[29]

By 1902 both Bruce and Manson had become Fellows of the Royal Society and members of its Malaria Committee and both were present at the meeting that recommended that Bruce be chosen to investigate Rhodesian redwater, as was Charles Sherrington, one of the greatest neurophysiologists of all time, who had been interested in bacteriology early in his career and had joined the Malaria Committee in 1901.

The full story of the Tsetse Fly Committee, the Malaria Committee, their successor, the Tropical Disease Committee and its successor, the Medical Research Committee of the Royal Society,[30] remains to be told. The support by the Royal Society of Bruce was of enormous importance and Chamberlain certainly deserves at least some credit, and perhaps major credit, for involving the Royal Society in medical research. When Chamberlain directed the Colonial Office to seek the advice of the Royal Society he knew exactly what he was doing and had good reason to anticipate an intelligent reply. Tropical medicine in the nineteenth century *was* colonial medicine. But there was no need for a Colonial Secretary to have a personal interest in medicine and science. Joseph Chamberlain's original forays in the field of public health preceded his appointment as Colonial Secretary by more than 20 years and the insights he acquired in the mid-1870s unquestionably influenced him during the years that he was Colonial Secretary.

Chamberlain and the "professionalization" of government

The late Victorian period saw a transformation of the British government, a transformation that was characterized by an increasing ability of the Civil Service to identify and rely on the advice of experts.[31] Chamberlain seems to have tried to make that transformation at the Colonial Office, e.g. by forming the Tsetse Fly Committee and the Malaria Committee, by appointing a Medical Advisor to the Colonial Office and by appointing Thiselton-Dyer as "Botanical Adviser to the Secretary of State for the Colonies." In spite of the increasingly important role of expert advice in other branches of the government and in spite of Chamberlain's commitment to science and technology, he did not change the bureaucracy of the Colonial Office. His personal interest in tropical medicine and his connections with Lister, Manson, Kew and the Royal Society seem to have had little effect on the day-to-day institutional machinery of the Colonial Office. As we have seen in chapter 4, the Colonial Office did not consult the Royal Society as to McFadyean's qualifications: it instead consulted the Board of Agriculture; when McFadyean, Delépine and Woodhead declined to go to Rhodesia, the Colonial Office seemed to have no idea of what to do other than to leave the search in the hands of Woodhead. And when Chamberlain demanded, on October 27, 1902, that the Royal Society be asked to find an alternative to Koch, the staff of the Colonial Office complied, but only reluctantly.

One cannot, to be sure, lay too much blame on the Colonial Office for its role in the search for an expert. It always acted on instructions; it was instructed by Milner to approach McFadyean and it was instructed by Chamberlain to consult the Royal Society. And it did verify McFadyean's qualifications by asking the Board of Agriculture about him. Had Milner asked the Colonial Office to approach McFadyean via the Board of Agriculture and to take the advice of that Board thereafter, the search might have proceeded differently.

But in 1902 even the Board of Agriculture had no division devoted to research on diseases of animals. As to the Colonial Office, it was not until 1919 that Milner, by then Colonial Secretary, appointed a committee "to examine and report on the agricultural services of the colonies." An Agricultural Advisor to the Colonial Secretary was not appointed until 1929; in the same year a Colonial Advisory Council of Agriculture and Animal Health was appointed to give expert advice to the Colonial Secretary.[32]

Chamberlain was an unusually forceful minister and a great believer in expert advice. Yet his efforts to induce the Colonial Office to rely on experts were at most only partially successful. Chamberlain strengthened the Colonial Office's reliance on Kew for advice on agricultural questions and he promoted the formation of "voluntary" organizations capable of giving advice on tropical medicine. But Chamberlain's role was a transitional one: the full professionalization of the British government in these and other areas of science did not occur until the 1920s, and did so then partly because of various shortcomings revealed during the First World War. The eventual professionalization of the British government in the field of agriculture was heavily influenced by four of the men who had dealt with East Coast fever in the Transvaal: Milner, F. B. Smith, Stewart Stockman and Arnold Theiler.[33]

October 27, 1902

Chamberlain's note of October 27 requires further comment. Chamberlain had never liked or trusted Rhodes and must have come to like and trust him much less after the scandal that followed the Jameson raid had come close to destroying Chamberlain's career and after Rhodes had blackmailed Chamberlain with the "missing telegrams." Rhodes was dead by October 27, 1902 but Chamberlain had not come to love the Chartered Company simply because Rhodes was dead.

As to Germany, Koch was not only a German; he had long been a government man and the Kaiser's man. (As E. H. Ackerknecht has written to me:[34] "In all Koch's assignments, e.g. his cholera mission, is a political element, also in his discussions with Virchow, Koch the man of the government, Virchow the democratic opposition deputy.") Germany and England had for many years been competing over the colonization of Africa. The German public and the German press had been pro-Boer; the Boer War was barely over; the Kaiser was, to the displeasure of the British government, about to pay what proved to be a very unpopular visit to England; and Chamberlain was about to leave for South Africa on a journey of reconciliation. Chamberlain did not leave for South Africa until November 25, but his plan to make that visit of reconciliation was announced in the press, to widespread approval, on October 27 – on the same day that he was asked to secure a *German* bacteriologist to study a disease that was raging in Rhodesia and the Transvaal.

Above all, Chamberlain's long-standing attempt to form an alliance with Germany against France and Russia had collapsed only weeks before the request for Koch's services came to his attention. On September 14, 1902, a high-ranking official of the German Embassy, Eckardstein, reported on a visit he had paid to Chamberlain at his country home on September 1:[35]

[Chamberlain's] repugnance to Germany has struck deeper roots and bears a far more dangerous character than I had thought . . . Mr. Chamberlain spoke of the attitude of German public opinion and of the German press during the Boer War . . . he . . . had been slow to realize the significance of the . . . German hatred against England. The German people had . . . the idea that . . . Germany would easily succeed in bringing down England and its Colonial Empire . . . English policy would, henceforth, have to reckon with the seemingly incorrigible hatred of the German nation . . . At the time of the Kruger telegram [the Jameson raid again] . . . and the Zanzibar affair in 1896, the two nations had stood close to war . . . today much lesser challenges . . . would be enough to set everything ablaze. He hopes . . . it would never come to that for he was clear . . . that . . . an Anglo-German conflict would have injurious results for England as well as Germany . . . [but, were that to happen] England could count with certainty on France and . . . one or more allies [*Kaiser's marginal note*: Very interesting for Petersburg].

Chamberlain had begun his career as a radical reformer, dedicated to improving public health. He ended his career as a dedicated imperialist, alarmed by the growing industrial power of the United

States and Germany, convinced that a trading policy that gave preference to trade between Great Britain and its empire was the best hope for the relief of poverty in Great Britain[36] and convinced that medicine and science had as crucial a role to play in the empire as they had played in Birmingham. He had given Milner all but unlimited resources for the restoration and modernization of the Transvaal (and for its new Department of Agriculture). He had struggled with the problems posed by Rhodesia and South Africa for seven years. He had opposed German colonial ambitions in Africa and he had just seen his hopes for an alliance with Germany collapse. And, both as a member of the government and as a former factory owner, he was all but obsessed by the increase in exports that were "made in Germany."

Small wonder, then, that some seven weeks after his conversation with Eckardstein, on the same day that his own visit to South Africa had been announced and acclaimed, and on the very day that Gray was urging Orpen to get Koch, Chamberlain wrote a note insisting that the Royal Society be consulted and, if they had a suitable candidate, that the Rhodesian government be told who that candidate was *and* be told that bacteriology is not "entirely 'made in Germany.'" *And* that if there were such a candidate and the Rhodesian government still wanted Koch, they could get him themselves!

7

Arnold Theiler, Charles Lounsbury and Duncan Hutcheon

During a time when figures of great international reputation such as Laveran and Nocard were claiming that the new disease was only a form of redwater, and while Koch was claiming that the disease, though new, was transmitted by the blue tick and that he had found a way to immunize against it, two young men who were hardly known outside of South Africa were at work establishing the facts. They were the Swiss-born veterinarian Arnold Theiler and the American-born entomologist Charles Lounsbury; both worked closely with and had the strong support of the senior veterinarian of South Africa, Duncan Hutcheon.

Arnold Theiler

Arnold Theiler was born in Switzerland on March 26, 1867 and obtained his diploma as a veterinarian in Zurich in 1889.[1] He found little work in Switzerland and decided to go to the Transvaal, where he arrived in March, 1891, in time to celebrate his twenty-fourth birthday. While working as "supervisor of cattle and forage" on a large farm, he lost his left hand in a farm-machinery accident; thus handicapped, he set up a private practice in Pretoria in September, 1891. That practice was so unsuccessful that Theiler was unable to send Christmas gifts to his family in Switzerland and was reduced to advertising a proprietary cure for horse sickness (for which there was and is no cure). While struggling to build a practice he imported expensive equipment from Switzerland, on credit, and taught himself bacteriology in his home, as Koch had done fifteen years before. Not until the middle of 1893 did Theiler feel justified in bringing his fiancée to South Africa, and even then they did not marry. Suddenly, in late July, 1893 he got a job in Johannesburg, supervising the production of smallpox vaccine: his financial condition can be judged by the fact that he immediately accepted that job at a salary of £50 a month, even though the initial appointment was for one month only. He finally married in October 1893, but his wife had to supplement the family income by working as a dressmaker and by taking in two boarders. Theiler again laid the ground for a private practice and continued to do bacteriological research on his own, in his home laboratory. (His job making vaccine lasted only five months, but he did get £25 severance pay!) In January, 1894, in his first month of private practice, he collected less than £4, but by June he was fairly prosperous and was on excellent terms with important government officials, partly because he had learned to speak both Dutch and the Taal. (*Taal* actually means language but "the Taal" meant the local colloquial form of Dutch. The Taal was later to be upgraded into the written and literary language now known as Afrikaans.)

The career that was to make Theiler world famous finally began in March, 1896 when the government of the Transvaal sent him to Matabeleland to see if the cattle there were afflicted with rinderpest or with some other lethal disease. In Bulawayo he spent three days with Charles E. Gray; by then, however, there was no doubt that the disease was rinderpest. Theiler left Bulawayo during a dangerous period of the 1896 uprising; on his return to Pretoria he reported directly to Kruger, speaking the Taal.

Having hoped for three years to become the Veterinarian of the Transvaal, Theiler finally got his wish: that post was created in May, 1896 and he was appointed to it at an annual salary of £500, ready for his first encounter with Robert Koch. On October 1, 1896, Theiler and Watkins-Pitchford left for a site near the Bechuanaland border to begin experiments aimed at finding an inoculation that would prevent rinderpest. Robert Koch sailed for South Africa for the same purpose the following month. By December, Watkins-Pitchford and Theiler had developed a serum that they believed would immunize animals against rinderpest, but before they had fully tested and perfected it, Koch announced, on February 10, 1897, that cattle could be immunized by injecting them with serum and with bile taken from the gall bladder of an animal that had died of rinderpest. It later turned out that Koch's method confers only an uncertain and temporary immunity, but Koch received credit for finding a means of preventing rinderpest. The method that Theiler and Watkins-Pitchford had worked on was later perfected by several workers, including Theiler himself, and came to be widely used, but neither Theiler nor Watkins-Pitchford got the credit for it that they felt they deserved. Most of the credit went to a Frenchman, M. J. Danysz, and a Belgian, Jules Bordet, and the whole experience was a frustrating one for Theiler. Meanwhile, Koch had left South Africa for India. On his way back from India, he stopped off at Dar-es-Salaam to investigate several diseases, among them a cattle disease that he decided was Texas fever.

David Bruce and his wife had also been in South Africa, working on the tsetse-fly disease of cattle. A brief stay in Natal in 1894 was followed by another stay that began in December, 1896, and lasted over two years. Bruce and Theiler met for the first time when Watkins-Pitchford and Bruce visited Theiler's laboratory in Pretoria in January, 1899. Three days later Bruce was recalled to active duty in the army: the Boer War, with all its disasters, was only nine months away.

As a loyal citizen of his new homeland, Theiler had been prepared to take up arms in defense of the Transvaal at the time of the Jameson raid and he did serve the Transvaal during the Boer War. He was present, with the Boer army, at the four-month-long siege of Ladysmith. Among the besieged, suffering great hardships, were David Bruce and his wife and Watkins-Pitchford. The siege of Ladysmith ended in late February, 1900, and Theiler was released from active service to return to his laboratory at Daspoort, near Pretoria. On June 6, 1900, long before the end of the Boer War, Pretoria fell to the British and Theiler was again temporarily unemployed. But the British almost immediately reinstated him at his laboratory and by July 1, he was back at work at a good salary.[2] He continued to serve the British in the Transvaal throughout the rest of the war, which officially ended on May 31, 1902.

On June 21, 1902, High Commissioner Milner took over as civilian Governor of the Transvaal and, as we saw in chapter 4, F. B. Smith, with Milner's support, began to build the new Department of Agriculture of the Transvaal in mid-September. Milner, who had already been asked to secure the services of McFadyean, and was soon to become embroiled in the problem of whether to hire Koch or Bruce, could hardly have known that Arnold Theiler, who was to correct so many of Koch's errors and oversights, had been hard at work on the new disease since June, 1902.

Charles P. Lounsbury

Charles Pugsley Lounsbury (1872–1955) was, like Arnold Theiler, an immigrant to South Africa. Born in Brooklyn, N.Y., he was taken as a child to Boston and later studied at the Massachusetts Agricultural College, where he stayed on as a graduate student and instructor. In 1893, when the Department of Agriculture of the Cape decided to create the post of Government Entomologist because of the invasion of the Cape vineyards by phylloxera, they asked the Colonial Secretary (not Chamberlain but his predecessor) to obtain recommendations from L. O. Howard, the head of the Division of Entomology of the U.S. Department of Agriculture. Howard eventually recommended Lounsbury who by then had not only studied entomology as an undergraduate and as a graduate student but had had practical experience at the Massachusetts Experimental Station. Several older men had turned the job down either because the salary was too low or because their wives refused to move to South Africa. By the time the job was offered to Lounsbury in 1895, the salary had been raised to £600 a year. Lounsbury accepted, married Rose Davis who was an assistant to the New York State Entomologist at Albany, and arrived in Cape Town shortly before his twenty-third birthday. He seems to have been an immediate success: he was only on the job for the last four months of 1895 but his annual report for 1895 "covered 51 pages and an enormous amount of work."

As soon as he arrived in Cape Town he asked for funds to buy a typewriter and a bicycle: told that there was enough money for only one or the other, he bought the typewriter with government funds and a bicycle with his own. During his first two or three years in the Cape Lounsbury did a great deal of work on the control of insect pests of plants. By 1896 he had built a fumigation house at the Cape where imported plants would be fumigated with hydrogen cyanide – said to have been the first such government facility in the world. By 1898, Lounsbury had begun to study ticks as vectors of animal diseases. When he arrived in 1895, Lounsbury had a one-room office, no assistant, no secretary, not even an office boy, and he says that he was the only full-time government entomologist in the continent of Africa. In 1902, when he began to study East Coast fever, he had just turned thirty and actually had one assistant. When he retired in 1927 he was Chief of the Division of Entomology of the Union of South Africa, supervising twenty-five professional entomologists, and had a world-wide reputation.

In his brief history of economic entomology in South Africa, Lounsbury mentions East Coast fever only in passing, in a description of his early facilities for research. "Much rearing of ladybirds and other insects was carried out [in the one-room office] and much in my bedroom at the boarding house." Lounsbury later moved to his own house but the study of ticks required animals for them to feed on. No stables were available so he used

the outbuildings of the private residences of fellow officers and friends, and in several instances the family cows of these generous people served as hosts for the ticks. Later . . . experiments were . . . in rough wood and iron sheds intended for the housing of builders' supplies . . . on a site in the heart of Cape Town . . . The first deliberate transmission of heartwater by ticks took place in my own back yard, and that of east coast fever at the aforesaid building site. The life cycle of the dog tick was followed through on a pup confined in the office . . . the life cycle of the fowl tick was traced on fowls imprisoned in the office.

Of the builders' sheds in the heart of Cape Town, Lounsbury said "though some cattle, and many goats, sheep, and dogs were kept there until they died . . . there were no serious complaints about them. Perhaps the S.P.C.A. people and the city fathers never even suspected what went on behind the high fence." (In his annual report for 1903 Lounsbury tactfully described those sheds as "our experimental station".) In one of his early studies of ticks he accidentally infected Duncan Hutcheon's family cow with redwater. Hutcheon's veterinary skills saved the cow but it stopped giving milk for a time. This episode did not prevent Hutcheon from giving Lounsbury generous support and cooperation. The combination of youthful enthusiasm and primitive facilities survived until 1903 when a stable designed for tick experiments was built four miles out of town; that is where most of the experiments on East Coast fever were done.[3]

East Coast fever invades the Transvaal

East Coast fever appeared in Umtali in October, 1901. Less than seven months later it invaded the Transvaal, but not from Rhodesia. It might have done so, since rail service had been established all the way from Cape Town to Bulawayo in 1897, but the disease came into the Transvaal from the coast, just as it had done in

Rhodesia. The Rhodesian farmers had insisted that the disease was a new one while the local veterinarians stubbornly insisted that it was only a virulent form of redwater. In the Transvaal, although they took a little while to decide, it was the veterinarians who were to insist that the disease was a new one while the farmers stubbornly insisted that it was not. In both places the farmers and the experts were completely at odds.

According to Theiler[4] the disease entered the Transvaal via Delagoa Bay, in Portuguese East Africa (Mozambique). It was first seen near Komati Poort (which is on the Transvaal–Mozambique border, about 75 km inland from the Mozambique port of Maputo) and, at about the same time, in Nelspruit (60 km east of Komati Poort, and on the main route to Johannesburg and Pretoria). Residents of Komati Poort and of Nelspruit had told Theiler that the disease had first appeared there in May, 1902. Also in May, 1902, an outbreak of redwater occurred in Daspoort, outside Pretoria, in a herd of forty cattle that had been brought from the Orange River Colony. In Theiler's words:[5] "The epidemic started with cases of ordinary South African redwater and ended with forms similar to the Rhodesian infection." Theiler saw the new disease for the first time on June 22, 1902, in cattle that had been brought from Nelspruit for use in the serum station in Pretoria.[4] (The warning had not been heeded: in spite of the experience in Rhodesia, cattle were being moved freely in the Transvaal, even by the Veterinary Department.) In the first ox that died in Pretoria, Theiler found "the typical parasites which Professor Koch had described in German East Africa, and which Robertson and Gray found in Rhodesian Redwater."[4] More cattle were brought to Pretoria in early July, from another infected region in the Elands River Valley. On July 12, 1902 one of them died; its blood cells also contained the typical parasites. During June and July, repeated reports were received that rinderpest was raging in Nelspruit and other parts of the Elands River Valley and "farmers and transport riders began to realize that some unknown disease, not rinderpest, had made its appearance in the Eastern part of the Transvaal."[4]

Since the new Department of Agriculture had not yet been formed, Theiler was working with the Public Health Department and with its Chief Medical Officer, George Turner. In early August, 1902, another outbreak occurred in Komati Poort, among some "repatriation" cattle, i.e. cattle intended to restock the Boer farms. Turner and Theiler arrived in Komati Poort on August 15; on August 29 Turner reported their findings to the Colonial Secretary G. V. Fiddes, in Pretoria.[6] He said that the disease was definitely not rinderpest and that the presence of pear-shaped parasites in the blood showed that it was redwater. "On the other hand we saw all of the forms of the redwater organism, including that which has caused so much loss in Rhodesia, first described by Professor Koch in 1898." Turner recommended that no cattle be brought to the area unless they had been immunized against both redwater and rinderpest; in a minute attached to Turner's letter, the Agricultural Advisor F. B. Smith said "I believe the precautions mentioned to be *absolutely necessary*."

A few days later, on September 15, Turner wrote to the Assistant Colonial Secretary in Pretoria to say that it was desirable for Theiler to go to Rhodesia so that he could see cases of the disease there and see post-mortems "to establish or otherwise the correctness of our opinion that the disease in Rhodesia is one and the same with that which prevailed in this country." Theiler left for Rhodesia on or immediately after September 18; he left Salisbury for Pretoria on October 2.[7] Theiler's first published article on East Coast fever was a preliminary report of the results of that visit; it appeared in October, 1902, in the first issue of the new *Transvaal Agricultural Journal*.[5] In his report Theiler said that he had no doubt that the new disease belonged to "the group of diseases . . . commonly known . . . as Texas fever or tick fever, and, particularly in South Africa, as redwater. I wish however, to emphasize the fact that this Rhodesian form of redwater does not represent itself under the form hitherto familiar to the South African observer." Theiler had no doubt that the disease he saw in Rhodesia and the disease he had seen in Pretoria in June, 1902 and in Komati Poort in late August, 1902 were identical. *However*, he saw only one case of *typical* redwater in Rhodesia. In all the other cases the "parasites were not round or oval but bacilliform or rod-shaped, and the urine was not discoloured." In one case, Theiler found "many pyroplasma, all of different shapes namely: Pyriform, spherical, ring formed, and bacilliform. The deduction I drew from this peculiarity is that the different shapes observed are only different stages of one and the same parasite." He added that: "I was, at one time of the opinion that the bacilliform pyroplasma, which was first described by Koch as redwater on the East coast, represents another species . . . of parasite." But, Theiler went on, he had sent slides to Professor Laveran, who did not agree and he was now "inclined to the opinion that . . . they merely represent different stages of the parasite's development."

Having described the clinical and post-mortem findings, Theiler remarked that his findings entirely agreed with those of Gray, Robertson and Hutcheon as presented in the joint report of Gray and Robertson: "Mr. Robertson especially emphasizes the constant presence of the bacilliform pyrosomas and, by their presence, explains the uncommon virulency of the disease." Theiler noted that Koch had regarded the bacilliform parasites as juvenile forms. "This would indicate that the animals died before the parasites had time to become fully grown, and thus Mr. Robertson's opinion, viz. – that the constant presence of the bacilliform pyrosomas accounts for the uncommon virulency of the disease, is confirmed." Theiler found a further rationalization for his conclusion: "In the newly observed Rhodesian form of redwater . . . I am inclined to believe that it is principally from the location of the parasite [in the tissues] that the cause of the difference in symptoms arises."

Theiler probably sent blood smears to Nocard and Laveran soon after he saw his first case of East Coast fever on June 22, 1902.[8] Theiler wrote to Laveran on August 3, 1902 (when Milner had just begun to ask the colonies to cooperate in securing an outside expert). Laveran replied promptly enough to allow Theiler to refer to his reply in his article of October, 1902. I have not located either side of the correspondence, but Laveran's published article, based on the proceedings of the March 16, 1903 meeting of the Académie des Sciences,[9] excerpts Theiler's letters.

Laveran, who was the discoverer of the parasite that causes malaria, began his report by saying that Theiler had sent him preparations of blood obtained from cattle, and that those preparations contained an atypical form of the pear-shaped parasite. In his letter of August 3, Theiler had told Laveran that the atypical parasites resembled bacteria and that the specimens of blood had been obtained from cattle that were suffering from what seemed to be Texas fever. But, he said, the disease was very virulent, the afflicted cattle showed no hemoglobinuria, and often suffered from disorders of the lungs. Laveran says that Theiler wrote to him again, on December 28, 1902, to say that the parasites seemed to be

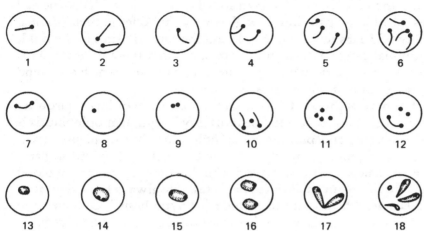

Fig. 2 Laveran's illustration of what he regarded as the atypical and typical forms of *Piroplasma bigeminum*. The "formes atypiques" are shown in 1–12, the "formes typiques" are shown in 13–17, and 18 shows all typical and atypical forms in a single red blood cell. The "rods" in 1–7, 10, 12 and 18 are *Theileria parva*, the "dots" in 8–12 and 18 are *Anaplasma marginale* and the large parasites in 13–18 are *Piroplasma bigeminum*, i.e. *Babesia bigemina*. (Reprinted, with permission, from A. Laveran, Sur la Piroplasme bovine bacilliform, *Comptes rendus Académie des Sciences*, 136: 648–53, 1903.)

different from those that had been seen before the Boer War. Theiler again said that the disease was more virulent and that its victims did not display hemoglobinuria, the constant sign of ordinary redwater. He added that the disease had recently been imported from the east coast of Africa and that cattle immune to redwater were not immune to this new form of Texas fever.

Laveran had also received specimens of blood from Dr. Loir. He found the same typical and "atypical" forms of the Texas fever parasite in both specimens: bacilliform or pin-shaped parasites, resembling a bacillus with a spore at one end; secondly, tiny round elements, resembling "micrococci"; thirdly, typical pear-shaped parasites (see figure 2). He remarked that the "atypical" forms were characteristic of the disease in Africa: not only had Koch seen them at Dar-es-Salaam, Gray and Robertson had seen them in Rhodesia, as had a Dr. Deixonne, who, according to Laveran, had studied them in Bulawayo.[10] All of those observers had seen the parasites in acute and severe cases. Laveran added that Smith and Kilborne had described large parasites as well as very tiny ones in their original study of Texas fever, but had found the tiny parasites in the mild, autumnal cases "which suffices to show that these little elements have nothing to do with the bacilliform parasites, which are found in Africa only in the most serious cases."

The new outbreak, Laveran said, differs from ordinary piroplas-mosis: the cases are severe, the mortality is high, hemoglobinuria is often absent, and pulmonary complications are frequently seen. These differences naturally lead one to ask if the bacilliform para-sites are a new and distinct species but "in the preparations of blood that are richest in bacilliform parasites, one always finds typical *P. bigeminum*, which seems to exclude that hypothesis." Only that and nothing more: for Laveran, because both parasites could always be found in any given blood smear, one must be the atypical form of the other. The bacilliform variety was, he said, nevertheless of great interest and was of prognostic value since its presence indicated that the disease was virulent.

Theiler was thus misled in October, 1902 not only by the views of Koch and Robertson but also because "Professor Laveran . . . to whom I had sent specimens of pyrosomes which I thought were not identical with the ordinary form of redwater informed me . . . that there was nothing to warrant an opinion that they were of a new species." Moreover, "Lignières . . . writes me . . . that he has found that there exist several varieties of pyroplasma, and although an animal may prove to be immune against one variety . . . such immunity will not protect . . . against another more virulent var-iety." Since calves, which resist ordinary redwater, contract the new form of the disease and since many of the animals that died in the Transvaal were probably immune to ordinary redwater, "we have before us the fact that redwater has assumed unusual viru-lency." Twice in this early report,[5] written before Koch had been suggested as a candidate to investigate the new disease, Theiler said that he had been inclined to regard the bacilliform parasite as a new species. He drew back because of Koch's views of 1898, because of Robertson's views, and, above all, because of the advice of Laveran, Nocard and Lignières. But by late August Theiler had already begun his own studies of immunity.

Immunity and immunization

In his interim report[11] Robert Koch said

bearing out my opinion that the Rhodesian fever is a specific disease I may instance another fact considered of considerable importance at the present day in the classification of infective diseases, and this is that it has been proved that cattle . . . which are . . . immune against Texas fever . . . will catch the Rhodesian fever and die of it.

In support of that statement Koch referred to the work of Gray, Robertson, Watkins-Pitchford and Theiler. As we saw in chapter 4, Watkins-Pitchford brought eight cattle from Natal to Rhodesia. The death of those cattle, presumably immune to Texas fever, had been described in the joint report by Gray and Robertson.

Theiler's proof that cattle immune to Texas fever are not immune to East Coast fever was obtained in mid-February, 1903, but had not been published when Koch wrote his interim report. Koch presumably learned of it from Gray. In reporting his findings, in an article[12] that was published in July, 1903, Theiler suggested that the term "Rhodesian Redwater" be dropped and replaced either by "Rhodesian Tick Fever" or "Coast Tick Fever." There is, he said, no doubt that

the disease . . . [belongs to] that group of diseases of which common . . . Redwater is the principal one . . . Professor Koch . . . in 1898 . . . identified it with Texas Fever, alias our common South African Redwater. This, and the fact that a certain percentage of the affected animals show red urine, explains the first use of the very term 'Redwater.' This, however, is of slight importance, as long as it is clearly understood that Rhodesian Redwater is by no means identical with the common South African Redwater . . . At the beginning of the outbreak . . . experts [thought] that this Rhodesian Redwater might be a more virulent form of ordinary Redwater . . . in addition . . . came Professor Koch's authority. He described the disease in the first instance as Texas Fever. The evidence [has] accumulated daily that the disease, although related closely to our common redwater, was a new disease altogether.

At this point Theiler stated that he had devised a series of experiments "which removed the last doubt on the subject." He did those experiments with the approval and support of Milner's new regime, i.e. with the backing of the Director of Stock of the Repatriation Department and of the Director of the Land Settlement Department and with the permission of F. B. Smith.

Between August and November 1902, as the first step in his

experiment, Theiler obtained twenty-eight head of cattle of various breeds. Some were from Texas, some were from the Cape, some were from Madagascar, and some were local Afrikander cattle. Of the fourteen Texas cattle, all presumably immune to Texas fever, nine received no special treatment, one was inoculated against ordinary redwater, two were injected with blood taken from animals suffering from "Rhodesian Tick Fever" and two were injected with blood from an animal that had *survived* an attack of Rhodesian Tick Fever. Of the five Cape cattle, also presumably immune to Texas fever, two were untreated, three were inoculated against ordinary redwater, and one was inoculated with blood both from an animal suffering from redwater and from an animal suffering from Rhodesian Tick Fever. Four animals were obtained from Madagascar. One was inoculated with ordinary redwater and one with blood from an animal that had *survived* Rhodesian Tick Fever *and* had been inoculated against redwater. One was injected only with blood from an animal that had survived Rhodesian Tick Fever. The final animal was injected first with blood from an animal that had survived Rhodesian Tick Fever and then with blood from an animal suffering from Rhodesian Tick Fever.

Three Afrikander cattle were used. One was hyperimmunized against rinderpest and one was injected with 100 cc of ordinary redwater blood. The third received the maximum imaginable immunization against redwater: it received 2,000 cc of ordinary redwater blood on August 27, another 2,000 cc on October 3, another 2,000 cc on October 14, a final 2,000 cc on November 14, and finally, on November 27, 10 cc of blood from an animal suffering from Rhodesian Tick Fever.

Twenty-seven animals, of four different breeds, were thus exposed either to immunizations known to protect against ordinary redwater or to procedures that might protect against Rhodesian Tick Fever. The final ox of the twenty-eight had already survived an attack of Rhodesian Tick Fever and had served as the source of the inoculations of blood from an animal that had survived the new disease.

On January 15, 1903 (a few days after Koch had left Berlin *en route* to Rhodesia), all twenty-eight cattle were exposed to "natural infection," i.e. to the infected veld, at Nelspruit. By February 12, 1903 all of the cattle were dead, with the sole exception of the ox that had previously survived an attack of Rhodesian Tick Fever.

Four showed only the typical large forms of the parasite, whereas the remainder had the typical small parasites of Rhodesian Tick Fever. Theiler remarks that this experiment had many interesting implications but "What interests us most at the present time is the fact that no breed of animals either naturally immune against ordinary Redwater or Texas Fever resisted the infection! Nor did any of the animals which were treated by inoculation with either ordinary Redwater or Rhodesian Tick Fever!" Even the ox that had been hyperimmunized against ordinary redwater by the injection of eight liters of blood had succumbed to the new disease. Thus "the strongest immunity against our common redwater gives no protection against the new Rhodesian Tick Fever – Hence we arrive at the definite conclusion, namely that Rhodesian Tick Fever is an entirely new and distinct disease."

Theiler's conclusion was of scientific importance. It was also of great and immediate practical importance: the new disease was a serious threat to all of the cattle of the Transvaal whether they were or were not immune to Texas fever. No one has ever doubted since then that immunity to Texas fever confers no immunity whatever to East Coast fever. What about the induction of immunity by inoculation or other methods?

All early attempts to induce immunity in a healthy animal by the inoculation of blood from an animal suffering from East Coast fever were frustrated by the fact that such inoculations never produced either a mild or a severe attack of the disease. As we will see in chapter 11, one reason why inoculation of blood does not ordinarily transmit East Coast fever is that the stage of the parasite by which the disease can be transmitted mechanically is not the "bacillary" form that is found in the red blood cells but another form, a form found in some of the white blood cells, the lymphocytes. There are very few lymphocytes in the blood, compared to the number of red blood cells. In 1909 K. F. Meyer did succeed in transmitting the disease by implanting tissue from the spleen.[13] Meyer noted that both Koch and Theiler had attempted to transmit the disease not only by the inoculation of blood but also by the inoculation of tissue obtained from the spleen or from lymph nodes. They had used that material "because these organs contain an enormous number of Koch's granules, which they consider to be a stage in the life cycle of the piroplasm." Since those attempts did not succeed, "hitherto the only known method of reproducing the disease has been by the agency of infected ticks." But Meyer did succeed in infecting two animals. Into one he implanted the entire spleen of an animal that had died of East Coast fever; into the other he implanted large strips of the spleen of an animal that had died of East Coast fever. Both of the animals contracted East Coast fever and died from it. In 1911 Theiler obtained the same result[14] and in the late 1920s it was found that the disease could even be transmitted by inoculation with blood, provided that blood was injected both subcutaneously and intradermally. But inoculation of either spleen or blood did not always cause the disease and never led to a satisfactory method for inducing immunity.[15]

In 1953, Neitz[16] showed that if aureomycin is administered during a period beginning 24 hours after East Coast fever is induced by the application of a tick, the onset of the disease "was followed by recovery and the development of solid immunity." In 1975, Radley and his colleagues showed that the injection of material prepared from infected ticks, together with the injection of a long-acting tetracycline, also induces immunity.[17] But according to Wilde,[18] that method is "cumbersome . . . does not show, at present, characteristics that are optimally desirable in a good field vaccine . . . [and] would be expensive to apply on a large scale."

In a recent review of efforts to develop a procedure for immunizing cattle against East Coast fever, Doherty and Nussenzweig[19] say that, despite its disadvantages, the "infection-treatment" method "could be economically feasible as there would be less need for costly dipping to control ticks." Less encouragingly, they add that "unfortunately early indications are that a reduction in dipping of E.C.F.-immune cattle leads to the emergence of other tick-borne diseases."[20] Thus the tick remains the enemy and East Coast fever remains endemic in areas where it has always been endemic, such as Kenya, Tanzania and parts of central Africa.

Charles Lounsbury, Arnold Theiler and the brown tick

The discovery that the brown tick transmits East Coast fever was of such fundamental importance that one would assume that it grew out of a systematic effort to determine which tick transmits the disease. But that was not how the discovery came about. Charles Gray had long been convinced that he was dealing with "virulent" redwater and he knew that redwater is transmitted by the blue tick.

But he had difficulty in persuading the farmers to reduce tick infestation by dipping their cattle and he thought he could make a stronger argument for dipping once the disease had been deliberately evoked by allowing ticks to feed on healthy cattle. That is why he kept sending ticks to Charles Lounsbury in Cape Town. But to everyone's surprise ticks sent to Cape Town from Rhodesia never caused any disease when allowed to feed on healthy cattle. On September, 30, 1902 Hutcheon cabled to Gray[21] "Lounsbury wires me that ticks hatched out from those sent have not communicated disease try if possible to send some more & see that [they] come from really affected animals." On October 2 Robertson wired Gray[21] " . . . quite unable to offer any explanation as to failure of experiments stop can you forward Lounsbury more ticks to repeat experiments." Since it had long been known that redwater is readily transmitted by the bite of the blue tick, the failure to evoke the disease in Cape Town was quite unexpected. Not only had the disease not been evoked by ticks, dipping did not seem to prevent cattle from contracting it. As a result Gray began to doubt that the disease really was redwater and he began to doubt that it was transmitted by ticks. He said as much on October 30, 1902, in a letter to Robertson:[21] "I think . . . we will find that some insect other than the tick may act as the intermediary of this disease." ("This disease": not this virulent form of redwater, simply "this disease.") He also sent Robertson smears from some "Kerrimuir [sic] cattle" that had sickened and died in spite of having been dipped on a regular basis: "evidence is piling up to indicate that dipping is not going to help us much." He ended his letter by saying "Excuse hurried scribble, but I can tell you my hair is beginning to fall out over this business."

Gray sent a copy of that letter to Watkins-Pitchford, who replied on November 12[21] that larval ticks might get on cattle and infect them before the cattle had been dipped, that the animals Lounsbury had used might already have been immune to redwater, that Lounsbury's experiments were as yet inconclusive, and that it would be premature to conclude that the disease was not transmitted by ticks. He ended his letter by recommending a proprietary remedy for loss of hair (Tatcho), "with my sympathy."

Watkins-Pitchford was right: Gray's conclusion was premature. In his letter of October 30 Gray mentioned that he had taken some ticks from the Kirriemuir cattle and had recently sent them to

Lounsbury. On December 17 Hutcheon sent an exciting telegram to Gray:[21]

the ticks sent by you on Octr. 16 said to have been taken from Kirriemuir cattle that sickened after dipping were placed on a two year old beast on Novr 27th on the evening Dec. 12 temp. was 104.8 . . . last night 106.4 . . . blood shows rod like intracorpuscular forms immature pyriform bodies and also spherical closely resembling the intracorpuscular bodies met with in blood of Rhodesian cattle disease the animal still feeds but is falling off in condition . . . no discolouration of urine has been observed.

On December 28 Hutcheon followed up his telegram with a seven-page-long letter:[21] "the ox . . . died about 5 PM on the 25th . . . Robertson and I made a [post-mortem] examination . . . 15 hours after death . . . kidneys contained numerous infarcts . . . the lymphatic glands were much enlarged . . films from the blood, liver, kidney and spleen shewed . . . parasites in immense numbers – bacillary and spherical." Hutcheon went on to ask how it was that only some ticks seem capable of communicating certain specific diseases? "Heat and moisture are the atmospheric conditions. What are the others I wish I knew." Gray received this letter on January 12, 1903, the day that Koch sailed for Africa. The new disease had finally been evoked under controlled conditions, and by the bite of a tick. And although Lounsbury could not identify those ticks, he knew that they were not blue ticks.

Lounsbury reported these findings in his annual report for the year 1902 in a section headed "Ticks and the Rhodesian Cattle Disease." This minor masterpiece,[22] which is about 1,000 words long, begins

During the latter half of the year [1902] continuous attention was given to experimental work bearing on the transmission of the serious cattle disease that since the latter part of 1901 has been raging in Rhodesia. The disease is considered to be redwater by the various veterinary authorities who have thus far studied it, but several marked distinctions can be drawn between it and typical redwater, and therefore a distinctive name for it . . . is deemed desirable.

Scientific studies in America and Australia, practical experience in South Africa and Dr. Koch's studies in German East Africa, six years ago, all pointed to the blue tick as the transmitter of ordinary redwater, but:

Through the kind services of Mr. William Robertson . . . [and] Mr. C. E. Gray . . . this office has received many lots of living ticks taken from cattle suffering from the Rhodesian disease. Most of the ticks have been of the common blue species, and it was quite expected that the progeny of these would give rise to the malady. But although five different lots, received at different times from different parts of Rhodesia, have been tested on what are unquestionably susceptible cattle, *this common tick (Rhipicephalus decoloratus) has failed to produce any fever* [Lounsbury's italics].

In general, Lounsbury used the *progeny* of the ticks that he received in his tests, presumably because he knew that the redwater parasite is passed on to the next generation of ticks via the egg. The progeny of the blue tick never transmitted the disease nor did the progeny of other species of ticks that Lounsbury was sent. But, Lounsbury said, about the middle of October, 1902 he received two batches of ticks that contained a few nymphs of a species that he could not identify; he thought they might be the red tick (*Rhipicephalus evertsi*). Lounsbury combined the two lots of nymphs, allowed them to mature into adults and, on November 27, 1902, placed five females and two males on the leg of an ox. Both males and one of the females attached themselves to the ox. Fifteen days later, fever appeared and, another four days later, "*organisms characteristic of Rhodesian cattle disease* were found in the capillary blood by Mr. Robertson." After the ox died, a post-mortem led Robertson and Hutcheon to pronounce that the appearances of the organs were

typical of the Rhodesian malady as opposed to ordinary redwater. Thus it has been demonstrated that the disease is communicated from animal to animal through the medium of ticks. Whether the infection in the one case produced was derived by the transmitting ticks in their nymphal feeding stage or whether it came to them through the egg stage is not known. But, however the infection was derived, the facts remain that *adults* transmitted it and that these were of a species having no close affinities with the common species presumed to be the carrier of ordinary redwater.

Lounsbury ended his report with a refreshing statement: "There is no need now to speculate on the significance of these facts as further investigations are in progress."

This brief article is intriguing for several reasons. For one thing, it contains the first report of the transmission of East Coast fever under controlled conditions; for another it is striking that Lounsbury could not positively identify the tick, although he was positive that it was not the blue tick. Lounsbury had to send specimens of the "brown tick" to L. G. Neumann, the world's leading authority on the taxonomy of ticks, who identified it as *Rhipicephalus appendiculatus*. Neumann had described that tick as a new species only the year before, in 1901; his original description had been based in part on specimens that Lounsbury had sent him at an earlier date.[23]

The phrase "organisms characteristic of Rhodesian cattle disease" is particularly interesting. As we will see below, by October, 1902, Gray had written to both Lounsbury and to Robertson to say that he was no longer sure that the epidemic was simply one of ordinary redwater. Lounsbury's remark, his comment that "several marked distinctions can be drawn" between the disease and typical redwater, his use of a new name (Rhodesian cattle disease) and his demonstration that the brown tick was the vector, certainly justify his later statement that it was "strongly suspected" in Cape Town as early as December, 1902, that the disease "was quite different to redwater."

As we will see below in the section on Duncan Hutcheon, in January, 1903, the government of the Transvaal sent an urgent message to the Cape to ask that Hutcheon come to the Transvaal to work with Arnold Theiler. Hutcheon spent all of February and half of March with Theiler; during that period Theiler completed his proof that cattle immune to redwater were not immune to the new disease. Just before he returned to the Cape, Hutcheon urged that Lounsbury be sent to join Theiler.

As a result, in March and April, 1903, at the request and at the expense of the government of the Transvaal, Lounsbury spent four weeks in the Transvaal working with Theiler. The government of the Transvaal asked Lounsbury to publish his findings and he did so in October, 1903.[24] He had, he said, obtained species of ticks with which he proposed to do further experiments, but those experiments would take a long time to complete, thus this preliminary report of his work up to July, 1903. Lounsbury went on to discuss the history of "the differentiation of African Coast Fever and Redwater": I will return to that part of his article later.

Having offered his analysis of how Texas fever and East Coast fever came to be regarded as different diseases, Lounsbury turned to his next topic: "African Coast Disease evidently a tick-transmitted infection." Lounsbury noted that the Rhodesian veterinary staff had suspected from the beginning that the disease was tick-borne because "the way in which it attacked one animal here and another there in the herd, often sparing for the time being those in immediate contact with sick and dying beasts, . . . [and] the way it appeared along the main traffic routes after a lapse of weeks from the passing of infected spans of oxen, all suggested the agency of ticks."

The original object of trying to transmit the disease by means of ticks, Lounsbury said, was to lessen public opposition to measures aimed at suppressing the ticks. Because Lounsbury had studied other tick-borne diseases "the work naturally drifted into my hands at Cape Town." Various lots of ticks were sent to Lounsbury in the latter half of 1902 and in early 1903. Since the disease was assumed to be redwater, most of the early specimens sent to Lounsbury were blue ticks, but they never produced the disease. But "it chanced that . . . in early October . . . [there] were a few engorged nymphs of a species of Rhipicephalus, which for the present will be designated simply 'brown tick.'" After those nymphs had shed their skins, the resulting mature ticks were placed on an ox on November 27, 1902, and, as we have seen, the animal died of East Coast fever in late December. The next successful induction of the disease occurred in April, 1903, using adult ticks brought from Nelspruit when Lounsbury returned to the Cape from the Transvaal. "Thus the direct evidence is good that the disease is transmitted by ticks. It should be observed, however, that there is no proof that the infection was derived from the animals off which the ticks were taken in either of the two cases; the significance of this remark will be appreciated later." (Lounsbury thus again alluded to the question of whether the parasite is transmitted via the egg or is only acquired by feeding.) Lounsbury remarked that Koch had said in his first report that he had transmitted the disease by the blue tick "But a perusal of his original report in the light of more recent knowledge makes it very clear that he was mistaken. The disease that he transmitted was evidently not African Coast Fever but Redwater and that of an exceptionally mild strain."

Lounsbury went on to discuss malaria and yellow fever, pointing out that the parasite of malaria must spend part of its life cycle developing within the mosquito. As to yellow fever, "the organism of yellow fever has not been discovered; but that it undergoes a development in its mosquito host is indicated by the fact that the mosquito cannot transmit the disease until ten days or more have elapsed from the time it became infected." Moreover, both yellow fever and malaria are transmitted only by particular kinds of mosquitoes, not by all mosquitoes.

In redwater, the parasite is carried forward via the egg of the tick. Another tick-borne disease, heartwater, is now known to be caused by a rickettsia. Although the causal organism was not discovered until 1925, Lounsbury had shown as early as 1900 that heartwater is transmitted by a tick *and* that the causal organism is not carried in the tick's eggs. It is transmitted by a tick that feeds on an infected animal as a larva and then transmits the disease to another animal on which it feeds as an adult. As to malignant jaundice, a piroplasm-caused disease of dogs, Lounsbury had just shown that it is transmitted only by an adult that developed from an egg laid by a female tick that had fed on an infected dog.[22] In other words, the piroplasm that causes canine malignant jaundice is transmitted from an infected female tick to her eggs and from those eggs to the larvae that hatch from them. Those larvae pass the infection on to the nymphs and the nymphs pass it on to the adults, which alone become able to infect a dog. Since the larvae and nymphs are not infectious and since they can feed both on dogs and on animals other than dogs, they can be carried over a considerable distance if they happen to attach to animals that are on the move. If that happens, the disease can suddenly appear in a previously disease-free region after the nymph has dropped off and matured and the resulting mature tick has fed on and infected a dog. Even worse, dogs that have recovered from malignant jaundice remain carriers of a virulent form of the disease. Thus, Lounsbury said, it is of the utmost importance to learn exactly how the tick that transmits East Coast fever does so and whether there are immune carriers: if the spread of East Coast fever resembles that of malignant jaundice, quarantine will be almost worthless and the spread of the disease will be almost impossible to check.

During the second half of 1902, Lounsbury had received a "score of sendings" of ticks. Some had been sent from the Transvaal; some from Salisbury, by Gray; some from Umtali, by Jarvis; some from Bulawayo, by Edmonds; and some from Melsetter by the local cattle inspector, C. E. Orpen. Lounsbury remarked that the ticks had been selected merely by plucking whatever tick came to hand, which meant that the samples that he received probably reflected the frequency with which the various kinds of ticks appeared on the cattle. The great majority of the ticks that Lounsbury received were blue ticks; the next most common were brown ticks. The bont leg tick, the red tick and the black pitted tick turned up occasionally.

The blue tick never transmitted the disease. On the other hand, the disease had not invariably been transmitted by the brown tick. Nor had it yet been established whether the brown tick could pass the infection forward via its eggs. Moreover, the "failures to transmit African Coast Fever ... with brown nymphs which as larvae fed on sick cattle ... naturally arouses the suspicion that this disease is transmitted like Malignant Jaundice, that is that the infection is taken up by the adult of one generation and transmitted by the adult of the next."[24] Experiments to test this were, he said, in progress, but they were very difficult because of the minute size of the early stages of the tick.

Lounsbury began his annual report for 1903[25] by pointing out that it had proved difficult for him to study "African Coast fever" because it could not be transmitted by inoculation, because it was difficult for him to obtain infected ticks, and because there was no source of infection nearby. He had therefore visited Bulawayo and its vicinity between mid-November and mid-December, 1903, to obtain a supply of infected nymphs in order to set up and maintain a source of infection in his laboratory. As of January 1, 1904, Lounsbury said only that: "The results of the tests have been somewhat conflicting and the only deduction which I yet (January 1st) feel safe in drawing is that the Brown Tick (*Rhipicephalus appendiculatus Neumann*) is a transmitter of the disease." (This was the first time Lounsbury gave a specific species name to the "brown tick"; he added that the identification had been made by Prof. Neumann to whom he had sent "abundant material.") Three more cases of the disease had occurred at the experimental station in Cape Town, all induced by brown ticks.

In his next article, Lounsbury gave a more detailed description of his visit to Bulawayo in November and December, 1903, to obtain infected larvae and told how he had shown that ticks normally present in the Cape Colony could transmit the disease.[26] Larvae were obtained in East London and were

taken as hungry nymphs to Rhodesia and there fed by the writer on a cow while it was in high fever with the disease ... when full fed upon the diseased animal the nymphs were brought back to Cape Town. Soon they moulted. Then, on the day after Christmas [1903], about a dozen were placed on one ox, a few days later, about a dozen more on another, and a few days later still, about the same number on a third beast. The results were most decisive. The three animals sickened, each in its turn, about a fortnight after the infestation, and all succumbed.

The diagnosis, both during life and post-mortem, had been confirmed by Robertson. A later experiment had shown that a *single tick* could transmit the disease. (Lounsbury's finding that the animals sickened "each in its turn," is interesting as an argument for causality.)

Lounsbury was invited to appear at one session of the Cape Town Inter-Colonial Veterinary Conference of May, 1904,[27] at which Hutcheon noted that Theiler had said the brown tick was the principal carrier of African Coast fever and asked for Lounsbury's views on that point. Lounsbury replied that he had made tests with at least a dozen lots of blue ticks and that the results had made it very clear that the blue tick could not transmit East Coast fever. Since the blue tick spent its entire life on one animal the only way it could transmit any disease would be via its eggs. As to the brown tick, it very clearly did transmit East Coast fever but the "transmission, however, was in every case by specimens which in the previous stage of their own life cycle had fed on a diseased animal. Because this tick drops off to moult its skin twice in its life cycle, it gets an opportunity to feed on more than one animal, which the Blue Tick does not get." On the other hand, larvae bred from the eggs of an infected brown tick were harmless: the parasite was not transmitted via the egg. He said that he had not been able to make any reliable tests with the pitted black tick, but that Dr. Theiler had shown that it too could transmit the disease. As to ticks feeding on animals that had recovered from East Coast fever, he said that they could not transmit the disease. One of the animals he used was certainly immune to East Coast fever because it remained completely healthy when very virulent ticks were allowed to feed on it. When uninfected larvae fed on that animal the nymphs or ticks into which those larvae developed were not infectious. On the whole, however, it was difficult to produce the infection using nymphs; they were far more likely to transmit the disease after they became adult ticks. Larvae taken from cattle near East London, on the Indian Ocean coast of the Cape Colony, and fed on infected cattle in Bulawayo, had turned out to be virulently infective when they became adults, so there was, unfortunately, no doubt that "the Cape had the right tick to spread the disease."

After some remarks by Theiler to the effect that adult ticks seemed better able to transmit the disease than nymphs, Hutcheon asked "if he was to understand that the most successful way of getting the disease experimentally was to feed the ticks as nymphs on an exposed animal and to put them on a susceptible animal as adults?" Lounsbury agreed. (Much later research, cited by Barnett[28] in 1977, showed that it takes time for the parasite to multiply in the salivary glands of the nymph or the mature tick. Nymphs reach their peak of infectivity more quickly than do mature ticks; apparent differences in their infectivity may reflect the time at which they are allowed to feed on uninfected cattle.)

Theiler's annual report for 1904 included a section with the title "The Transmission of East Coast Fever by Ticks."[29] By then Lounsbury had shown that the brown tick could transmit East Coast fever, and Theiler had found that nymphs of the brown tick that had fed on infected cattle while they were larvae could also transmit the disease. But Theiler had by now studied some other species of ticks, to see if they could also transmit East Coast fever. In Theiler's experiments, ticks were collected at every stage of their life cycle. Some were collected from infected animals, others were allowed to feed on infected animals.

Blue tick larvae were collected from animals suffering from East Coast fever and were placed on six healthy animals, all of which remained healthy. Larvae of red ticks also failed to transmit the disease in two trials, as did the larvae of brown ticks and black pitted ticks. (In those experiments the larvae were allowed to feed on infected animals and then moved to healthy animals. Since the tick must moult before its next stage becomes infectious, larvae that are moved from an infected animal to an uninfected one while they are still larvae cannot transmit the disease.) In the next set of experiments, nymphs were used, the larval precursors of which had been feeding on infected cattle. Five animals that were fed upon by brown tick nymphs died of East Coast fever, confirmed by post-mortem examination. A single animal exposed to an infected nymph of the black pitted tick had died of East Coast fever, confirmed by post-mortem examination. In the next set of studies, engorged nymphs were removed from infected cattle and allowed to moult into adults, which were placed on healthy animals. Blue ticks and red ticks did not transmit the disease. But eight of nine animals exposed to brown ticks obtained in this way died of East Coast fever, confirmed by post-mortem examination. One animal became infected when only two ticks were placed on it; one animal that did not become infected also had had only two ticks placed upon it.

Theiler confirmed Lounsbury's finding that infectious nymphs, once they had transmitted the disease, developed into mature ticks that could not transmit the disease. In addition, he removed adult ticks from cattle that they had infected and found that they could feed again on another animal without infecting that second animal. Thus "we may further conclude that the pathogenic tick produces the disease only once." As Barnett put it in 1968:[30] "the act of feeding is necessary for the final development of the parasite in the salivary gland, and then every parasitic element in the tick either passes to the mammalian host in the process of the tick feeding or it perishes, since no infection passes over into the next instar [stage of the life cycle]." Theiler listed forty-six separate animals that were tested; some of them were tested many times with successive infestations of the same species of tick. Theiler also gave the dates of each experiment, which ranged from April 24, 1903 through March 30, 1904. His conclusion, long since amply confirmed, was that East Coast fever can be transmitted by the black pitted tick but that the brown tick is the principal carrier of the infection. If we recall that East Coast fever has an incubation period of up to two weeks and that each animal had to be followed for at least that long, and much longer if it fell ill, and then died and was subjected to post-mortem studies, we get some idea of the amount of work and expense that the experiments of Lounsbury and Theiler entailed.

In his report for the first half of 1904,[25] Lounsbury said that

tick experiments with African Coast Fever are being continued. The objects in view are: 1, to ascertain certain factors which have led to the failures to propagate the disease from the cases experimentally produced, in the hope that the knowledge may throw new and important light on the natural transmission of the infection; 2, to ascertain if ticks fed in the first or larval stage on sick cattle may transmit the disease when they become adult if in the intervening stage they are fed on non-infected animals; and 3, to determine if the Red Tick . . . the Capensis Tick and other ticks . . . may transmit the disease.

Later in the report Lounsbury gave the details of seven successful attempts to transmit the disease using the brown ticks that he had infected in Bulawayo.

Lounsbury returned to the subject in 1906, in an article[31] which had proved to be too long to be included in his annual report for 1905. It reported all the work that Lounsbury had done between October, 1903 and February, 1906. By then Lounsbury had shown that the red tick can, in fact, transmit East Coast fever. So can the black pitted tick, the shiny brown tick (*Rhipicephalus nitens*), and the Capensis tick (*Rhipicephalus capensis*). They all, like the brown tick, feed on three animals during their life cycle, except for the red tick which feeds on only two animals. Lounsbury had kept the disease going experimentally ever since he had brought infected ticks to Cape Town from Bulawayo in 1903. He did that by transmitting the disease from one animal to another with ticks, both to test the infectivity of the ticks and to keep a reservoir of animals infected with East Coast fever available as a source of the infection. This sounds like a risky procedure, from the point of view of possibly introducing the disease into the Cape, and one case did arise by accident. Thereafter, "all the stable litter, manure and carcasses" were destroyed in an incinerator. Altogether, "the disease was communicated by twelve sick animals to thirty-five healthy ones." Only two of those thirty-five survived (once again, a 95 per cent mortality rate). From the first tick bite to the first sign of illness took an average of 13.5 days. It took an average of another 12 days before the animal died, but few of the animals appeared seriously ill until they were within a few days of death. It followed, Lounsbury said, that there were generally a number of days when a sick animal in the veld might be scattering infective ticks.

This article of 1906 contains tables that give the date and the result of every experiment that Lounsbury did. It is an impressive list. A total of 175 trials were made on 48 oxen; the number of ticks applied in a single experiment ranged from one to thousands. In table I Lounsbury listed 35 instances in which East Coast fever was induced by ticks, 24 times by the brown tick and 11 times by other ticks. Table II listed 71 experiments in which presumably pathogenic ticks failed to infect cattle. In 13 tests summarized in table III, Lounsbury had used nymphs that developed from larvae that had fed on sick animals. In every case, those nymphs were infectious but, having transmitted the infection as nymphs, they developed into mature ticks that were *not* infectious. The tick, it seemed, could transmit the disease only once. Table IV laid to rest the fear that East Coast fever might resemble malignant jaundice, in which ticks born of infected eggs become infective not as larvae or nymphs but only as adults. At the beginning of 1905 it was still felt that "the possibility of infection passing through the egg stage had not been fully disproven." The fact that in other kinds of experiments ticks that should have been infective sometimes were not infective made Lounsbury unwilling to draw conclusions from negative results obtained only in a limited number of tests. Thus "large numbers of the progeny of Brown Tick females pulled from sick cattle were reared on susceptible cattle through all three of the feeding stages. The adult progeny in all stages proved as innocuous as the larvae and nymphs and the suspicion was thus stilled."

Table V reported fifteen experiments in which ticks that fed on animals that had *recovered* from East Coast fever failed to transmit the disease when allowed to feed on healthy cattle. Lounsbury cautioned that "Owing, however, to our ignorance of the nature of African Coast Fever infection, and the shortness of the period in which the disease has been under careful observation, it seems to me rash to definitely conclude from present evidence that ticks never become infective through feeding on recovered animals." (They can become infective but do not always do so.)

Table VI showed that six oxen that had recovered from East Coast fever remained immune when again exposed to pathogenic ticks. Lounsbury said that "Ox 19 had experienced a very mild attack of the disease, so mild that its appetite and condition had not been noticeably affected, yet the immunity which it had gained proved ample nine months later to protect it against the infection from about 250 Brown ticks of a lot from which smaller numbers applied to five cattle transmitted fatal fever in every case."

Of the thirty-five cases in which Lounsbury transmitted the disease, thirty-two occurred after Christmas, 1903. Only three occurred at a time when they might have influenced Koch's thinking, had he known about them. In the first of those experiments, the ticks were applied on November 27, 1902 and the animal died 28 days later. In the other two experiments, the ticks were applied on April 8 and April 23, 1903. Since Gray, who was by then working with Koch, had supplied the ticks that Lounsbury used in November, 1902, he surely knew the result of that experiment, but he may not have known about the experiments done in April, 1903, which used ticks from the Transvaal, obtained by Lounsbury while he was working with Theiler. And so Koch was able to say, at the Bloemfontein conference[32] of early December, 1903, that "He would not say other ticks did not carry the disease but he had never been able to produce infection with any but the blue tick ... The disease produced at Cape Town by the agency of the brown tick was not necessarily conclusive. Only one case was not sufficient."

The dates of Lounsbury's experiments allow us to relate his work to that of Theiler. Lounsbury was the first person to evoke East Coast fever by use of the brown tick. Lounsbury's first successful transmission of the disease, in November–December, 1902, and his second and third (in April, 1903, using ticks he obtained while working with Theiler at Nelspruit), were followed by many failures to transmit the disease by the blue tick (as expected) and, as not expected, by two failures to transmit it by the brown tick. In an important series of experiments in July, August and September, 1903, he finally showed that larvae born from the eggs of infected brown ticks do not transmit East Coast fever. The experiments that suggested that the brown tick cannot transmit East Coast fever if it has fed on animals that have *recovered* from that disease were done in December, 1903. But the vast majority of instances of actual transmission of the disease were obtained in 1904 and early 1905.

As to Theiler, his studies that showed that "Nymphae of the Brown Tick which have been feeding as larvae carried the infection" had been done sometime prior to December, 1903, since he reported them at the Bloemfontein conference. The work of Lounsbury and Theiler thus overlapped; the findings of each supported, corroborated and extended the findings of the other. By the time that Koch left Rhodesia in April, 1904, both Lounsbury and Theiler had proven beyond any doubt that East Coast fever could not be transmitted by the blue tick but could be and usually was transmitted by the brown tick.

Duncan Hutcheon

Duncan Hutcheon had spent most of August, 1902 in Salisbury with Gray and Robertson, observing sick animals, studying slides of blood and other tissues and observing post-mortem examinations. In a letter written to Orpen on August 25, he said that "I have just read Messrs. Gray and Robertson's final report" and that "I entirely agree with the views which they have expressed with respect to the nature of the disease, its origin, the manner in which it has been spread, and the reasons advanced to account for its peculiar virulence."[33] As we have seen, Hutcheon then returned to Cape Town and was present when Lounsbury first succeeded in transmitting East Coast fever by brown ticks.

In early November, 1902 another serious outbreak occurred in the Lydenburg district, which included Komati Poort and Nelspruit. George Turner and Arnold Theiler soon confirmed that the outbreak was not rinderpest but "Rhodesian redwater." On January 22, 1903, the authorities in the Transvaal sent an urgent telegram to the Governor of the Cape Colony:[34]

We are suffering from a severe outbreak of disease of cattle and cannot ascertain positively what its nature may be ... I should be extremely obliged if you would request your minister to allow Chief Veterinary Officer Hutcheon to come up to Pretoria immediately ... His assistance would be of greatest value to us ... these cattle have been freshly imported and this may be a new disease in which the interest of the whole of South Africa may be seriously affected.

The Cape complied somewhat reluctantly but it did comply[34] and Hutcheon left for Pretoria on January 28, 1903. He remained in the Transvaal, working with Arnold Theiler, until March 16.

In his annual report for the year ending March 31, 1902, Hutcheon again discussed the work he had done with Gray and Robertson in 1902.[35] He also presented some preliminary conclusions from the work he had been doing with Theiler in the Transvaal. Hutcheon ended that report with the remark "Dr. Koch ... has commenced his investigation at the time of writing." Much of the letter to Orpen of August 25, 1902 is incorporated more or less verbatim into the second report, but there are significant additions. Hutcheon had by then studied specimens in the Transvaal and was able to say that those specimens, like those of Gray and Robertson, contained parasites identical to those that Koch had described in 1898. In addition, Hutcheon now mentioned Theiler's studies on immunity, completed in January and February, 1903, which had shown that cattle immune to redwater died of the new disease. As Theiler had done earlier, Hutcheon quoted Lignières to the effect that "There exist several varieties of pyroplasma, and although an animal may prove to be immune against one variety, such immunity will not protect against another variety."

But he added:

This, however, leaves us just where we were, as we do not yet know whether the variety of the pyroplasma is the cause of the particular character of the disease and its modification in type, or whether the character or the intensity of the disease is the cause of the variety and modifications in the appearance of the pyroplasma.

Even more shrewdly, he said

If the various forms of microparasite . . . are merely different varieties of the same species of pyroplasma, as expert bacteriologists assure us, we would expect the diseases . . . would be but varieties of the same disease. . . . We would not, however, expect that the disease would manifest a distinct type against which the most severe attack of the ordinary form of Redwater gives no perceptible immunity whatever, which this new disease manifestly does.

Toward the end of his report Hutcheon said that if the disease

is a form of Texas fever or Redwater . . . then it is a form of that disease which is not alone intensified in virulence . . . but is also altered in type and character so that for the present it should be treated as a new disease, and every precaution taken to prevent its introduction into any part of the Cape.

Hutcheon dealt with the results of his visit to the Transvaal at length in a special report to the Department of Agriculture of the Transvaal, which was published in April, 1903.[36] That report was completed by March 6, before Koch's interim report was published.[37] Hutcheon repeated much from his previous reports, but he added a great deal. He and Theiler had spent six weeks together, investigating the outbreak in the Transvaal, and Hutcheon began by saying that he and Theiler "had consulted together on every point . . . we are perfectly satisfied that this is the same disease which has been prevalent in Rhodesia . . . and . . . that it was the same disease that Dr. Koch met with in German East Africa, in 1897." Hutcheon then quoted nearly a quarter of Koch's report of 1898 "in order to show that the virulent disease of cattle which he met with in the coast districts of German East Africa, and which he described as undoubted Redwater or Texas fever is the same disease which has for some time been prevalent in Rhodesia, and is at the present time prevalent in certain districts of the Transvaal." Hutcheon also quoted Gray and Robertson's description of the parasite and said "I have no hesitation in stating that the description of the various forms of this micro-parasite as given by Dr. Koch, Messrs. Robertson and Gray, corresponds exactly . . . [to those seen in the Transvaal]." He said, as he had said in both preliminary reports, that it was unfortunate that Koch had not described the post-mortem findings in more detail in 1898, since they "diverge considerably from the usual lesions . . . [of] ordinary Redwater."

Hutcheon described the post-mortem findings in detail and then traced the early history of ordinary redwater in the South African colonies, beginning with its appearance in Natal in 1870. Ordinary redwater had then assumed a virulent form, as it invariably does when it first invades a new territory, yet we have "no information to lead us to believe that the disease ever assumed the peculiar type or character which it had manifested in Rhodesia and the Transvaal." Moreover, Hutcheon said, Theiler had immunized twenty-eight cattle against redwater and they all had died when exposed to the new disease, apart from one that had already contracted and survived it. Hutcheon then traced the spread of the new disease in Rhodesia and the Transvaal and commented that although redwater was capable of increasing in virulence when it passed through a series of susceptible animals "we had no previous experience that when redwater increased in virulence it also altered in type." He repeated the passage from Lignières that he had quoted in his second report, and repeated his own comment that varieties of the same parasite might produce varieties of the same disease but would not be expected to produce a disease that was altered in character and against which recovery from the most severe type of redwater gave no perceptible immunity whatever. Moreover, he added, Lounsbury had produced the disease "not by the blue tick but by another species not yet determined."

Hutcheon thought the initial increase in virulence must have come about when the disease swept through susceptible cattle, including the Australian cattle. But, he asked, how could passage through susceptible animals "so completely alter the type of disease" especially since "there is no evidence . . . that the disease ever assumed its present type during its first invasion . . . of the Transvaal," when the cattle, he said, must have been more susceptible than they are now. He said "I have a strong conviction that the original source of this particular form of Redwater in Rhodesia is the East Africa Coast districts to the north of the Portuguese territory" and said "I am of opinion that this . . . disease . . . was imported into the Transvaal from the East Coast . . . seven or eight months ago." Hutcheon repeated his earlier statement that:

The Blue Tick . . . is recognized as the transmitter of the ordinary form of Redwater . . . [but] Mr. Lounsbury . . . succeeded in communicating the

Rhodesian cattle disease to a young ox . . . by . . . another species of *Rhipicephalus*, not yet determined. I am of opinion, therefore, that the altered type of the disease can be conveyed by this particular tick. It has to be shown whether its various complications are due to mixed tick infection."

Throughout his article, Hutcheon spoke of "this new form of disease," "this new type of the disease," "this peculiar form of Redwater," and "this severe form and altered type of Redwater," but he never went beyond that. On the contrary, having repeatedly contrasted the behavior of the new disease with that of ordinary redwater, Hutcheon finally said that he had very little doubt that it was a "form of Texas fever – Redwater – intensified in virulence and also altered in type and character."

Why had the disease altered in type and character? Since Mr. Lounsbury had communicated the disease with a tick other than the blue tick, "the altered type of the disease [is] due to mixed tick infection." Having almost persuaded himself that the disease was a new one, carried by a new tick, Hutcheon thus persuaded himself that it was Texas fever after all, altered by being caused by a *mixed* tick infection. But, prophetically, he added "it is through the study of the tick side of the question that the problem is to be solved." Near the end of this long article Hutcheon listed eight features of Texas fever as described by Smith and Kilborne and *again* emphasized certain differences between redwater and the new disease! On March 16, 1903 another telegram went to the Governor of the Cape, to say that Hutcheon was about to leave and that his services had been of enormous help:

at the same time we are still at the threshold of successful research and have reached a stage where the book [*sic*: work?] of such an entomologist as Mr. Lomsbury [*sic*] would be of great possible aid . . . This is Dr. Hutcheon's opinion . . . Specimens . . . sent to him . . . are useless . . . after transmission . . . if he could visit the infected areas he might discover solution in the field . . . matter is of much importance.

The reply said "Ministers having regard to . . . importance of interests at stake . . . have pleasure in acceding . . . Mr. Lounsbury . . . will leave . . . on the 18th."[38] (We have already seen the results of Lounsbury's collaboration with Theiler. The study of East Coast fever owed a great deal to Hutcheon: he had sent Robertson to Gray, he had spent a month with Robertson and Gray, he helped

Robertson and Lounsbury in the studies of the tick in Cape Town, he spent six weeks in the Transvaal with Theiler, and he was instrumental in arranging for Lounsbury to work with Theiler in the Transvaal.)

The next publication on East Coast fever was Koch's interim report,[39] in which Koch declared Rhodesian redwater to be entirely distinct from ordinary redwater. As we have seen in chapter 5, in reaching that conclusion Koch relied heavily on the absence of immunity to the new disease: on the subject of immunity he had had far more experience than Robertson, Hutcheon or Theiler. Koch's interim report was reprinted in the July, 1903 issue of the *Agricultural Journal of the Cape of Good Hope*, and was followed in the same issue by a reprinting of the report by Hutcheon that I have just summarized.[40] Hutcheon made a few interesting changes in that reprinted version. He added an explicit citation of Koch's 1898 report: "vide *Agricultural Journal*, Vol. XIV, No. 10, p. 658." He added a footnote: "Dr. Koch in his preliminary report states that it is a distinct disease but closely allied to Texas fever." He added another footnote indicating that Lounsbury had again transmitted the new disease by using a tick other than the blue tick: "This experiment has been repeated with the same positive results." And, finally, he *omitted* the section near the end of the original version in which he had called attention to certain differences between Texas fever and the new disease. In that section Hutcheon had pointed out that calves, which are not susceptible to redwater, are susceptible to the new disease and that the lung, liver and kidney lesions seen in the new disease are rarely seen in the ordinary form of redwater.

It is not clear why Hutcheon omitted that part of the original version of his article, nor is it clear why he, like Theiler, held back from saying that Rhodesian redwater was a new disease. Hutcheon was aware of the different microscopic appearance of the parasites, he was aware that animals immune to redwater were not immune to Rhodesian redwater, and he was aware that the clinical and post-mortem findings in redwater and Rhodesian redwater were different. But Hutcheon was neither a bacteriologist nor a parasitologist; he was a skilled practical veterinarian. Besides, the "expert bacteriologists" had misled him. For him, presumably, the more important point, which he made repeatedly, was that Rhodesian redwater was unusually virulent, required urgent and special attention as a serious threat to the cattle of the Transvaal and must be kept out of the Cape.

As we have seen in the section on immunity above, Theiler began his experiments on immunity in late September, 1902 and completed them in February, 1903. He reported his findings in an article that was not published until July, 1903, well after Koch's interim report had appeared.[41] In that article, without mentioning Koch's assertion that the disease was a new one which should be called African Coast fever, Theiler said that his experiments on immunity had proved that "Rhodesian Tick Fever is an entirely new and distinct disease."

Some responses to Koch

Lounsbury reviewed these events in October, 1903, while Koch was still hard at work in Bulawayo:

When African Coast Fever appeared in Rhodesia over a year ago it was classed by investigators as Redwater. So the Chief Veterinary Surgeon of Rhodesia (Mr. C. E. Gray) and the Bacteriologist of the Cape Agricultural Department (Mr. W. Robertson) call it in their joint report, dated August 1902. Almost from the first, however, certain differences from Redwater as previously known in South Africa were observed in the lesions produced, and in the form of the intracorpuscular organisms seen in the blood. These differences were pointed out by Gray and Robertson in their report. Various factors were suggested as the cause of them, such as the high altitude of Rhodesia and intensification of the virulence of the disease by its passage through a large number of highly susceptible animals.

The two diseases are still considered closely related, but it is highly probable that they would have been differentiated at the outset, or very soon afterwards, despite their close association, were it not that Dr. R. Koch, in a report on cattle troubles in German East Africa made in 1897, had previously confounded them. Dr. Koch at that time described the organism[s] associated with African Coast Fever, and unqualifiedly considered the disease occasioned by them identical with Texas Fever – that is Redwater. His error was very naturally perpetuated by those who studied the disease in Rhodesia, no one presuming to question the correctness of the diagnosis by so eminent an authority.

It is possible, too, that both diseases were present in the same herds at the same time in the early Rhodesian outbreaks, and that since [then] the epizootic has consisted almost exclusively of African Coast Fever. *Within three months of his signing the report with Mr. Robertson that the epizootic was only a very severe type of Redwater, Mr. Gray, in letters written to Mr. Robertson*

170   *Theiler, Lounsbury and Hutcheon*

and to me, was gravely questioning the conclusions that they had then reached, the admixture with Redwater having become less [emphasis added].

From Dr. Koch's German East Africa report it seems very probable that the two diseases existed coincidentally about Dar-es-Salaam in 1897 amongst cattle recently brought to the coast just as it appears to have done in Rhodesia. Dr. Koch describes what are unmistakably the lesions of Redwater, and then, going on to speak of the microscopical examination of the blood, he dwells at length on the organisms now considered peculiar to African Coast Fever.

That the Rhodesian disease was quite different to Redwater was at once strongly suspected in Capetown when a case produced by ticks in December, 1902, yielded post-mortem lesions dissimilar to those of Redwater, but identical with those found in what had become to be considered the typical Rhodesian disease, and when the examination of the blood disclosed only the new organisms. There was no longer any high altitude to offer as an explanation of differences, and the duration of the incubation period and prolonged course of fever precluded the idea of extreme virulence. Evidence that the disease was not Redwater was meanwhile accruing in Rhodesia, and also in the Transvaal. Redwater has long been known in the latter Colony, and when the new disease appeared, Dr. Theiler was at once able to distinguish between the two by microscopical examination of blood smears. Moreover, early in the present year he demonstrated by exposing cattle on infected veld at Nelspruit that a very high degree of immunity against Redwater gave no protection whatever against the new disease, and, what was still more significant, that the inoculation of even large quantities of virulent blood into susceptible animals was followed by no perceptible reaction. Dr. D. Hutcheon, the Chief Veterinary Surgeon of the Cape, was called to investigate the Transvaal outbreaks, and in his report, written about March 1st, while discussing the disease as 'a severe and altered form of Redwater' he shows that it is so distinct in its behaviour that it must be treated essentially as a new disease and he makes suggestions for the prevention of its spread in accordance with this idea. Altogether, therefore, the way was well paved for Dr. Koch, in his first report (about April 1st), to reverse his East African conclusion by definitely stating that Redwater and the new disease are specifically distinct.[42]

In chapters 3 and 5, I suggested that Gray and Robertson may have been held back from recognizing that they were dealing with a new disease because Koch had said, in 1898, that the small forms of the parasite were merely the juvenile forms of the Texas fever parasite and that the disease in which they appeared was only a virulent form of Texas fever. I wrote those passages before I located C. D. Alexander's "The Inconsistency of Dr. Koch," which is quoted in chapter 5, and before I located Lounsbury's more temperate remarks. Both articles advanced suggestions similar to my own and did so at a time very close to the event. I have not revised my comments in chapter 5 in the light of Lounsbury's comments or of Alexander's, with which they certainly agree. Lounsbury's comments do, however, raise two questions. If Gray changed his mind in October, 1902 and decided that the disease was a new one, might he have told Koch as much? Whether Gray said anything of that sort to Koch, we do not know. And, if Gray had changed his mind, why did he never say so in print? His only comment seems to have been that made in his annual report for the year ending March 31, 1903[43] in which he said that Koch was now of the opinion that Rhodesian Redwater presented certain differences from Texas fever and

> that these differences, and the outcome of experiments which have been conducted at Salisbury and Bulawayo, and also at Pretoria by Dr. Theiler must be accepted as proof that the Rhodesian disease is a specific tick-communicated disease, which he proposes shall be called 'African Coast Fever' for reasons which are eminently sound.

If Gray had decided as early as October, 1902, that the diseases were different and had said so publicly, he would have become known as the discoverer of that new disease. Perhaps he was not fully convinced; perhaps, not being a professional scientist, he saw no reason to claim priority. Or, perhaps, he had changed his mind and did not say so publicly because to do so struck him not as an opportunity to gain credit but as a confession that he had been wrong in his long wrangle with the farming community of Rhodesia. That seems possible, because while Bevan was attending McFadyean's postgraduate course in London, he met

> Mr C. E. Gray, the Chief Veterinary Surgeon of Southern Rhodesia, who recently by reason of his lack of knowledge of protozoology had made a most serious mistake in identifying a new disease, East Coast Fever, as Redwater of cattle, with disastrous results to the country. That I did not know at the time, but it was his reason for attending the course.[44]

We might also note that Gray, in October, 1902, may not have decided that "Rhodesian Redwater" was a single new disease but only that it was, as Kotzé telegraphed to Milner "a mixed infection of redwater and some previously unclassified disease."

The new parasite

In 1897 and 1898, Koch saw the parasite that causes East Coast fever. Following a suggestion of Smith and Kilborne, which is discussed in chapter 10, he concluded that it was the juvenile form of the parasite that causes Texas fever. Koch's conclusion was accepted by Gray and Robertson in 1902, although they were impressed by the fact that they saw the small form of the parasite far more often than they saw the "adult" form, and, as we have seen, it misled all subsequent investigators to a greater or lesser degree.

In his article of July, 1903, published *after* Koch had announced that both the disease and its causal parasite were new, Theiler described three forms of parasite:[45] (1) elongated forms, straight or curved, very fine, inflated at one end [the 'pin' shape], the curved elements sometimes taking the form of a ring; (2) the coccus or spherical forms which may reach about half the diameter of the pear-shaped parasite; and (3) "the typical forms of *Piroplasma bigeminum* ... the parasites ... constantly found in our common ... Redwater. They are pear-shaped, spindle-shaped, or spherical. The first two forms vary in length from 2.5 to 3.5 [microns], the spherical ones have a shorter diameter [1.5 to 2 microns]." Moreover, "The three forms may exist in one and the same animal and even in one and the same red corpuscle."

In his experiments on immunity, two animals died three days after exposure to the infection, and two more died eight days after exposure. Those animals must, Theiler said, be supposed to have already been infected by ordinary redwater and to have died of it, since the incubation period of the new disease is more than eight days; moreover no bacillary or spherical parasites were found in the blood. (Three of those animals had been imported from Texas and one from the Cape; none had been treated with injections of any kind.) That left twenty-three cattle to be considered further. Of those twenty-three cattle, fourteen showed only the parasite of Rhodesian Tick fever whereas nine showed both that parasite *and* the typical Texas fever parasite, *Piroplasma bigeminum*.

And so, Theiler said, the question now arose: was the *Piroplasma bigeminum* part of the life cycle of the Rhodesian Tick Fever parasite or was it a separate species which accompanied Rhodesian Tick Fever as a secondary infection? Theiler noted that Professor Koch had thought, in 1898, that the "small organisms were really the first forms in the development of *Piroplasma bigeminum*." But, Theiler argued, there actually were three distinct possibilities. The first was that the *Piroplasma bigeminum* was indeed the last stage of development of the small parasite, but if that were so we should expect to find it in all sick animals, which was not what we found. The second possibility was that, in animals previously immune to ordinary redwater, infection with the small parasite caused the *Piroplasma bigeminum* to reappear. We knew, Theiler argued, that infection with rinderpest might cause the large parasite to reappear in animals that had previously recovered from ordinary redwater. The third possibility was that animals immune against neither disease could be simultaneously infected by ordinary redwater and by Rhodesian Tick Fever.

Although he had spoken of "this new cattle disease" in the first sentence of his article and had said that the results of his experiments on immunity had "removed the last doubt on the subject," Theiler was meticulously careful to say that the question of the causal parasite had *not* been resolved. The small parasite might indeed be the juvenile form of the large parasite; on the other hand infection with the small parasite might cause a relapse of Texas fever, with the reappearance of the large parasite. And, finally, the two infections might be contracted simultaneously. The question, Theiler said, was of scientific importance, and the answer remained to be found. How was that answer to be found? "By the study of the agency by which the disease is produced. It is, as Dr. Hutcheon stated in his recent report, through the study of the tick that the problem will finally be sorted out. The evidence, so far collected, points to the fact that the *Piroplasma bigeminum* has nothing to do with the piroplasma of Rhodesian Tick Fever."

As we have seen, Lounsbury and Theiler had provided what seems to us convincing proof that East Coast fever was a new disease. They had done that by repeatedly transferring the disease from one animal to another, using infected brown ticks, which readily transmitted East Coast fever but never transmitted Texas fever. Moreover, the blue tick, which readily induced Texas fever, never induced East Coast fever. Convincing as this argument may seem to the reader of today, Theiler did not rely on it.

Theiler's formal claim to have identified the parasite appeared in the first section of his annual report for 1904.[46] In that article, which was entitled "The Piroplasma bigeminum of the Immune Ox," he did not even mention his tick experiments. He began by pointing out that until recently only one disease of cattle caused by a piroplasm had been known, namely Texas fever. But Koch had noticed a new malady, in 1897 and 1898, and again in Rhodesia, and

Dschunkowsky and Luhs had also seen that disease in the Transcaucasus and called it "tropical piroplasmosis" (that disease turned out not to be East Coast fever). In 1898, Theiler said, Koch had thought that the small piroplasma was the first stage of *Piroplasma bigeminum*. Morover

> after the disease had been introduced in Rhodesia and the Transvaal, it was repeatedly observed that the blood of the sick animals contains the *Piroplasma bigeminum* along with the parasite of tropical piroplasmosis. And the opinion of Dr. Koch, which it may be said was also shared by Laveran, of the identity of these two parasites, was for some time maintained.

But "the examination of many hundreds of smears ... revealed [that] ... in the majority of cases the small piroplasma was exclusively present." It also, Theiler said, had soon become clear that there were really two distinct diseases, with a different clinical course and different post-mortem lesions; moreover, cattle immune against Texas fever were not immune against the new malady.

> The main feature was, however, that the tropical piroplasmosis could not be inoculated into susceptible cattle, even with large quantities of blood containing the small piroplasma in great numbers. This fact clearly marks the two diseases, since Texas Fever is easily inoculable into susceptible cattle.
> Thus, as the new piroplasma must be considered to be a species of its own, I propose to call it by the name of '*Piroplasma parvum*' (*n. spec.*).

How did Theiler reach this conclusion? By showing that the diseases were distinct, that there was no cross-immunity, and that one can be caused by the injection of blood from a victim whereas the other cannot. The parasites, which look different under the microscope, must therefore actually be different.

In a brief note entitled "East Coast Fever,"[47] Theiler summarized the results of early experiments and again argued that a distinction must be made between piroplasm-induced diseases in which the blood is infective (Texas fever, malignant jaundice of dogs, biliary fever of horses) and those in which the blood is not infective. Theiler listed fifteen results that showed that "The disease has nothing to do with Texas fever ... it is a new disease due to a piroplasma, different to the one found in Texas fever." He ended this brief article by again saying: "The Coast Fever piroplasma ... represents therefore, quite a different species, and I propose to call it by the name of *Piroplasma parvum* (*n. spec.*)." The logical structure of this brief article is the same as that of the preceding article: (1) the diseases are different, (2) the parasites look different, (3) one disease is inoculable and the other is not, (4) therefore the parasites are different. Nothing is said about the tick.

Reprise

In 1893 Smith and Kilborne announced that Texas fever is transmitted by ticks and that acute cases of Texas fever are caused by large, twinned, pear-shaped parasites which they called *Pyrosoma bigeminum*. They also described *mild* cases associated with a tiny round parasite which they thought was the juvenile form of the large pear-shaped parasite.

In 1897 and 1898, Koch studied a serious disease of cattle in East Africa and decided that it was Texas fever. He saw large pear-shaped parasites in some cases of the disease. In *severe* cases of the disease he saw small rod-like parasites. Influenced by Smith and Kilborne, he decided that these small parasites were the juvenile form of the large parasites. As Lounsbury later put it, he confounded the two diseases; he also confounded the parasites.

In October, 1901, East Coast fever was introduced into Rhodesia, a country where Texas fever or redwater had long been prevalent. The problem had become so serious in Umtali by January, 1902, that E. M. Jarvis asked Gray to come there to investigate the outbreak. Gray immediately noted the absence of hemoglobinuria and the presence of pulmonary edema, as well as the unusual virulence; but he concluded that the outbreak was only one of an unusually severe form of Texas fever (ordinary redwater). He said as much in a pamphlet published later that month, and said so again in his annual report for the year ending March 31, 1902, which was written in April, 1902, although it was probably not published until early 1903.

Partly because the disease was so virulent and partly in order to reassure the public, a veterinary bacteriologist, William Robertson, was brought up from the Cape in April, 1902. On May 21, 1902, Robertson and Gray completed separate interim reports which were published in pamphlet form in June. Robertson described the small forms of the parasite but cited Koch as having said that they were only the juvenile forms of the parasite of ordinary redwater.

Gray and Robertson agreed that the disease was only a virulent form of redwater, i.e. Texas fever.

In mid-May, 1902, the disease appeared in the Transvaal, at a time when the Boer War had not ended, and long before its devastations had been repaired. Milner was installed as civilian Governor of the Transvaal on June 21, 1902 and Theiler saw his first case of East Coast fever the next day. A few days earlier, on June 16, 1902, Watkins-Pitchford brought eight Natal cattle to Rhodesia. They died between July 11 and July 16, just as Gray and Robertson were finishing their final joint report. The death of the Natal cattle convinced both the Resident Commissioner and Milner that outside expert advice was needed.

In August, 1902, while Milner was asking the various colonies to agree to hire an expert, the joint report by Gray and Robertson was published in Cape Town. It gave a detailed description of the clinical course of both typical and 'atypical' redwater and of the differences in the post-mortem findings. It also gave detailed descriptions and figures of the parasites, and it reported the death of the "immune" Natal cattle. Gray and Robertson again said the disease was not a new one and Duncan Hutcheon agreed with them. The report was widely reprinted, in the Cape, in the Transvaal and in two British veterinary journals. And, finally, we know that both Laveran and Koch studied it. On August 3, 1902, before that report had appeared, Theiler sent a letter and specimens of blood to Laveran who advised Theiler that the parasites were only those of Texas fever. Nocard did the same, and Lignières advised Theiler that animals immune to one variety of redwater might succumb to another.

On September 2, 1902, Milner cabled the Colonial Office to ask it to secure the help of Professor John McFadyean. Confronted by the demands of the citizens of Bulawayo that the charter of the British South Africa Company be revoked, Kotzé promised both that an expert would be brought out and that he would work in Bulawayo. The Colonial Office finally suggested Strangeways as an alternative to McFadyean on October 15, but by October 11 Gray began to suspect that the disease was not simply a virulent form of Texas fever. He said as much in letters to Lounsbury and to Robertson, letters which Lounsbury described as having been sent within three months of the signing of the joint report. He presumably also advised either Orpen or Kotzé, because on October 11,

Kotzé cabled to Milner to say that the disease was "probably a mixed infection of redwater and some hitherto unknown unclassified disease." The same cable recommended getting the services of Koch because he had studied a similar situation in German East Africa. Partly because of the gravity of the situation and partly because Milner failed to advise the Chartered Company of the steps he was taking, the search was accompanied by bad feelings between the Colonial Office and the Chartered Company. Partly because of bureaucratic delays and partly because Koch's services proved to be very expensive, he was not employed until December 19, 1902.

Even before Gray had changed his mind, Theiler had begun to collect oxen of various breeds and to immunize them in various ways to see if they could withstand exposure to the new disease. (The "hyperimmune" ox received its first injection of "redwater blood" on August 27, 1902 and its last injection, of Rhodesian Tick Fever blood, on November 27, 1902.) In a short article published in October, 1902, Theiler warned that the disease was not the familiar form of redwater and said that he had been inclined to regard the parasite as a new one but had changed his mind because of advice he had received from Laveran and Lignières.

Milner asked the Colonial Office to secure Koch's services on October 22, and Chamberlain attempted to prevent the employment of Koch on October 27, 1902; the Royal Society recommended David Bruce as an alternative on November 5. On December 6, 1902, Bruce said that if he were to be employed he would require the assistance of a veterinary surgeon, preferably Arnold Theiler. On December 7, Nocard, in declining an offer to go to Rhodesia, mentioned that he had studied specimens sent to him by Theiler and had concluded that the disease was only virulent Texas fever.

Throughout the latter half of 1902, ticks were repeatedly sent from Rhodesia to Lounsbury in Cape Town. Blue ticks never caused the infection but brown ticks, placed on an ox on November 27, 1902, caused the ox to fall ill on December 12 and to die of East Coast fever in late December. In Lounsbury's words, this and other findings immediately led to the fact that there is a difference between the Rhodesian disease and redwater being "strongly suspected in Capetown." After that ox had fallen ill, but before it had died, Koch accepted the offer of the Chartered Company, on December 20, 1902. He left for Rhodesia on January 12, 1903, in possession of the joint report by Gray and Robertson which described the clinical findings, the post-mortem findings, the small parasites, and the fact that the supposedly immune Natal cattle had died. Because of Kotzé's demand, Koch went to Bulawayo rather than to Pretoria, where he might well have worked with Theiler, or, at a minimum, been in regular communication with him.

In February and March, 1903, Hutcheon spent some six weeks in the Transvaal, studying the new disease with Theiler. On January 15, 1903, the oxen that Theiler had begun immunizing as early as August, 1902, were exposed to "natural infection" at Nelspruit. One animal that had already recovered from East Coast fever survived; the other twenty-seven were dead by February 12, six days before Koch reached Beira.

Because of the many delays that had occurred during the search for an expert, and because he took a time-consuming route along the east coast of Africa, Koch arrived in Bulawayo near the end of the rainy season. From April through October he had to work in a period when both the ticks and the disease were relatively rare. Nevertheless, on March 21, 1903, Koch correctly announced, in his interim report, that Rhodesian Redwater was a new disease and that the parasite that caused it was different from the parasite that caused Texas fever. Koch based this assertion on his own experiences, at Dar-es-Salaam (in 1897 and 1898) and in Bulawayo, on the differences in clinical and post-mortem findings as described by Gray and Robertson, and on the fact that animals immune to ordinary redwater were not immune to the new disease. In his interim report Koch placed special weight on the findings regarding immunity as representing "another fact considered of considerable importance at the present day in the classification of infective diseases." Koch presumably knew of Watkins-Pitchford's results before he reached Rhodesia, since they were mentioned in the joint report by Gray and Robertson. But he could have learned of Theiler's more conclusive studies only after he reached Rhodesia.

From April, 1903 onwards, Koch devoted himself to attempting to immunize cattle against East Coast fever by inoculating them with blood from other animals. During the same period, Theiler and Lounsbury studied the brown tick and Theiler also studied the effects of the inoculation of blood. At the Bloemfontein conference, in early December, 1903, Theiler had no hesitation in contradicting Koch on every point. Koch argued that the blue tick carried the disease; Theiler said it was the brown tick. Koch had said that the disease would sweep through all of South Africa; Theiler said no, only through those regions where the brown tick flourishes. Koch said that the presence of a "ring-shaped" parasite in the red blood cells of an animal proves that the animal is immune to East Coast fever; Theiler said, no, not at all, such parasites have nothing to do with East Coast fever. Koch announced the virtues of his method of immunization, produced by the injection of blood; Theiler said that the Transvaal had no intention of using any kind of inoculation. Most importantly of all, Theiler was able to state not only that he and Lounsbury had incriminated the brown tick, but that he had himself shown that nymphal forms of the brown tick could convey the disease provided that they had fed upon infected cattle as larvae.

Koch left Rhodesia in April, 1904, believing that he had found a way to immunize cattle against East Coast fever, but Gray reported, in late May, 1904, that Koch's method had failed to produce immunity. Also in 1904, Theiler reported that the "ring forms" of the parasite that Koch took as a sign that cattle were immune to East Coast fever had nothing to do with East Coast fever. Theiler wrongly suggested that they were an "immune form" of the Texas fever parasite.

Theiler's work on East Coast fever was done in many different parts of the Transvaal, and even in Rhodesia, from mid-1902 to mid-1904, some of it before the new Department of Agriculture had been created and all of it during a period when he was constantly called upon to deal with other serious diseases of livestock and when he was also investigating equine piroplasmosis, bovine spirochetosis, trypanosomiasis in cattle and in camels, bluetongue in sheep, bovine heartwater, rinderpest, lung sickness and horse sickness, subjects on which he published articles in 1902, 1903, 1904 and 1905. The bibliography of Theiler's work, provided by Du Toit and Jackson,[48] shows that Theiler published some fifty articles in that period. Theiler's study of East Coast fever was a remarkable "part-time" achievement; Lounsbury's work was equally brilliant. And, by and large, their results stood up. As we will see in chapter 10, the only serious confusion still present in 1904, the confusion about the various small parasites, was resolved in 1910, again by Theiler.

By the end of 1904, after three years of intensive study, the main picture had become clear. Although two more parasites remained to be identified, the differences between the clinical and post-mortem findings in Texas fever and East Coast fever had been described (by Gray and Robertson). Watkins–Pitchford and Theiler had shown that cattle undoubtedly immune to Texas fever had no immunity whatever to East Coast fever. Koch had correctly asserted that the diseases were different and it had come to be generally accepted that East Coast fever had been imported from Tanganyika, where it had long been endemic. The principal vector of East Coast fever had been shown (by Lounsbury and by Theiler) to be the brown tick. Koch had asserted that the small forms of the parasite were a new species. The new species of parasite had been transferred from one animal to another via the brown tick (by Theiler), named (by Theiler) and been shown (by Theiler) to cause the disease, to be present when the disease was present and absent when the disease was absent (thus fulfilling Koch's postulates, which Theiler did not mention). As we will see in the next chapter, the length of time needed for an infected field to cleanse itself of infectious ticks had been determined (by Theiler and Stockman). Finally, in spite of Koch's heroic efforts, it had been found by Gray, Theiler and Stockman that inoculation does not induce immunity.

The next step was to find some way to check the spread of the disease and, if possible, to eradicate it, with no effective treatment and no preventive inoculation available to help in that task.

8

The fight against East Coast fever

Throughout most of 1902, Charles Gray and the Rhodesian government took the position that the new disease was only a form of redwater and that cattle that had once been immune to redwater had lost their immunity and were now liable to reinfection. As Orpen said on April 17, 1902,[1] since a general infection of Rhodesia by redwater had taken place long ago, the disease would break out again, wherever local conditions were favorable. Thus no legislation could check its spread. On May 22, Robertson reported[2] that since "all Rhodesia is infected with ticks, I do not think any cordon or barrier can be of any avail." In the same report Gray attacked those who "lay all blame for the spread of the disease at the door of the Agricultural Department without taking into consideration the fact that the apparent epidemic nature of the disease may be the natural cumulative result of long established infection." On May 12, 1902,[3] Gray had even written to Orpen that the cordon between Salisbury and Bulawayo "was instituted temporarily to allay public unrest in Bulawayo, fomented by those who declined to accept . . . that the disease was redwater." Thus, Gray said, as soon as Robertson had confirmed his views, the cordon was withdrawn.

The disease was new, at least in Rhodesia, and it was spread by a tick, the brown tick. Its spread could, perhaps, have been checked, if vigorous action had been taken the moment the first case was seen in Umtali. But the brown tick was as dispersed throughout Rhodesia as the blue tick, and it seems certain that the spread of the disease could not have been checked once it had reached not only Salisbury but half way from Salisbury to Bulawayo.

The situation was a little different in the Transvaal, since the authorities there were inclined to think that whether the disease was a new one or not, it should be handled as if it were a new one. On August 22, 1902, Ordinance No. 17 of 1902 appeared in the *Trans-*

vaal Government Gazette. It dealt explicitly with what it called "Rhodesian Redwater." The ordinance required that all outbreaks be reported to the Resident Magistrate, and that the Resident Magistrate, once satisfied that an area was infected, should inform the Colonial Secretary "who shall by notice in the Gazette declare such farm or place to be an infected area." No cattle were to be moved from an infected area nor kept near a public road and all animals dying from Rhodesian Redwater were to be buried or burnt. Moreover, the Governor was given the power to make regulations designed to prevent the spread of the disease or to require the isolation, inoculation, removal and slaughter of stock "suffering or suspected to be suffering from the said disease." As early as October, 1902[4] Theiler warned that "this Rhodesian form of redwater does not represent itself under the form hitherto familiar to the South African observer" and said that "I think it advisable to consider the uncommon virulency of the . . . outbreak as serious, and I recommend that the disease should be dealt with vigorously and drastically."

In spite of Theiler's recommendation and in spite of the sweeping powers to stop the movement of animals granted by Ordinance 17, East Coast fever was probably as entrenched in the Transvaal by October, 1902 as it was in Rhodesia. Even if it were not too late to arrest its spread, the farmers in the Transvaal were convinced that the disease was not a new one and they bitterly opposed all attempts to control it.

Stewart Stockman and Arnold Theiler

Stewart Stockman had taken a position in India after the end of the Boer War. In May, 1903, he returned to Africa to become Government Veterinary Surgeon of the Transvaal and immediately joined forces with Arnold Theiler. Their first move against East Coast fever was to begin a census of the infected farms and roads. One year later Stockman was able to say that "since May, 1903, careful records had been kept regarding infected farms and roads, and the dates of infection. The places infected before that date had been carefully sought out, and they were now in a position to say that for practical purposes the infected places were nearly all earmarked."[5]

Almost as soon as they began the census Theiler and Stockman initiated a permit system designed to control the movement of cattle. "They never for a single moment believed that [the permit system] would bring the matter to a final issue,"[5] but they hoped that it would retard the spread of the disease until they obtained the power to fence in infected farms "for the purpose of keeping cattle on trek off of them."[6] Around September, 1903, they urged the government to pass a fencing ordinance that would compel the fencing of infected areas but "the farmers objected strongly to it, and said they could not afford it."[5] Since the government was not prepared to bear the cost, the "Fencing Ordinance was still-born ... it did not assist the Veterinary Department at all ... there was nothing [in it] whereby an infected farm could be fenced."[5] By late November it was clear that the fencing of infected areas was not going to occur and it was clear that the permit system was not working. Theiler and Stockman then turned their attention to a new possibility, that of "cleansing" infected areas by keeping them free of cattle until all the ticks in those areas had died. Theiler alluded to this plan at the Bloemfontein conference.

The Bloemfontein conference

At the Bloemfontein conference[7] of early December, 1903, Koch opposed quarantine as useless. His opposition was based on practical grounds. "I am sure that under the present conditions of trekking and communication ... the disease will spread throughout South Africa ... quarantine regulations ... would stop it for a time ... but there would be considerable expense and the disease would come again." Koch offered a better solution: the use of his "protective inoculation." Texas fever, he said, had been present in South Africa for forty or fifty years and the country eventually became immune. "In the same way South Africa will become immune from this [new] disease in a certain time. But we can make it so in a very short time in an artificial way with very small loss (Loud applause)."

Theiler responded that he did not think that the disease would travel throughout the whole of South Africa, but only through areas in which ordinary redwater occurred. The question of which tick carries the disease was, however, of great importance to their work in the Transvaal. They had not been able to induce the disease by the blue tick, "but it was demonstrated by Mr. Lounsbury in the Cape Colony that it was produced by the Adult Brown Tick."

After Koch had replied that he still believed that the blue tick was the carrier, Theiler said

with regard to the isolation of farms . . . it was not exactly their intention to destroy the ticks but to prevent them from becoming infected, by removing the cattle until the infection had died out. If, as Professor Koch believed, the blue tick was the principal carrier of the disease, then the chances of getting rid of the disease would be more hopeful as the blue tick undergoes all its changes on one and the same animal.

As to artificially-induced immunity, Theiler said that the inoculation of blood, as recommended by Dr. Koch, would transmit other diseases "like Heartwater, ordinary Redwater, and Trypanosomas . . . The time had not arrived to start inoculations in the Transvaal." They intended, until they had obtained more experience, only to recommend the fencing of farms. "The tick does not travel and a fence is a good barrier against the inroads of the infection."

Stewart Stockman argued that the kind of immunity obtained in bacterial infections differs from the kind of immunity developed against infection by animal parasites, "Immunity against infection by animal parasites is, at best, a tolerance of the infection." He said that, if Koch's method were to be widely used, all of the cattle in southern Africa would become carriers of the disease. "Not only would all the cattle in the country have to pay tribute to it, but all imported cattle would have to do the same."

The conference adopted four resolutions none of which mentioned inoculation:

That this Conference is of opinion that the fencing of farms is one of the best methods to prevent the spread of contagious disease, and that Governments should be recommended to carry it out immediately on all farms where African Coast Fever had broken out.

To retard the spread of African Coast Fever all reasonable measures should be taken to check the movements of cattle in those districts threatened by an invasion of the disease, or which have been declared infected.

In cases of isolated outbreaks of the disease the whole of the infected cattle to be destroyed (with payment of compensation) the infected veldt quarantined and fenced, and the cattle in the immediate vicinity dipped or cleansed from ticks.

That this Conference is of opinion that the different Governments should be requested to collect information and conduct experiments with regard to the possibility of eradicating the tick plague.

Cleansing the fields

By the time of the Bloemfontein conference both Theiler and Stockman knew that fencing was not going to occur on any large scale and they knew that the permit system was working less and less well. They had therefore already begun new experiments designed to determine how long it took for all the ticks on infested ground to die. In the annual report of the veterinary department for 1904, Stockman explained the motive for undertaking that study:[8] "The situation which stared us in the face, and which has still to be faced, is as follows:– The Transvaal is debarred on account of Rhodesian Redwater from exporting a single head of cattle to any adjoining Colony; ox transport between our territory and that of our neighbours is therefore impossible, and likely to remain impossible for years to come." It had also become apparent that dipping for the destruction of ticks held out no promise for furnishing a final solution of the problem, although it might be a valuable auxiliary. The fencing of farms, particularly infected farms, had been advised and rejected in the early part of the year.

"During the time Dr. Koch was engaged on his investigations in Rhodesia we were bound to provide for the contingency of these investigations proving unsuccessful." Stockman and Theiler therefore investigated the possibility of cleansing infected ground: "It appeared to us that since the life period of all living things is limited, the infected ticks were bound to die out in time, provided all cattle were kept off the pastures."

Theiler and Stockman[9] selected a field that had been heavily infested in May and June, 1902, when all the cattle on it had died. A few cattle were introduced in September, 1902 and they soon died. Since then no cattle had been on the farm. A particular area was chosen and marked off by a double fence; "the fenced area abutted on the railway line, and we were therefore able to introduce cattle from trucks without their having to pass over any portion of suspected ground." On December 5, 1903, about fourteen and a half months after the death of the last ox on the farm, ten Texas heifers were placed in the fenced camp. "These cattle came overseas from a country in which East Coast Fever is unknown . . . some of their fellows, exposed on ground known to be infected, died in the usual time . . . [the cattle] were received by ourselves from the ship, and were kept inside clean kraals and fed on imported forage" before being released on the field. One of the animals thus tested was found dead in a water hole, apparently having been overpowered by a crocodile, but its blood contained no parasites. The other nine cattle were kept in the field until the end of May, 1904 [i.e. for just short of six months] and remained healthy the whole time. Theiler and Stockman concluded that "an area which at one time was badly infected . . . does purify itself after a reasonably short period . . . on average 15 months" and that other evidence showed that pathogenic ticks may remain active for at least six and possibly eight months. The next section of Theiler's report was headed "Inoculation experiments according to the methods of Professor Koch."[10] It described studies made on nine calves that had been brought from Texas and had never been on Transvaal pastures. The animals were inoculated according to Koch's method, four times at seven-day intervals. They were then exposed to infected veld, where a fifth inoculation was made. All of the animals but one died, after being on the infected veld from twenty-four to seventy days. One was alive six months later and had normal blood smears. Theiler and Stockman concluded that inoculation would be of little value, although they could not refute Koch's claim that injections must be made for five months to produce immunity. They noted, however, that the only cattle that Koch had inoculated for that long had not yet been exposed to infected veld (when they were, as we learned from Gray, they died).

Theiler and Stockman next turned to "Dipping experiments."[10] Their conclusion was that because the larvae and nymphs so rapidly re-infest dipped cattle and because dipping so rarely kills all of the ticks on an animal "the application of dips in a badly infected area gives no guarantee against the further spread of the disease and no hope of extinguishing an outbreak unless the animals be also removed to fresh pastures." But such removal risks infecting the "route over which the animals are removed, not to speak of the new pastures."

But "we do not wish it to be understood that we are foes to the general idea of dipping cattle." However, it is not practical to dip cattle every fourth or fifth day.

Those who are inclined to trust to dipping to keep tick fever off their farms are leaning on a broken reed. If a man fences a clean farm, keeps his cattle on the place, and only brings in fresh animals after they have undergone a period of quarantine in a shed or special paddock, we do not think he need greatly fear tick fever even in an infected district. If however, he insists on doing transport with his oxen on dangerous roads, his animals will sooner or later pick up the disease and bring it on to his farm in spite of dipping.

Neither Theiler nor Stockman thought very highly of dipping, but that was because they knew that the larvae and nymphs drop off infected cattle and reattach themselves to new animals so often that dipping would have to be very thorough and would have to be repeated every few days, which seemed entirely impractical. It is now widely used, and it *is* repeated every five days.

Stockman versus the Department of Agriculture

On May 9, 1904, Stockman sent a thirteen-page-long letter to F. B. Smith[11] in which he enclosed a copy of remarks he had made the month before at a meeting of the South African Association for the Advancement of Science.[12] At that meeting he had expressed the hope that the high veld might remain free from the disease because of "the inability of the special ticks of Rhodesian Tick Fever to live in the high country." He added that it was too soon to be sure of that and that it would be unwise to move infected herds to the high veld because they might carry ticks with them. As to inoculation, he said that "our trials so far with [Koch's] method have shown that it does not protect." He warned that even if inoculation did prove to be protective it might also produce carriers of the disease which would mean that "we shall have made up our mind to have this disease always with us . . . I do not think the time has yet arrived for us to say the disease is going all over the country and therefore the sooner we let it go and get the nucleus for an immune race the better." He pointed out that the surviving nucleus would be only 5 percent of the cattle now in the country and "we should have to contemplate the task which lay before Noah . . . with the important distinction that this flood threatens to carry off the cattle only, whilst the people are being left stranded." Finally, he mentioned his new plan to make infected fields free of ticks. Stockman's letter to Smith began "I have the honour to submit a scheme for stamping out the disease known as Rhodesian Red Water." Stockman reminded Smith that the permit system had been introduced "in order to delay the advance of the disease until legislation could be obtained requiring that infected farms be fenced." But the fencing legislation had contained nothing of use, "moreover, by the time it became law the infected areas were of such extent that the initial expenditure would have been beyond the reach of the country."

The essential feature of Stockman's plan was that cattle be removed from infected land for at least a year, to allow time for the ticks to die out. What about the cattle that had originally been on or near infected land? One possibility would be to slaughter all such cattle; but Stockman had a second plan, one that he hoped would save many of them. Cattle from severely infected farms would be killed, but cattle from "slightly infected farms" or "farms under suspicion" might be moved to clean areas once they had been quarantined at an intermediate stop to be sure they were free from the disease. (As eventually put into operation, cattle in the quarantine area were monitored daily to be sure they had no fever, hence those areas came to be called "temperature camps.")

Smith's deputy, William Macdonald, objected to the plan[13] because he doubted that it would be possible to spray large herds and move them safely from slightly infected areas to safe areas without spreading the disease. He also doubted that farmers in clean areas would "tolerate the passage of large herds of suspected cattle through their preserves." Macdonald conceded that if Stockman's proposal to fence an infected area and allow no cattle to be moved from them had been adopted nine months before it might have checked the spread of the disease and added "even at this late date, I hold that fencing is the most practical solution." Even if fencing did not check the spread of East Coast fever, "it would still be a valuable and permanent asset to the Colony." Smith raised his own objections (which I have not located) and sent them to Stockman along with Macdonald's.

Stockman sent a long and almost acerbic reply to Smith on May 25,[14] presumably written just as he was leaving for the Cape Town conference:

I feel bound to join issue with yourself and Mr. Macdonald on almost all the most important points which you have raised ... I do not hesitate to state that only the veterinarians fully realize the gravity of the situation ... I must again place on record ... that this is a disease which will ruin the cattle industry of the Colony for an indefinite period of years, if it be not immediately tackled by drastic measures.

As to fencing, if it

was financially impossible nearly a year ago, it is doubly impossible now owing to the further spread of the disease . . . you seem to have overlooked the fact that fencing in of infected farms was merely for the purpose of keeping cattle on trek off them . . . it would also have been necessary to remove all cattle from the fenced farm itself before the ground could become purified.

If fencing was too costly a year ago, to add fencing to the temperature camp method now would be enormously more expensive. Smith had apparently argued that the present regulations had checked the spread of the disease, to which Stockman replied, "I have always warned you . . . that these tactics . . . can never achieve anything in the shape of finality." He added "I cannot agree with you that there is not much time to be gained by 'precipitate action' which I take to mean immediate action. Everything is to be gained by immediate action."

Stockman added that he could devise no other solution, that "if we do not act now, we shall have to do the same thing next year at much greater expense" and ended by insisting that the scheme, if adopted, must be mandatory; if it were voluntary the refusal of a single farmer to take part could prevent the cleansing of a large area. Long passages in Stockman's two letters to Smith are very similar to long passages in Stockman's remarks at the Cape Town conference and it seems certain that Stockman used that conference as a platform to put pressure on the Transvaal authorities. He enjoyed a degree of independence because he had already accepted the post of Chief Veterinary Officer of Great Britain, a post he took up on January 1, 1905.

The Cape conference

The Bloemfontein conference adjourned on December 5, 1903, with the intention of meeting again in about a year. The next Inter-Colonial Veterinary Conference was held less than six months later, at the end of the rainy season. It convened in Cape Town on May 25–31, 1904 and was opened by the Secretary for Agriculture of the Cape Colony.[15] He told the delegates that the

Government looked for great results from their deliberations "especially with regard to the checking of that wretched scourge ... Rhodesian fever." The Secretary apologized to the delegates for "calling them together so hurriedly but they felt, on the outbreak of the disease in Natal, that they had better ... secure some action ... to stop its further spread." Duncan Hutcheon welcomed the delegates in his role as head of the Veterinary Department of the Cape Colony. He apologized for the fact that the conference was being held before the proceedings of the previous meeting had been printed, but since the experiments of Dr. Koch "were not so satisfactory as expected ... the Government was anxious to have some really trustworthy opinion to go upon in dealing with the disease from a professional as well as an administrative point of view."

The same regions were represented at both conferences: Rhodesia, the South African colonies (Cape Colony, Natal, the Transvaal and the Orange River Colony), Basutoland (now Lesotho), Bechuanaland (now Botswana), Portuguese East Africa (now Mozambique) and German South West Africa[16] (now Namibia). The conference was immediately advised by Gray that Koch's method of immunization had failed and it was advised by Theiler that Koch's "ring forms" were not a variety of the East Coast fever parasite. Both Theiler and Lounsbury told the delegates that the brown tick was undoubtedly the major vector of the disease.

How was the spread of the disease to be stopped? Gray said that in Rhodesia the disease was extending gradually. They had tried to prevent the moving of stock but they could not wholly enforce that, besides which the Africans would move stock no matter what the government did. The disease was spreading relatively slowly only because the government had stopped the moving of stock as much as they could. Stockman said that the same was true in the Transvaal where "they blamed transport ... much more than anything else ... people insisted on going into the market [centres] with infected cattle, despite orders and advice to the contrary, with the result that they took the disease back with them ... and infected many of the bye roads." The government had tried to persuade farmers to leave their oxen on clean land and complete their journey to town with donkeys supplied by the government but that had failed to work in many areas. They had used a permit system to limit the movement of cattle while they waited for a law to require fencing and while they still hoped that Koch would succeed in finding a way to immunize cattle. The permit system was only directed at holding the disease in check while waiting for weapons with which to fight it. But Koch had not succeeded and the fencing law had been still-born because the farmers said they could not afford it. There was nothing in the law that enabled the Veterinary Department to require that an infected farm be fenced to keep the infection inside. Meanwhile the permit system was working less and less well. If things went on as they were doing then, the disease would ultimately completely ruin the cattle industry of the country.

Nine months earlier, Stockman said, he and Theiler had recommended that all farms be fenced. They were told that that was impossible and were ordered to find another approach. That is why they had begun experiments to see how soon an infected area would cleanse itself if kept free from cattle. In May, 1903 they had started keeping careful records of infected areas and roads and they had obtained a pretty good idea which areas were infected. They now proposed a scheme to eradicate the disease on badly infected farms, by removing the cattle via routes which would then be closed and placarded. Those cattle would be killed and the land left to cleanse itself. They planned to deal with slightly infected farms, and with farms that were suspicious, in a different way, namely by removing the cattle to clean areas and keeping them there until the farms had purified themselves. But the cattle would first have to be moved to observation areas, where any sick cattle could be separated from the healthy cattle. Meanwhile those areas from which cattle had been removed would need other kinds of transport, such as camels and donkeys. But all of this would cost a great deal of money, especially if the farmers were compensated for the cattle that were killed. Stockman came up with various figures based on different assumptions about the value of the carcasses; one of his figures was £100,000. Stockman concluded by saying that if this scheme were introduced it must be compulsory "and there must be no optional clause. If it is not to be made compulsory, my advice is to leave the whole scheme alone." (Nearly all of Stockman's detailed suggestions to the Cape conference had already been put to Smith in nearly the same words in his letter of May 9;[17] his rebuttal of May 25[17] actually ended with the words "I must, therefore, advise that if the Government is not prepared to make the scheme compulsory it should be left alone.")

Duncan Hutcheon followed up on Stockman's remarks by saying that he thought the governments involved would support a scheme that cost £100,000 if it seemed certain to work. "Judging from past experiences with Rinderpest, he feared they were going to have a great deal of trouble not only with Natives, but also with the Dutch farmers, with regard to the slaughtering of stock." Dr. Smartt interjected "And with the English farmers, too," and Hutcheon rejoined that he thought "the farmers of Cape Colony would rather join in killing cattle in the Transvaal than kill their own."

Gray objected to Stockman's scheme on the grounds that the proposal to salvage cattle from "slightly infected" and "suspicious" farms was a major weakness. The scheme could work only if *all* of the cattle in infected *and* suspicious areas were killed, all the roads in those areas were closed to cattle and new kinds of transport animals were provided. And that extreme measure would cost far more than the measure Stockman had suggested and certainly far more than Rhodesia could afford, which would prevent the scheme from being uniform. Stockman then said that he "would heartily approve of Mr. Gray's suggestion to slaughter off all the stock in the infected areas . . . but he feared it was not financially feasible . . . and they had to make a compromise." As to Rhodesia, he had assumed that it might not be able to adopt his plan, which was why he had proposed it only for the Transvaal. Gray responded that as far as protecting the Cape Colony they should fence all the farms "in a belt of the country to the South of that which was infected, and absolutely prevent the employment of oxen for transport in these belts."

Theiler returned to the attack the next morning. He said that Stockman's proposal was aimed at the whole of the Transvaal and that it was based on scientific principles and on experiments that had already been made in the Transvaal. Those who had not as yet experienced the disease in their own countries did not realize what a scourge it was. It was not the business of the conference to discuss the cost, it was their business to advise their governments what should be done. The choice was plain: remove the animals from infected land for long enough for it to become clean or allow the disease to spread until 95% of the cattle had died. "If the disease is allowed to rip, they would never be able to restock the country." They had a pretty good idea where the infection was now to be found. The central infected areas should be handled first, "after a year or fifteen months they would know the results." Theiler went on to say that "Experiments had proved that it only required one single tick to spread the disease ... it was easier to remove cattle from infected areas than to kill off the infected ticks, and by removing the cattle the infection must die out."

The argument went on and on. The delegate from Natal pointed out that the "native stock-owners ... would move their cattle if they had made up their mind to do so, not withstanding the restrictions." Moreover, those "who were subjected to the regulations would think that they were being made a buffet [*sic*] for the rest of the community. Farmers could understand restrictions for a time but would not submit to indefinite quarantine." As to the African-owned cattle, "The average native did not believe in accepting payment for cattle. He would allow his cattle to be killed on condition that he would get other cattle in their place. He would not usually take money for them."

The delegates from as yet unaffected areas duly expressed their doubts. The delegate from the Cape Colony asked what good it would do to deal with the disease in the Transvaal if it remained unchecked in Rhodesia? The delegate from Bechuanaland said they had not yet had a single case of the disease and that the Africans there were very fond of moving about with their cattle. The delegate from German South West Africa noted that so far not a single case had occurred in that region. Gray responded that he was in the unfortunate position of objecting to the scheme without having an alternative to propose. There was no way in which Rhodesia could recover the costs of slaughtering cattle by selling the carcasses. Moreover, in spite of all precautions, the natives would move cattle about. Hutcheon finally commented that they had to do something, because if the disease was not stopped, the cattle industry of South Africa was threatened with the most serious disaster that had ever overtaken it.

After prolonged discussion, Theiler proposed that the conference recommend the most radical remedy and resolve that "the only effective method of eradicating African Coast Fever is to kill off all cattle in infected areas and to leave such areas free of cattle for a period of not less than eighteen months." The conference agreed, thus going well beyond Stockman's original scheme, which had envisaged saving as many cattle as possible from slightly infected or merely suspicious farms. Theiler also proposed that the adjoining, and as yet uninfected, colonies should be asked to contribute to the expense of carrying out this policy; Hutcheon commented that "it was really cheaper for them to fight the disease in the Transvaal than to fight it later in their own Colony." He added that "They had already waited a long time for the results of Dr. Koch's experiments, during which time the disease was gradually gaining ground. They had waited in the hope that they would have a practical scheme to fall back upon, but now ... inoculation was a broken reed [and] the only practicable scheme ... was the one brought forward by Mr. Stockman."

Asked whether the Transvaal would undertake the scheme if the other governments would bear their share of the expense, Stockman said that he "believed it would be so." (A somewhat surprising reply in view of his recent exchanges with Smith, but see below.) Asked whether Rhodesia would also undertake the scheme if given financial assistance Gray said that "he did not think so." After more discussion the words "as an experiment" were added to Theiler's second resolution and it was adopted:

... the Government of the Transvaal is invited to undertake the purification of the Territory involved in the Southern outbreaks first, as an experiment, as these are the centres which more immediately menace the adjoining Colonies, and that these [adjoining] Colonies ... be asked to contribute a *pro-rata* share towards the expenses ...

The conference went on to pass resolutions recommending fencing "on all farms where African Coast fever has broken out," the adopting of "all reasonable measures to check the movement of cattle in those districts threatened by an invasion of the disease or those which have been declared infected," and recommending that in cases of "isolated outbreaks ... [all] cattle should be destroyed ... with payment of compensation, [and] the infected veldt quarantined." Another resolution, one that is only too familiar to the modern reader, was adopted, one calling for more research.

Why was dipping not emphasized? Mostly because both Theiler and Stockman doubted that it could control the disease. Theiler admitted that dipping every third week could control the blue tick, but the brown tick may drop off an animal after only three days. It would take a long time to clean a farm from the brown tick and the dipping would have to be carried out at much shorter intervals than are needed to control the blue tick. Moreover the dips that were available were sometimes injurious to cattle. Stockman said that the only effective dip was the arsenical dip, but that dip often killed cattle, sometimes because they swallowed it. After much further debate, Gray proposed a resolution that "dipping is the most effective means of eradicating ticks [but that] experiments should still be conducted with the object of perfecting the dip to be used ..." Stockman seconded the motion and it was adopted.

Stockman's original "scheme" had involved fencing, quarantine and the slaughter only of heavily infected herds. Possibly sick cattle in slightly infected herds were to be slaughtered but the rest were to be saved. The conference went far beyond that by agreeing with Gray that *all* cattle in infected or suspicious districts must be slaughtered.

The Cape conference probably had no expectation that its recommendation would be carried out. Duncan Hutcheon had already advised the Cape to build a fence to prevent movement of cattle from the Transvaal into the Cape, and on July 1, 1904 he wrote "This Government has urged the Government of the Transvaal to adopt the stamping out policy – at present, however, the farmers there are strongly opposed to it."[18] A few days earlier, on June 27, 1904, Milner had written to the Colonial Secretary, Alfred Lyttelton,[18] to tell him that "in anticipation of your concurrence" he had authorized the erection of a fence along the border of the Bechuanaland Protectorate. He enclosed a copy of the "scheme for slaughtering cattle wholesale" that had been recommended at the Cape conference and added "Whether that scheme be adopted or not, and in the last few days the opposition which has arisen to it among the Boers makes it doubtful, it is clear that the fence which is being erected by the Cape Government along the Transvaal border, is still more necessary along the Protectorate Border." Milner added that the disease was advancing "straight towards the Protectorate and if it once gets into the Chief's Reserves it will be next to impossible to stop it traversing the whole territory where you are aware the only wealth, if such can be said to exist at all, is in stock." Opposition by the Boer farmers had obstructed plans for fencing and had interfered with the operation of the permit system. Less than a month after the Cape conference had adjourned it was obvious to Hutcheon and Milner that the same opposition would block any proposal to slaughter herds.

That radical measure, which might have succeeded and which Stockman and Theiler voted for, was indeed overruled in the Transvaal itself, as Stockman's annual report for the year ending June 30, 1904 reveals. The government decided that the slaughtering of large numbers of animals should not be undertaken, since it was "repulsive . . . to the stock owners."[8] On the other hand, virtually all of the measures that Smith had opposed in May were adopted by legislation on August 12, 1904. That legislation provided for "(a) the fencing in of infected farms, places, and towns, lands or roads, on generous terms; (b) the compulsory slaughter of stock, with compensation, in the case of isolated outbreaks; (c) the optional slaughter of stocks on infected farms; (d) the removal of all oxen from infected or suspected farms; (e) the stabling of milch cows in infected areas."[19]

What had actually happened and where did Smith really stand in the matter? In September, 1903, Stockman had proposed what amounted to a slaughter scheme: all infected areas were to be fenced in and no cattle were to be removed from those areas except those destined for the slaughter house. His compromise plan abandoned fencing but proposed to keep infected areas free of cattle until all the ticks on the fields had died. Some cattle would be slaughtered but others would be saved by use of the quarantine and temperature camp system. The slaughter of *all* animals from infected areas was then proposed again, by the Cape conference, at Theiler's urging.

The proposing and rejecting of the extreme measure did, however, pave the way for the acceptance of the previously rejected temperature camp scheme. About two months after the end of the Cape conference the government did accept the plan that Smith had rejected in May. If Stockman and Theiler used the Cape conference to put pressure on the government, they may have done so with Smith's approval; Smith himself had to deal with the farmers and may have welcomed having his hand strengthened. One thing is certain: Smith remained on good terms with Stockman. On leave in London only eighteen months later, on December 12, 1905, Smith wrote to Macdonald[20] that "I have seen Stockman & many old friends. The Board is backing Stockman well & I think he is going to be a great success & exercise a valuable influence on the Department, by infusing them with fresh ideas."

In his annual report for the year ending June 30, 1904,[8] Stockman
commented that "It would be futile to deny that under [these
provisions] the final eradicating of the disease will be a much slower
process than it would have been under a scheme of general compulsory slaughter of all bovine animals on or near infected ground."
How much it would have speeded things up to slaughter all animals
on infected ground we will never know. The methods that were
adopted took exactly fifty years to eradicate East Coast fever in
Rhodesia, and more than fifty years to do the same in South Africa,
and the last stage in each country involved the slaughter of infected
herds.

Both Koch and Stockman suspected that animals that had recovered from East Coast fever continued to carry the disease. Had
Stockman been able to prove that, his call for the slaughter of all
herds in infected areas would have been much more persuasive. But
Lounsbury, Theiler and most other investigators believed that
animals that had recovered from East Coast fever no longer har-
bored the causal parasite, so that ticks that fed on recovered animals
could not infect healthy animals. It is now known that many
animals that have recovered from East Coast fever do in fact
become carriers of the disease. That is probably why the disease
broke out again and again until, nearly fifty years later, the slaughter of infected herds was added to other control measures.[21]

The Transvaal farmers versus the veterinarians

In July, 1903, Theiler said[22] "although we do not know every thing
about the disease, the knowledge we have gained warrants us
sufficiently to prophesy a bad outlook for the future of cattle
breeding in the Transvaal." (As this Germanic construction suggests, Theiler was still mastering English, his third or fourth
language.) The disease was spreading rapidly, partly because of
indifference and negligence and partly because of "wilful disbelief"
on the part of the farmers. "The disease came from the Eastern
Boundary of the Transvaal, and can in nearly every instance be
traced to cattle introduced from these parts." These facts should
convince "any observer that we have to do with a new disease . . .
[but] there are . . . many . . . who cannot be convinced . . . if we have
to wait until every man is satisfied . . . this scourge will have carried
off the majority of our cattle."

Speaking to the Second Annual Meeting of the South African Association for the Advancement of Science, held in Johannesburg in April, 1904, Theiler delivered an indictment of both the farmers and the transport riders.[23] As to the farmers, Theiler said that they should naturally be particularly interested from an economic point of view. "But as a rule they only begin to be on the alert when the disease has touched their pockets." He went on to say that the Department of Agriculture had tried to educate the farming population but had, by and large, failed. "The cause of this indolence and distrust is an ignorant unbelief in science in general, and in particular in that branch which my department represents."

Later in his report, Theiler spoke of the transport riders.

A transport rider, who went with his cattle into an infected locality where the disease was raging, naturally lost his whole span . . . later experience taught him that the disease . . . was liable to appear several weeks later . . . he must have recognized the abnormal symptoms . . . yet, not withstanding these hard facts, he would not believe, nor does he still, that he has to do with a completely new disease.

As to the farmer who believed that the disease attacked only cattle newly imported into the country, what he

failed to see was that the native cattle had died off . . . But as usual he had his argument . . . the untimely burning off of the grass [which was a result of the Boer War].

But the Boer farmer, basing his argument exclusively on local experience, will not believe that the same conditions [hold in places] where the disease has not yet appeared . . . the advance which we have made has not met with the sympathetic support of those for whom it has been . . . intended . . . all legislation against the disease which is based on scientific observations, is scouted.

At the end of his article, Theiler said that "so far we have failed in the majority of cases in convincing our farming population of the seriousness of the situation."

In his annual report for the year ending June 30, 1904, Stockman devoted twenty-five pages to East Coast fever; much of that section was devoted to attempts to limit the spread of the disease.[24] Stockman said that early efforts to check the spread of the disease had been hampered by the Boer War and its aftermath. Since then,

One of the greatest obstacles we have had to contend with . . . [is] the mistaken confidence of the Boer farmer in his own prowess as a pathologist. He has constantly and assiduously advanced the argument that, because he has spent his life amongst cattle he must know everything about their ailments and how to cure them, even in the case of a disease which only entered the country some two years ago.

Insisting that the disease was gall sickness, the farmers moved cattle freely and helped spread the disease.

The native, too has helped much to spread the disease, but he has done so to a less extent than the traders who visited his locations with ox-transport for the purposes of commerce . . . In spite of lectures, pamphlets, and even ocular demonstration,[25] it has taken two years to convince even a reasonable proportion of the farming population that the disease is spread by ticks. Like the Pharisees of old, they cried out for a sign, which was already staring them in the face.

Stockman went on to say that when the farmers finally realized that the disease was "one of location" they also realized that "if they moved their cattle on to fresh ground after each outbreak, the sick ones dropped out, and they eventually left the disease behind them." Even this might have been done safely, but "each man was a law unto himself, and he left a trail of infection behind him for the cattle of his unsuspecting neighbours to pick up." Although an infected animal might travel on the roads for 20 days and carry the disease for 200 miles, observation had shown that the disease did not ordinarily take longer leaps than 65 miles, except by rail. Since that distance corresponds nearly with the limit that a sick animal could be trekked, we must conclude that "the omniscient farmer . . . did not know that his oxen were sick, in spite of the fact that he has been used to cattle all his life, or that he did know and moved them all the same over his neighbour's ground." Later in the report Stockman said

One must admit that the Stock-owner will do everything in his power to protect his property once he knows how to do it . . . [but] he cannot see at a glance what it takes experts months to discover by laborious investigation on scientific lines. The existence, then, of a central authority with powers to hold the destructive unbelievers in check while the teachings of science are being imbibed is a necessity.

The opinions of Stockman and Theiler about the Boer farmers were amply confirmed on March 10, 1905, when a group of Boer leaders went over the heads of the veterinarians and the officials of the Department of Agriculture to complain to the Lieutenant-Governor of the Transvaal (Sir Arthur Lawley).[26] The Boer delegation was headed by two men who were to become the first and second Prime Ministers of the Union of South Africa, Louis Botha and J. C. Smuts. Smuts began the discussion by saying that the fencing regulations and the permit system were causing great hardship. "The farmers were very poor and were becoming more and more impoverished every day." They could not bring their produce to market because of the lack of transport. Botha said that the farmers in his district had "thousands of bags of produce and rolls of tobacco husbanded since the first year after the war but they could not get anything away. He had seen the girls and married women walking barefoot – there was no more credit at the shops."

Smuts argued that it would be a better policy to allow the disease "to work its way through the country and die out"; then the country could be re-stocked. Fencing was a heavy burden on already impoverished small holders and the "remedy employed by the Government was worse than the disease." Smuts said that although farmers could not get permits, cattle traders could and that "they knew of cases where Jews got permits and farmers could not." (Botha repeated this allegation and added that "Jews who were peddlers before the war had now become cattle buyers . . . such men do not mind who are infected as long as they make a profit." As we will see below, Stirling said exactly the same thing about the Afrikaner farmers in Rhodesia.)

The Commissioner of Lands said the complaint about the Jews was a common one, for which there was no proof, and challenged the Boer delegation to produce examples and evidence. They did not do so. As to relaxing the regulations, the Commissioner said "They were facing a tremendous evil. The Government were not playing with it. If the Government fail, woe betide. If the Government fail, this country is absolutely lost. The disease would spread like wild-fire."

The government officials made it clear that the fencing regulations were to remain in place; Smuts made it equally clear that the transport problem had to be solved, perhaps by supplying the farmers with donkeys. The farmers have "kept this up for two years, they cannot go on for another two years. They will have to trek to other parts of the Transvaal or to other parts of the world. They will have to trek within the next two or three years."

The Lieutenant-Governor said that if the government were to do away with the regulation of transport the whole of the cattle in the Transvaal would disappear within four or five years. The Commissioner of Lands added that it was not just the government that was preventing the movement of cattle, it was the farmers into whose area cattle might be moved. How could the government force cattle in on people against their will? If the government did away with the regulations there would be civil warfare. He hoped that it would be shown that when the disease had spread it had done so because the regulations had been disobeyed – if it turned out that the disease had been spread as the result of the regulations then "the country may be shut forever."

Asked why the government would not help pay the cost of fencing clean farms but only the cost of fencing affected areas, the Commissioner said that "the people refused to have the fencing Ordinance [for clean farms]. This Ordinance had become practically a dead letter." Nothing was resolved by this long argument, although the government agreed to look into the question of supplying donkeys to certain areas. Nothing in the minutes of the meeting suggests that the Boer delegation accepted any of the government's arguments: at best they became convinced that the government was not going to change its policies. Those policies, too strict to be acceptable to the farmers, were far too lax to be acceptable to the veterinarians. The Boer farmers not only still opposed fencing and the permit system in 1905; as we have seen, in 1904, it took them about two months to block the only measure that might have arrested the spread of the disease, the systematic slaughter of all herds in infected areas.

Between mid-1904 and 1910, when short-interval dipping began to come into use, efforts to control East Coast fever in the Transvaal were dominated by the permit system and the temperature camps, and a limited slaughter policy was introduced. The farmers very slowly came to be more cooperative, since they eventually realized that the permit system was not intended to *prevent* the movement of cattle but to make it possible to move them safely. But there were not very many cattle left in the Transvaal by 1910.

The economy of Rhodesia

As we have seen, even the government of the Transvaal, backed by the resources of the gold mines of the Rand and by Chamberlain's earlier support of Milner's program of reconstruction, was unable to bear the costs of a full-scale effort to eradicate East Coast fever. Rhodesia was much poorer. Correspondence between the London office and the Salisbury office of the Chartered Company in 1904 and 1905[27] contains many suggestions for ways to combat East Coast fever, including fencing and dipping, and almost as many refusals by the London office to bear the expense. Even small expenditures were vetoed or questioned. The plain truth was that neither the settlers nor the Chartered Company could afford the costs of an all-out attack on East Coast fever. Few of the settlers arrived in Rhodesia as rich men and very few of them had made any money in Rhodesia. Nor had the Chartered Company made any money in the years since its occupation of Rhodesia. In October, 1903, H. Wilson Fox, the Managing Director of the Company, sent a 25-page-long analysis of the situation to Earl Grey.[28] Fox's letter was written to refute the criticisms of Sir George Farrar, who had urged Earl Grey to promote more locally-managed entrepreneurial activity in Rhodesia. Fox began by contrasting the situation in Rhodesia with that in Johannesburg. Johannesburg, he said, has a business community "largely composed of independent men, frequently of great wealth, managing their own businesses and generally helping ... to direct the affairs of the various mining companies. In Rhodesia ... there are no wealthy residents, and the leading inhabitants are the salaried officials of companies whose head offices are in London." This state of affairs, Fox said, had historical roots. In the early days of the Witwatersrand the mines quickly became of immense value; besides that they were often the property of men who had previously become rich at Kimberley, such as Eckstein, Barnato, Rhodes, Rudd and Robinson. Influx of capital from London came only later, when management was already in the hands of capable men on the spot, men who were prepared to remain: "Local management has been the rule from the beginning and has never been disturbed."

"Rhodesia on the other hand, has been from the start a poor man's country." Its pioneers have been

men who had failed to find fortune on the Rand ... and newcomers ... tempted principally by love of adventure to see what could be made of the new territory. No money flowed from the Rand to Rhodesia such as had flowed from Kimberley to the Rand. For some years commercial enterprise depended entirely upon Chartered funds, upon money wrung by the personal exertions of Mr. Rhodes from such corporations as the De Beers and the Goldfields of South Africa and upon capital raised in England.

The individual "broadly speaking has never made more than a living in Rhodesia . . . partly due to physical conditions and partly due to the successive misfortunes by which its progress has been retarded." This had made it impossible to raise capital in Rhodesia and difficult to raise it in London. "It must be remembered that Southern Rhodesia has lately experienced a serious loss of wealth through the destruction of cattle by the recent epidemic and that its industries have been handicapped by war, scarcity of labour and difficulties of transport." As a result, the Company had constantly endeavored to cut down its annual expenses, moreover the leading independent development companies were then "spending practically nothing." Sir George Farrar had urged Earl Grey "that more power should be given to the local men, but . . . the men do not exist in Rhodesia to whom it is safe to give power . . . very few first class men have been attracted to it . . . circumstances have tended to bring together a business community of far smaller average brain power than on the Rand." Fox pointed out that he had advised that Milton be given far greater responsibilities and a much higher salary because a man of his caliber might fill the gap but the Board had decided instead to give more power to Lewis Michell and Dr. Jameson. The people in Bulawayo had asked for "a real live Managing Director . . . [but] I do not think they know exactly what they do want . . . [perhaps a] 'Deus ex machina' who will substitute prosperity for depression." Fox then quoted from a letter from Maurice Heany: "the whole grievance consists in the general hard times that are prevailing . . . they are indeed desperately hard up. Businesses are being closed down, houses vacated, and many people, particularly mechanics and small tradesmen, leaving the country." Overall, Fox said, what Rhodesia needed was more money, both from the British South Africa Company and, if possible, from other corporations. Fox said that he had been urging this ever since he became Managing Director in 1898, but the Board had been cautious because of the depression in South Africa caused by the Boer War and because of the poor yield of the Rhodesian gold mines. In fact, as Baxter said in 1969, in his guide to the National Archives,[29] "from the incorporation of the Company in 1889 to granting of Responsible Government in 1923 the shareholders never received a single dividend for their investment."

What about the settlers, sometimes disparagingly described as "Rhodes' mercenaries?" Mercenary or not, many of the settlers were refugees from what General William Booth had not long before called "Darkest England." Booth spoke of the "sinking classes" of whom he said that

without some kind of extraordinary help, they must hunger and sin, and sin and hunger, until, having multiplied their kind, and filled up the measure of their miseries, the gaunt fingers of death will close upon them and terminate their wretchedness. And all this will happen this very winter, in the midst of the unparalleled wealth, and civilization, and philanthropy of this professedly most Christian land.

I do not suggest that many of the settlers in Rhodesia were members of what Booth called the "sinking classes," but they certainly came from a situation in which there was no "safety net" for the unemployed and not much help for many who were employed.[30]

As Apollon Davidson says of Rhodes' companions on his first sea voyage to South Africa:[31] "After all they are not travelling to foreign shores merely to while away the time, but because they are compelled to do so by their hard lot in life. God knows what awaits them at their destination." A poignant example of two young men "tempted by love of adventure" can be found in letters from a mother asking for news of her son:[32] "he had a banjo and a good silver watch, also a little money . . . I don't expect to get anything of that kind sent." The reply read, in part,

Madle died of fever at the Zambezi and his friend passed away from the same disease before reaching Bulawayo . . . It is with regret that we conclude from this information generally corresponding with yours that this must have been your son . . . P.S. The age given was about 19. Left for the Zambezi in April 1898, with chum, Anderson by name. Madle died and was buried the other side of the Zambezi . . . by Anderson, who eventually succumbed himself when nearing Bulawayo upon his return. Had blue eyes and was fair but not considered by Cooke to be called tall, as stated by yourself, but on this point opinions might differ.

Stanley Portal Hyatt was another refugee from Darkest England. Having tried to make a living in Australia for two years, he and his brother went to Rhodesia in 1897, when Hyatt was barely twenty. Seven years later, bankrupt, he and his brother, Amyas, went to the Philippines, where Amyas died. When Hyatt finally got back to England he was "only 28 in point of years but middle-aged in reality, penniless, weary and a broken man." He died less than nine years later, in 1914, the year in which *The Old Transport Road* was published.[33]

As we saw in chapter 2, even Charles Gray, already a trained veterinarian, and hardly a member of the "sinking classes," came to Rhodesia as a refugee not only from Darkest England but also from Philadelphia. Unable to earn a living as a veterinarian in England, Philadelphia, South Africa or Rhodesia, he was forced to revert, for a time, to his boyhood training as a telegraphist.

General Booth published *In Darkest England and the Way Out* in 1890; in 1903 Kingsley Fairbridge conceived the idea of the famous Fairbridge farm schools as a refuge for the poor and orphaned children of England. When the first of those children reached the first farm school (in Australia, in 1913)[34]

a more incongruous, desolate little bunch of humanity it would be hard to imagine. There they sat in the hot evening sunlight in their thick nailed boots, cheap woollen stockings, cheap smelly suits, the trousers half-mast to allow for growth, and tweed caps, each boy clutching an overcoat and a dirty white kitbag ... they had nothing suitable for wear in that climate. The Guardians had just fitted them out for life in an English work house.

Recruits for Rhodes' mercenaries?

Rhodesia in 1902 was very much a frontier community, not unlike the American West, with "tin boxes" for houses, furniture made from packing crates and empty coal-oil tins[35] and oxcarts for transport, but by 1903 there were no longer any oxen, and men who had fled from Darkest England hoping to find a better life in Rhodesia were now fleeing Rhodesia. The colonial settling of Rhodesia had not done the Africans any good, but in 1903 it looked like it might not do the settlers any good either. Small wonder that Charles Gray told the Cape Town conference that he did not think Rhodesia could or would support a costly program for the eradication of East Coast fever. (The story was replayed in Natal a few years later. The Zulu uprising of 1906, the Bambata uprising, allowed East Coast fever to run out of control. By 1910 the economy of Natal was in ruins because of the cost of suppressing the uprising and because of the effects of East Coast fever. Skilled mechanics and tradesmen were leaving for places as far away as the Argentine. In 1910 this severe economic depression played a role in persuading Natal to join the Union of South Africa.)[36]

Rhodesia 1904–1910

As we saw in chapter 3, throughout all of 1902 the Rhodesian veterinarians took the position that the new outbreak was only a form of redwater, transmitted by the blue tick and made more virulent by some unknown change in climatic conditions or by the abnormal number of ticks. Since the whole country was already infested with presumably infective blue ticks, there was no point in restricting the movement of cattle. Dipping might help if it reduced the number of ticks, but no other measure was recommended. By the time of the Cape conference, Rhodesia was, in fact, thoroughly infested with infective brown ticks, and nothing could be done to reverse that. Nor was the government willing or able to bear the cost of fencing or the cost of reimbursing farmers for the slaughter of herds. But it was willing to impose strict controls on the movement of cattle and the farmers were willing to accept those controls. In fact, in contrast to the farmers of the Transvaal, they were demanding strict regulation of the movement of cattle. On August 30, 1904, J. M. Sinclair[37] wrote to the Cape Colony to ask what measures were being taken there, since there was "strong agitation in Rhodesia – more especially in Matabeleland – for Government to absolutely prohibit the movement of cattle except animals brought to the towns for slaughter purposes, and breeding stock for veldt and water ... the few persons opposing this are those owning salted(?) transport oxen now on the road."[38]

After the government had consulted the farmers at a series of meetings held in different parts of the country, Rhodesia instituted stringent measures. According to Sinclair,[39] in August, 1904, the government of Rhodesia passed an Animal Diseases Consolidation Ordinance which replaced all earlier ordinances of that kind and provided for "wide and ample powers for dealing with existing diseases and others likely to appear or be introduced." Sinclair added that

shortly after the promulgation of this Ordinance,[40] regulations were published ... for controlling cattle movements, ... [to prevent] the spread of Coast Fever ... in ... Matabeleland. These regulations provided for (1) the prohibition of importation of cattle into Matabeleland for any purpose from beyond the border of Southern Rhodesia; (2) the movement of slaughter cattle to consuming centres, and control of same on arrival at such centres; (3) the movement of cattle required for milk supplies to Bulawayo and adjoining townships, such cattle to be confined in an enclosed paddock or stable from date of arrival; (4) the movement of working cattle (transport) within a radius of six miles of working mines ... The effect of these regulations was the almost complete stoppage of cattle movements in the greater part of the province, except those required at the large centres for food supplies. In January, 1905, regulations on similar lines were promulgated for the province of Mashonaland. Shortly afterwards power was obtained to compel the enclosure of all calves born at the large centres or areas of common grazing. This provision was applied to the commonage at Salisbury, Bulawayo, Gwelo, Selukwe, Umtali and Gwanda, where infection was being perpetuated from year to year by calves, and resulted in the complete eradication of infection from each of these centres. In most cases the calves were moved out to clean farms after weaning.

These regulations seem very drastic compared to those now [1922] in force, but they were instituted at the urgent request of the majority of cattle owners in both provinces. The fact was that those who had any cattle left were willing to undergo any hardship or restriction in an effort to save them.

The temperature camps

We have an eye-witness account of what it was like to operate temperature camps in Rhodesia. In October 1907, a young Scot named R. F. Stirling, then barely twenty-one, accepted a position in Rhodesia, where he spent the next few years dealing with East Coast fever. He left Rhodesia in 1911 and, in 1912, in order to become a Fellow of the Royal College of Veterinary Surgeons he submitted a thesis[41] entitled "East Coast fever in Rhodesia and its control." Here is his description of the temperature camps in use in Rhodesia between 1907 and 1910:

Immediately on the known outbreak of Coast Fever on any farm or kraal or group of farms and kraals, a Government Veterinary Surgeon with one or more Cattle Inspectors (laymen) and a squad of natives take over charge of the area.

The first thing done is to select a portion of grazing found on what can be considered as 'clean veldt', i.e. where no cattle have grazed for a considerable time before the outbreak, the longer the better, virgin veldt best of all.

This selection having been made the native 'boys' then hurriedly erect a kraal, made of poles, sufficiently large to hold the not-yet-infected animals which the Veterinary Staff are now separating from the infected. This selection is made purely on thermic grounds, every animal in an infected place and showing a rise in temperature is for purposes of control taken as infected.

All animals showing a rise in temperature are left behind at the original kraal and this place is then designated the Sick Camp. All the apparently healthy cattle are then driven one by one through a crush pen and thoroughly sprayed with a suitable fluid and they are then moved on to the 'New Camp' already prepared by the 'boys' and this 'New Camp' should be not less than 2 miles distant from the primary infected area.

These doings would occupy in most cases the first two days of the outbreak and by that time the Police Force will have been called into the struggle and they will then form, under Veterinary supervision, a cordon around all the area infected or suspected of being infected for a radius of from 7 to 10 miles in the average instance.

Pari passu with these doings all the cattle within the cordon are examined by the Cattle Inspectors and if any suspicious circumstances are reported by them the animals are examined by a Veterinarian and if necessary they are dealt with as in the main outbreak. Our cattle having now been separated into healthy and sick and segregated into different camps – temperatures are taken of the cattle in the healthy camp morning and evening and any animal showing a rise in temperature is immediately returned to the Sick Camp. In addition, the animals in the new camp are sprayed once a week during the three weeks that they remain in 'New Camp No. 1'. Three weeks being the maximum period of incubation it is held that provided the New Camp No. 1 was erected on clean veldt and temperatures were taken regularly and carefully, it can be held that the animals remaining, if they are free from ticks, are free from contagion.

A second camp is now selected, still working away from the infected place and at least a mile from No. 1 Camp and to this place the animals are then removed, and provided that all has been carefully carried out they are now safe from infection and the outbreak is so far conquered.

Stirling remarked that although "this reads well . . . the difficulties are immense." He cited one case in which thirty cattle were removed to the sick camp. Within three weeks fifty-one of the cattle in the "clean" camp had sickened and the sole survivor was slaughtered, as it was not worth the cost of guarding it. And what if the exercise succeeded? The healthy cattle had to be kept on clean veld for two years "provided that the unfortunate owner does not become so disgusted that he sells them off for butcher meat" much sooner. The infected area was supposed to be kept free of cattle for two years but there was little to prevent stock being driven through it since the police cordon had two- or three-mile intervals between its patrol tents. Fencing the infected area had succeeded in one instance, but the Chartered Company was not willing to make that a general policy because it cost too much. "In addition to this control, during an outbreak, there is [in] normal times, the prevention of movement of all cattle without a written permit from the

Veterinary Authorities (Local), systematic dipping of all cattle used for transport, and continual inspection of stock."

Stirling reported many difficulties arising from the long, unfenced border between Rhodesia and Portuguese East Africa, run

by a Company styled the 'Compagnia de Mozambique' . . . it is a common saying that the pay of a Portuguese African official is one third money and two thirds pumpkins . . . this Company's whole idea of Government or misgovernment is to get as much as possible out of the country which it possesses and to put as little as possible into it . . . to them a Veterinary Staff is a luxury not a necessity . . . With such a storehouse of infection on her very border and with illicit cattle traffic going on between the two countries, as will be shown later, is it anything to marvel at that Rhodesia is constantly suffering for the laxity of her neighbours?[42]

Stirling also had harsh words for what he called "Dutch racial peculiarities." "The average uneducated Dutchman and by such I do not necessarily mean the poorer class of Dutchman, is cunning, suspicious, avaricious and a marvel in the art of combining the singing of Psalms with the filling of his own pockets at the expense of others he cares not whom they may be." Stirling gave two examples of outbreaks that had been caused by the illegal movement of cattle by Dutch [i.e. Afrikaner] farmers. In one, a serious new outbreak appeared in Bulawayo which took years to subdue. The culprit, who made a profit of many hundreds of pounds, was detected and fined only £100. Stirling concluded that "our Dutch settlers in Rhodesia will evade all laws for monetary considerations, will conceal disease if it suits them to do so, and will try to hinder the work of our Profession in every way they can."

The Africans, Stirling said

on the first idea of disease and subsequent control of their cattle . . . betake themselves and their herds possibly already infected 'to green fields and pastures new far from the madding crowd' of Cattle Inspectors.

And thus, in many instances, arise those fresh foci of disease which seem to spring up at some considerable distance from the main outbreak without apparent reason.

On the other hand, Stirling said, the African,

although wary and suspicious of all the doings of the White Inspectors, . . . has a wholesome dread of the ruling Powers of the land, and can through this feeling be exercised upon so long as he is dealt with by firmness combined with such explanation of the necessity for the actions taken as he can understand, but no longer.

Stirling's views of the British South Africa Company unconsciously echoed much of what H. Wilson Fox had written to Earl Grey. He said that a boom in Rhodesian shares had been followed by a slump and the company was

then in the unhappy position of trying to run a country to the satisfaction of the share holders and in order to gain the approval of its Directors . . . there was retrenchment on every side; and although this retrenchment was certainly necessary in many instances, it has proved to be a costly one as far as the control of the disease we are considering was concerned.
Until 1907 there were in the whole of that huge country, Southern Rhodesia, ony 4 qualified Veterinary Surgeons and up till 1910 there were only 7 men to cope with the numerous diseases of the land, each of whom had to control a tract of country larger than England and Wales combined. Things have changed within the last two years and today it is satisfactory to learn that there is a sufficiently large staff to deal efficiently with disease amongst animals.[43]

Stirling's own prescription included fencing the Mozambique border (which would, at least in the mountainous parts, be impossible even today), restricting the importation of cattle, replacing fines for the illegal movement of cattle by jail sentences, taking a regular census of African-owned cattle, the compulsory fencing of farms, and the creation of a Veterinary Department independent of "lay Ministers of Agriculture." As to fencing,

the Government, conservative in this as in all else have replied 'No, we can't afford to supply you with the material, and we are afraid to make you supply it in case we shall frighten settlers away' or words to that effect.
And so they have gone on, have spent thousands in trying to cope with the disease, have chased settlers from the country on account of it, and have rejected the advice of their Veterinary experts until now.

As to the veterinarians, the government would, some day, listen to them and "When that day comes then will Rhodesia flourish and be started on the way to attain her great ideal:— to be a ranching country ranking with the great Plateau as is befitting to 'God's Outpost.'" Stirling signed his thesis "*Labor omnia vincit.*"

The 1910 enquiry in Rhodesia

In 1910, while Stirling was still in the country, the government of Rhodesia set up a Committee of Enquiry on African Coast Fever.

That committee held hearings in 12 towns, heard evidence from 125 witnesses during 25 sessions of public meetings and received a number of depositions.[44]

The deposition of the stock owners of Selukwe provides a sample of the testimony. The farmers and mining companies of Selukwe had often figured in clashes with the veterinarians, as shown by Gray's comment:[45] "Native cattle may die off wholesale – a native uprising may be precipitated but the Selukwe mines must not be deprived." The Selukwe stock owners recommended "(1) That the spot where an outbreak takes place should immediately be fenced to the extent of one square mile and all infected cattle destroyed and their carcasses burnt. (2) That the country for 10 miles round this fence be cleared of all stock for at least 18 months. (3) That periodical dipping and spraying be compulsory." So far, so good. But recommendation 4 read:

... we are entirely opposed to roads being closed and transport being stopped in clean areas; not only because such a measure would be contrary to all reason but that it would be the ruination of hundreds of small men who earn their living as carriers – many of them here having disposed of their donkeys and mules lately in exchange for oxen.

On the other hand, the Selukwe stock owners were willing that movement of cattle should be subject to permit "and ox-wagons be licensed if they need be ... [and] all movements of cattle be along recognized roads and not haphazard across country."

The Committee of Enquiry also heard from L. E. W. Bevan, who had recently rejoined the Veterinary Department.[46] Asked if the disease could be transmitted in any way other than by ticks, he replied: "the original cause is a sick beast and ... from that ox, the disease is transmitted to others by ticks." Was the tick the only way? "Yes." Had the disease originated from outside the country? "Yes, certainly." In that case, how had the recent outbreaks occurred? Had they been introduced from outside the country? Bevan replied that the recent Umtali outbreak might have come from outside and led to the other outbreaks.

If so, the committee asked Bevan, why should it break out in these places more than in others? Bevan said that local supervision must have been inadequate and that the "the machinery [for control] is not large enough." He added that when he was in charge of the Salisbury district the cattle inspector "used to go out fairly frequently and every now and then he would find a herd which had never been heard of before." Could 500 cattle be brought in? Probably not, but perhaps 100, and certainly a smaller herd, without being found out.

How far could an ox, travelling while infected with East Coast fever, spread the disease before it became too ill to travel any further? Bevan surmised that once an animal had picked up an infected tick, the animal would live about three weeks. But an infected animal would be too ill to travel after about 15 days, during which he might travel 150 miles. The chairman asked: "the first thing to do is to have more control of movement?" "Yes, that is it." As to the cattle traders, Bevan said "I am rather afraid of the trader. He is one of those men dealing in these unknown parts, where things are not under control." Bevan said that the commonest cause of a new outbreak was the illicit removal of a sick beast from an infected area to a clean one. Asked whether ox transport should be restricted, Bevan replied "I cannot say. It would be a counsel of perfection." Bevan also advocated the use of the police to give out permits so that the cattle inspectors would have more time to go out and inspect cattle instead of spending all their time in their offices issuing permits. As to central dipping tanks, Bevan was against them because cattle might have to cross infected areas to get to such tanks and, in general, the less movement of cattle the better.

The discussion made it clear that ox-drawn transport was back in a big way, from farm to town, from railway to mine, and even over long distances, just as in 1902. In Bevan's opinion, the chief sources of danger were the commonages, the cattle traders and the transport riders. After many questions about fencing and the temperature camps, the committee returned to the question of whether ticks could be spread other than by cattle, for example in blankets, or on railway trucks or by other animals; Bevan and the committee agreed that since the recent outbreaks had occurred near the railways more attention should be paid to the risks of moving cattle by railway.

Among other things, the committee finally concluded that mules and donkeys had not proved to be satisfactory substitutes for ox-drawn transport, which thus remained essential to the economy. To minimize the risk of spreading the disease, the committee recommended that although trek oxen could not be abolished, they should not be allowed to make long journeys but should be confined to local journeys. More dipping and careful regulation of trek oxen were also recommended.

As to fencing, "The time does not appear to be ripe for instituting a general measure of compulsory fencing," because (as Stirling had supposed) it would cost too much. On the other hand all commonages should be fenced and all cattle on commonages should be dipped regularly. But it did not seem feasible to make dipping compulsory throughout the country. The committee agreed with Stirling that "the punishments . . . for breaches of the cattle laws . . . are . . . entirely inadequate. Cases have been brought to our attention where the law has been broken deliberately, the profit to be gained thereby far exceeding any punishment to be feared." They did not go as far as Stirling, who thought such breaches should be made criminal offenses, punishable by imprisonment. As to the temperature camps, "A good deal of high feeling exists in and about the scenes of certain recent outbreaks owing to the action of the Veterinary Department directing the destruction of cattle on a rise of temperature." Since the belief that herds had been slaughtered without good cause could lead to outbreaks being concealed, "great care should be taken to prove to the owner, when it becomes necessary to destroy cattle, that the disease is actually present in his herd." As to Stirling's favorite subject, the veterinary profession, the committee said that there were not enough cattle inspectors; moreover, "we consider it essential that the country should be well supplied with men scientifically trained in stock diseases, and recommend that Veterinary Surgeons be appointed to take charge of districts and eventually replace the Cattle Inspectors."

Stirling's thesis and the report of the 1910 Committee of Enquiry make it clear that the measures in force in 1910 were far less stringent than those that had been adopted in 1904. The farmers and the mining community were as unwilling to be inconvenienced in 1910 as they had been strident in their demands of 1902 to 1904 that the government take drastic action. The situation deteriorated to the point that in 1911, E. M. Jarvis, then Acting Chief Veterinary Surgeon, found himself under great pressure to allow the removal of cattle from Selukwe, where the disease was endemic, to Hartley, where the disease had never occurred. Jarvis wrote to the Director of Agriculture that[47] "I view the situation with gravity, and the resumption of ox-transport with considerable alarm." But the regulations became steadily less restrictive and East Coast fever continued to recur, although the outbreaks were increasingly isolated.

More conferences and commissions

In 1909, the Transvaal convened a Pan-African Veterinary Conference.[48] It was more "Southern African" than "Pan-African," but it did include delegates from the Belgian Congo and Madagascar. It was chaired by Charles Gray, who had left Rhodesia in 1905 to succeed Stewart Stockman as Chief Veterinarian of the Transvaal. Gray's successor in Rhodesia, J. M. Sinclair, reported that he was cautiously optimistic about the progress being made in Rhodesia. But the disease was widespread in Swaziland and had gone dangerously out of control in Natal. The delegate from Portuguese East Africa confirmed Stirling's view of the situation in that country: he could give but little account of the disease in Portuguese East Africa as a whole, as the territory was a large one, and veterinary supervision had been established there only seven months before. According to Gray, large areas of the worst-infected parts of the Transvaal had been fenced, many cattle had in fact been slaughtered and "I have every reason to hope that we shall, before long, be able to confine the disease to the north-east part of the country, and ultimately stamp it out."

The delegates of both Bechuanaland and Basutoland reported that the Africans and their chiefs were well aware of the risks of allowing the disease to appear in their midst and were cooperating in preventing the entry of cattle into Bechuanaland from Rhodesia or the Transvaal and into Basutoland from Natal. As to the Cape, there was a fence running the whole length of the Bechuanaland border (over 200 miles) and a barbed wire fence from Basutoland to the sea (over 300 miles). Both borders were patrolled, by 130 mounted riflemen and 136 Africans. "These precautions are costing a great deal of money, but there is a very large number of cattle at stake." James Spreull wrote in 1914 that

The first steps taken by the . . . Cape government to prevent an inroad of the disease from Natal consisted of the formation of a cordon along the border. This took advantage of the three boundary rivers which form the dividing line . . . and these were further strengthened by a barbed wire fence extending from the Drakensberg Mountains to the sea, whilst a very efficient guard of Cape Mounted Riflemen and natives patrolled the fence.

Spreull added that

Natal fought the disease by the stoppage of all cattle movements, by a stamping out policy, and latterly with greatest success, by short-interval dipping for purposes of tick destruction; but the last procedure was only possible then in the European-owned blocks, the huge native-squatted areas having to be more or less abandoned to their fate.[49]

The Pan-African Veterinary Conference was held on an anniversary, an anniversary of which it took no official note. In January, 1902, Gray had begun to notice cases of "atypical" redwater in both Umtali and Salisbury. Only seven years later, in January, 1909, mounted riflemen were patrolling hundreds of miles of fence, trying to keep the disease out of the Cape Colony. They failed.

Very little enthusiasm was expressed for dipping at the congress, but radical changes in the role of dipping were at hand. In classic studies that began around 1909, Watkins-Pitchford showed that dipping cattle at three-day intervals, using a dip containing sodium arsenite, could greatly reduce the number of ticks and thus be a powerful weapon against East Coast fever. Watkins-Pitchford wrote a series of pamphlets advocating and describing his methods;[50] Charles Gray soon showed that, with a stronger dip, the interval could be extended to five days. Rhodesia passed a compulsory dipping law in 1914.[51]

But the addition of dipping to the other measures was not enough to control or eradicate East Coast fever, even after its use became widespread and even mandatory. Both in South Africa and Rhodesia, whenever the disease seemed to be under control it broke out again. Each new outbreak was, if it was serious enough, followed by another conference or Committee of Enquiry. We have already noted four between 1903 and 1910: Bloemfontein in 1903, Cape Colony in 1904, "Pan-African" in 1909, and the Rhodesian Committee of Enquiry in 1910; there had also been one in the Transvaal in 1905[52] and there were official enquiries in Rhodesia in 1917 and 1920 and in South Africa in 1920, 1924, 1926 and as late as 1943. The purpose was always the same – to enquire into the adequacy of the methods being used and to determine why the latest resurgence of the disease had occurred. The farmers tended to blame the veterinarians, the veterinarians tended to blame both the farmers (for not cooperating) *and* the government (for not hiring enough veterinarians), and the government tended to appoint Committees of Enquiry.

Analyzing an outbreak that had occurred near Melsetter in 1914, the 1917 committee[53] noted that the initial outbreak was quickly arrested and "the survivors . . . were retained for some five months on clean veld . . . [but they were returned] to infected ground and the disease again broke out." The committee said that the owner blamed the veterinarian for that movement: "This is strenuously disputed by the latter." The committee agreed that one would not expect an owner to endanger his valuable cattle; on the other hand, why would a veterinarian who had taken the trouble to stamp out the disease carelessly allow it to reappear? As to who had been at fault, the committee suggested that "There is evidence that the owner maintained that the disease was gall sickness, and threatened to shoot the officer in charge if he destroyed any of the cattle; it is not, therefore, improbable that a person holding these views would see any risk in removing the animals on to infected veld."

That single outbreak was followed, during the next two years, by thirty-nine widely separated episodes: "The Veterinary surgeon . . . attributes it to cattle straying or illicitly moved from infected veld . . . [whereas the local farmers] . . . regard the Veterinary officers and Police, with their retinues as most likely to have carried ticks . . . from the infected areas." Other outbreaks were blamed on inadequate dipping; the committee discounted the possible existence of immune carriers and commented that "The terms 'mysterious' and 'inexplicable,' so often applied to outbreaks of African Coast Fever, do not appear altogether appropriate, in view of the length of time which an infected tick remains a source of danger, and the ease with which it may be conveyed from place to place."

Overall, the 1917 committee saw no long-term solution other than eradication of the tick; it strongly urged the increased use of dipping and of much stronger laws to enforce dipping: the existing law of 1914 had not even mandated that the dip be of adequate strength. Interestingly enough, there were many areas containing African-owned cattle where dipping was accepted and practiced. Meanwhile, because of the First World War, Rhodesia was back down to a staff of only seven veterinarians. The committee said at least eight more were needed, who should be obtained as soon as the war was over. The committee also attacked the "usual suspects," the transport drivers and cattle traders, especially cattle traders who operated over long distances, and proposed new legislation to enforce dipping.

Another Rhodesian committee,[54] in 1920, again pointed to a lack of cooperation between the farmers, the veterinarians and the cattle inspectors, and to the need for more and better-trained cattle inspectors and for closer regulation of cattle traders. Once again it was noted that "No difficulty was experienced in persuading the natives to adopt the scheme of a fund from which further [dipping] tanks could be built, and their interest as cattle owners generally advanced and safeguarded."

Much the same picture was painted by the Select Committee that was appointed in 1920 in the Union of South Africa,[55] where Charles E. Gray had been Principal Veterinary Surgeon since 1911. Its report noted that "East Coast Fever in the Union and the adjoining Native territories has cost the country, and the cattle farmers . . . millions of pounds." As to previous remedial measures, in the Transvaal, "when it was realized that fencing was not effective, the government resorted to the expedient of killing off herds large and small, whenever there was an outbreak, and what the disease did not carry off the executioner's bullet exterminated to such an extent that the northern districts of the Transvaal became almost denuded of cattle." But this had all been changed by dipping, as introduced by Joseph Baynes and confirmed by Watkins-Pitchford and by Theiler.

However,

the administration and the carrying out of the East Coast Fever regulations leave much to be desired . . . it is difficult to determine whether this is caused by a want of interest in the subject, by fear of offending those farmers who have no faith in dipping, or by a want of funds . . . divided authority and consequent jealousy in the higher ranks of the Public Service entrusted with combating the disease, added to the employment of inefficient and unexperienced subordinate officials, such as cattle guards, etc., have made the administration of the East Coast Fever Regulations in some parts of the Union a rope of sand, of which fact the tick has not been slow to take advantage.

The Commission recommended that the veterinarians make "it their duty to go out amongst the farmers and acquaint them with the symptoms of the disease and to convince them of the established fact that constant and regular dipping and hand-dressing are the only remedies therefore."

Every witness had testified to "the absolute necessity of short interval dipping and hand-dressing" and the commission said that such dipping, combined with hand-dressing was imperative "if the country is to be rid of the terrible scourge of this disease which is proving such a loss to the agricultural community, and is such a set-back to the prosperity of the Union."

The final effort

In 1948, A. M. Diesel reviewed the situation in South Africa.[56] He divided the effort to control East Coast fever into three periods: "1) The period prior to the institution of short-interval dipping, i.e. between 1902 and 1910. 2) The short-interval dipping period, i.e. between 1910 and 1929. 3) The period of intensive control, i.e. between 1929 and the present time." Diesel began his review with a summary of the discussions that occurred at the Bloemfontein conference and included in that summary much of the disagreement between Koch and Theiler. He noted that the early measures, prior to short-interval dipping, had failed to control the spread of the disease.

Diesel went on to discuss the years between 1910 and 1929, the period of short-interval dipping. He commented that "H. Watkins-Pitchford performed an outstanding service to the country in proving the necessity of short-interval dipping." Nevertheless,

the period of short-interval dipping was almost characteristic [*sic*] of alternating optimism and pessimism. Official phases such as 'just when you think you have beaten the disease is the time to expect East Coast Fever' and 'there is something we still have to learn about East Coast Fever' were in daily use. All farmers recognized Joseph Baynes of Natal as the person who owned the first cattle dipping tank in Natal. The number who claimed to have owned the second, was legion. This was a very interesting period in the campaign against East Coast Fever, but finality in its ultimate eradication seemed by no means to be at hand ... In many outbreaks, cattle continued to die in spite of short-interval dipping, at least until this operation had been in progress long enough 'to wear down the infection.'

In 1913 there were 329 new outbreaks in South Africa; in 1918, 86; in 1921, 284; in 1925, 85; in 1929, 60; and in 1930, 85. "This fluctuating incidence was sufficient evidence to lead the authorities to the view that short-interval dipping *alone* could never hope to eradicate the disease.''

Slaughtering each outbreak as it arose seemed a sound method of approach. But the cattle farmers and the natives were against that.

By this time the Union cattle owners had been subjected to a compulsory dipping campaign of just on twenty years. From their point of view, the regulations were worse than the disease, and in their opinion, 'the Government should relinquish all restrictions, let the owner who valued his cattle look after them, and let the rest die' ... It was obvious that the campaign would be very long. While it was relatively easy for the Portuguese East African authorities to apply a slaughter policy to their country, having a cattle population of less than 300,000, such a policy would never be agreed to by the Union farmers ... There would, always, only be one opportunity when this policy could be applied, and that was in order to prevent further spread from isolated outbreaks.

What Diesel called a "final period of intensive control" began in 1930 and was still underway in 1948. After the period of heavy reliance on dipping, the new approach, which Diesel called the "counts and smears" policy, relied on early diagnosis (by microscopic examination of smears of blood and spleen), strict counting of all herds, with the registration of all births and deaths of cattle, close supervision of dipping of cattle and control over cattle movements under a permit system. Much of this sounds familiar, but there was another important change, a large increase in the number of people employed to *enforce* these measures. For example, in 1923, there were 64 "dipping inspectors" in Natal; in 1945, in the same province, there were over 500 "dipping inspectors" plus 154 stock inspectors. From 1928 to 1948, 3,476 head of cattle were slaughtered, on 130 farms. As to diagnostic smears, in one year (1945–6) nearly 900,000 diagnostic smears were made and examined! In spite of this level of activity a severe outbreak had occurred in Natal in 1942, an outbreak that led to yet another enquiry, the East Coast Fever Commission of 1943. In 1948 Diesel was able to write that "since 1944 the Transvaal has been completely free of the disease ... today Natal has only three infected centres ... and in [the Transkei and Eastern Cape] only three outbreaks have occurred over the past three years." In two of those three outbreaks the herds had been slaughtered but in the third "the cattle were successfully removed from the infected zones through temperature camps." Thus the temperature camp method was still in use, more than forty years after its introduction.

In 1977, J. K. H. Wilde[57] summed up the measures taken to control East Coast fever in South Africa: "It was recognized that dipping alone would not control [East Coast fever], and strict quarantine measures were brought into effect. The incidence of the disease was considerably reduced in both number and size of outbreaks. Eventually a slaughter policy was introduced in the remaining pockets of infection and [East Coast fever] was eradicated from South Africa." The slaughter policy was introduced in part because of a growing conviction that there might, after all, be immune carriers and in part, according to Professor John Lawrence,[58] to deal with areas in which very heavy tick infestation, combined with rough and uneven topography, made all other methods impractical.

In spite of all the difficulties and recurrences, the disease was eventually eradicated in Rhodesia. T. Lees-May,[59] writing in 1966, estimated that 19,720 cattle had died in the period 1903–5 (many had also died in 1902). But, in the ten-year period 1906–15, only about 5,000 deaths occurred, whereas the number of healthy cattle had increased enormously. The 1917 Rhodesian Committee of Enquiry[60] estimated that there were 30,369 European-owned cattle and 36,000 African-owned cattle in Rhodesia in 1905, whereas in 1916 the numbers were 468,504 and 491,522 respectively. Thus there were nearly 15 times as many cattle in Rhodesia in 1916 as there were in 1905, and far fewer deaths from East Coast fever. The economic burden had shifted from the cost of lost cattle to the cost of the control measures, plus, of course, the social cost of the always present fear of new outbreaks. As Lees-May said, "Few cattle ranchers living today remember the endless panics and many Commissions of Enquiry that eventuated on every new outbreak of African coast fever when approximately 90 percent of the cattle concerned were doomed to die if gross tick infestation of the veld were allowed to build up."

Some five to six thousand deaths occurred in the next ten-year period of 1916–25, and about the same number in the ten-year period of 1926–35, but the number of deaths fell to about 1,200 in the period 1936–45 and to only 47 in 1946–55. Even during the worst years of the war that led to the independence of Zimbabwe, that is in the late 1970s, when dipping was often neglected, the disease did not recur, although deaths from other tick-borne diseases and from a disease related to true East Coast fever did increase, especially during 1979. The brown tick had not been eradicated, but East Coast fever had been eradicated. As J. A. Lawrence wrote, in 1982,[61]

The success of the campaign was dependent on the control of the movement of cattle. No cattle anywhere in the country could be moved without a permit and permits could be withheld if the cattle were to move from, through or into an infected area. Having limited the spread of infection the next step was eradication and initially this was achieved by moving the cattle away from the disease. Healthy cattle were removed from an infected herd, monitored during the incubation period to confirm freedom from infection, and then transferred to clean grazing. Infected cattle were slaughtered and infected grazing was kept cattle free for 15 months, after which time all ticks on the pasture would have died. With the perfection of techniques for dipping with arsenic it was found that the disease could be dipped out by temporary eradication of the vector. Compulsory short interval dipping was introduced in the commonages in 1911 and in selected farming areas from 1914. The dipping network was gradually extended to cover the whole country and the final eradication of the disease was hastened by partial destocking of disease-prone areas and slaughter of infected herds. The last outbreak occurred in Melsetter in 1954.

With the addition of short-interval dipping, all of the measures endorsed by Stockman and Theiler at the 1904 Cape Town conference were eventually adopted, including the eradication of herds. If those measures had all been adopted in 1904, the disease might have been eradicated much sooner. Since neither the government nor the farmers were willing to adopt those methods in 1904, the disease lingered on in Rhodesia until 1954 and even longer in South Africa. As Stockman had said in his annual report for 1904,[62] "It would be futile to deny that . . . the final eradication of the disease will be a much slower process than it would have been under a scheme of general compulsory slaughter," but compulsory slaughter came into use only decades later, and only in isolated outbreaks that occurred after the disease had been almost completely controlled.

One could, I suppose, argue that Theiler's discovery of the parasite had not been of much practical use, but he had shown how to diagnose the disease, had shown that its control depended on control of the brown tick, and had shown how to cleanse fields of infectious ticks. Neither Koch, Theiler, nor anyone else succeeded in finding the most powerful preventive method, that of immunization, nor is any fully satisfactory form of immunization available even today. Cattle that have recovered from East Coast fever do become immune and it is possible to induce immunity by "simultaneous inoculation of a stabilate of infective forms derived from ticks together with a single dose of a long-acting oxytetracycline."[63] But, as we saw in chapter 7, this method has not come into widespread use. Meanwhile, according to Doherty and Nussenzweig,[64] East Coast fever kills approximately 500,000 cattle each year in East Africa and Central Africa, where it has never been eradicated, and there is still a risk that it might reappear in southern Africa, where the brown tick remains widespread. In Zimbabwe alone, some 5.5 million cattle are dipped weekly at an annual cost of some 15 million U.S. dollars, often using dips that must be purchased with scarce foreign exchange.[65]

9

The African-owned cattle in Rhodesia

The terms "native cattle" and "European cattle," as used in early reports, had, perhaps unintentionally, a double meaning. "Native cattle" meant the cattle owned by the African peoples of the country, but those herds were also made up of strains of cattle that had been in the country for many years. The "European cattle" were not only owned by the European settlers, they were, by and large, made up of imported strains.

The fate of the African-owned cattle concerns us for many reasons. The killing of the African-owned cattle during the outbreak of rinderpest unquestionably contributed to the uprising of 1896, and memories of that uprising led to fears that the appearance of a new lethal disease of cattle might provoke another uprising. Secondly, it concerns us because of the often expressed fear that, once the disease had invaded the African-owned cattle, those cattle would become a permanent and ineradicable reservoir of infection because of the insistence of the Africans on moving cattle when and where they would. And it concerns us because of the great importance of cattle to the Africans not only because cattle were a store of wealth but because the ownership of cattle was woven into the very fabric of their society.

The fear of an uprising provoked by the death of cattle was to last for a long time. Stirling, who did not arrive in Rhodesia until eleven years after the 1896 uprising, reflected its persistence by mentioning in his thesis[1] that "the Great Spirit of the Ancestors said that the White Man had brought Rinderpest into their land and that he must be driven out from it ere the plague would cease." When East Coast fever invaded Rhodesia in 1902, such beliefs and fears were still very much alive and caused at least some Europeans to fear that the death of cattle or any measures taken to combat the disease might provoke another uprising. Gray's rejoinder of July 9, 1902 to the

Chamber of Mines[2] provides a perfect example: in condemning the demand that trek oxen be used to supply the mines, Gray had said that the mine owners did not care what happened even though "native cattle may die off wholesale . . . a native uprising may be provoked." Gray had some basis for his concern since he had been in Bulawayo during the rinderpest epidemic and during the 1896 uprising. As he remarked in 1902, in his joint report with Robertson,[3] the "rinderpest which practically denuded the country of stock . . . was followed by a rebellion which at one time threatened to send the white settlers after the cattle."

There was no sign of an uprising as the result of East Coast fever, as we can learn from the reports of the Native Commissioners. The Chartered Company had divided Rhodesia into Native Districts and had appointed Native Commissioners or Assistant Native Commissioners whose duties included overseeing those districts, collecting taxes and filing annual reports. The reports of those commissioners for the years 1903, 1904 and 1905 contain no suggestion that there was ever any danger of such an uprising, or even that there was much anxiety about that possibility. Professor T. O. Ranger, who has read far more extensively in such records than I have, has told me that he has the same impression, but he agrees that the fear of such an uprising must always have been present in a general, diffuse way. The report of the Chief Native Commissioner for Mashonaland, for the year ended March 31, 1904, is to the point.[4] It begins:

A vague feeling of unrest has been noticed during the Spring and Summer in all Mashonaland with the exception of the Victoria District. It would be as difficult for the natives as for myself to account for this. During March, reports from unreliable sources were received to the effect that the natives in the Inyanga District [a mountainous region in the northeast] were to rise. I at once proceeded to that district accompanied by a patrol of police. Full investigations of the rumours and the sources from which they emanated, failed to elicit any reliable evidence substantiating them. The natives appeared to be thoroughly peaceful . . . at present everything is quiet.

The Commissioner's explanation for this state of affairs is interesting, if not entirely persuasive: he suggested that the Africans had come to accept the existence and authority of white rule, and were therefore paying less attention to the chiefs. Moreover, he suggested that the voice of the chiefs' "paid M'limo or Mhondoro [spirit medium], no longer terrorizes." The Commissioner listed a number of areas in which the Rhodesian government had intervened in the previous eighteen months: "The enforcement of the marriage laws – the Rabies Act – the great restrictions placed on all moving of large and small stock owing to various diseases – the general vaccination of natives [against smallpox] in outlying districts – and the new Tax Ordinance." The Commissioner, rather optimistically, suggested that all of this activity had convinced the average African that he was now living under "civilized government." He may have been nearer the·mark when he added that "they see that they, as well as their chiefs, have to obey the laws of the government."

The sudden appearance of East Coast fever had produced near panic in a large part of the European community; indeed it was the settlers who were on the edge of an uprising. Yet there was little or no unrest among the Africans, probably because their cattle were, in fact, little affected by the new disease, which invaded their territory only gradually. The Chartered Company had, long before, seized large areas of what it hoped would be good farm land and had seized other areas that offered promise for mining.[5] By 1902 several towns or small cities had grown up, among them Umtali, Salisbury, Fort Victoria (now Masvingo) and Bulawayo. The first railroad to be completed in Rhodesia connected Umtali and Salisbury in May, 1899; the next railroad to be completed did not connect Salisbury and Bulawayo until December, 1902.[6] But the railroads did not wholly supplant even long distance ox-drawn transport and all short-haul transport from regions served by the railway to other regions was still conducted by ox-drawn transport. Those regions were, by and large, the European-occupied regions, not the regions that remained to the Africans and to their cattle. As Robert Koch said, the Africans had drawn back from the Europeans. The remoteness of the African-owned cattle from the main roads used by the transport riders protected those cattle from the new disease for a surprisingly long time.

The reports of the Native Commissioners for the year ending March 31, 1902, show how long it took for East Coast fever to attack the African-owned cattle.[7] By that time, the disease was rampant in Umtali, Melsetter and Salisbury and was well on its way south towards Bulawayo. But the Chief Native Commissioner of Mashonaland noted in his report[8] that:

The natives have been warned about the various outbreaks of disease among the European cattle and instructed to keep their cattle away from all main roads and not to drive them about from district to district without first obtaining permission to do so. A serious disease has lately made its appearance in the Umtali and Salisbury districts and the number of European cattle that have died is considerable. I am pleased, however, to state that the native cattle in and around these districts have, so far, escaped infection.

The reports for the Salisbury and Umtali districts confirmed that statement. The report for the Salisbury district said: "Although . . . redwater is very prevalent in the district, I am pleased to report that as yet no case amongst the native cattle has been brought to my notice." The report from the Umtali district said that the number of African-owned cattle was actually increasing gradually, although it had been a very bad year for European cattle owners because "some peculiar disease has been rampant . . . herds have been more than decimated, and it has proved to be a most infectious and contagious disease, which was not the idea when it first made its appearance . . . the native cattle have escaped, most fortunately, this no doubt is owing to their not having come in contact with the white man's cattle."

A year later, by March 31, 1903, East Coast fever had devastated nearly all of the European-owned cattle in Rhodesia; when Koch had travelled through Umtali and Salisbury at the end of February, 1903, he had found very few cattle alive. It is thus remarkable to read, in the Report of Native Affairs for the year ended March 31, 1903 that:[9] "The disease known as redwater that has played havoc with most cattle in and around the different townships and mining centers in the country has not spread amongst the native herds to any great extent. In fact, in the outlying districts it has hardly made its appearance."

Apparently the Africans and their cattle had indeed drawn back (or been forced back) so far from the Europeans and their cattle that many of the African-owned cattle remained free from East Coast fever for nearly eighteen months after the disease had appeared in Umtali and for nearly a year after it had spread to Bulawayo. One could hardly ask for more convincing proof that those of the Africans who were still trying to conduct their old way of life were avoiding the Europeans as much as possible. But not completely. The report for the year ended March 31, 1903 added that "Many natives living near the towns and main roads have suffered a good deal and have lost most of their cattle." On the other hand, overall, the African-owned cattle had increased in number by

5,409 head during the past year, which is very satisfactory [and in remarkable contrast to what had happened to the European cattle] and a proof that the natives have been careful in observing the regulations regarding the removal of cattle indiscriminately about the country, as, had they done so, the whole of the native districts would have become infected and the numbers of stock would have been considerably reduced.

The situation was far from uniform. In the Charter district, ninety-six cattle had died in Chief Rangas' herd, but the disease had been confined by quarantine and isolation. In Chibi, six cattle had died in Mawalila's Kraal, but the disease had disappeared after the healthy cattle had been moved to clean veld. Three more small outbreaks had occurred, at Madamgompies' Kraal, at Tshombge's Kraal, and at Mr. Barker's trading post. "I feel convinced that the disease has been brought into this district from Selukwe [a mining area] but up to the present I have not been able to definitely ascertain this as the natives are very inclined to conceal information of this description."

In Chilimanzi "the total loss so far has not been great, 15 head or, on an average, 1% of all the cattle owned by the natives in the district." On the other hand, "the mortality of transport oxen along the Selukwe–Victoria road has been very great during the year."

In Cutu, redwater had been prevalent for five months, but "only at those kraals close to the highroad . . . the natives have lost from fifty to seventy head." In Hartley, "with the exception of Kwali, who has lost nine head . . . the stock has done splendidly. The judicious course of preventing cattle from being moved from one place to another has borne most excellent results. The natives themselves acknowledge this." In Inyanga, there had been "practically no disease among stock belonging to natives. Though most of the European farmers have been ruined by their losses in stock by redwater it is only within the last month that it has attacked [African-owned cattle]." Whereas there had been 1,850 head of African-owned cattle at the time of the annual report for 1901–2, there were now 2,040 head.

In Lomagondi (in the far north-west) the African-owned cattle were "singularly free from sickness," moreover cattle had been brought from Northern Rhodesia and were being kept there,

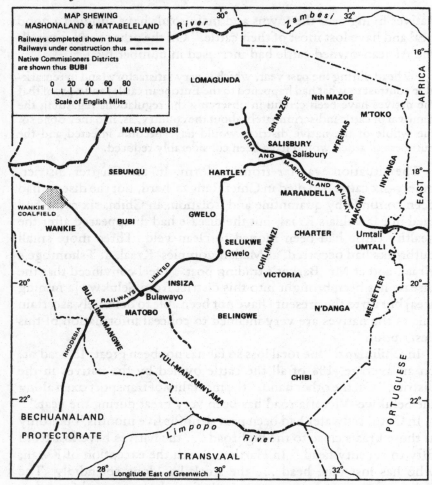

MAP SHEWING
MASHONALAND & MATABELELAND

Railways completed shown thus ━━━━
Railways under construction thus ━━━━
Native Commissioners Districts
are shown thus **BUBI**

0   20   40   60   80
Scale of English Miles

Fig. 3   Rhodesia: map showing the native districts in about
1902. The Fingo location is not shown; it was north of
Bulawayo. The Cutu district is not shown; it was merged with
Chilimanzi. The spelling of place names in the text follows that
of the Annual Reports and thus occasionally differs from that
on the map: for example, "Sebungwe" and "Sebungu";
"M'rewa" and "M'rewas." (Based on a map in *The British
South Africa Company Reports on the Administration of Rhodesia
1900–1902*. n.p., n.d. [London, 1903], by permission of
Charter Consolidated.)

"waiting until the present redwater is over [vain hope!]. They came
down in good condition and thrive well down here."

In Makoni, the big herds had been spared so far and the cattle had increased from 1,870 head in 1902 to 2,707 in 1903. In North Mazoe (in the north-east) "the stock does well," but there had been forty-seven deaths in the Marondella district (through which ran the main road from Umtali to Salisbury), and a number of deaths had appeared in the Southern Mazoe district (which was near Salisbury). Even worse, in the Salisbury district, which had been clean the year before, "the natives have lost a great number of cattle from . . . redwater [and] the disease appears to be on the increase." 137 deaths had been reported, but there had undoubtedly been many more. In M'toko and N'danga the disease had still not appeared, although there had been two small outbreaks in M'rewa.

In Melsetter, where the disease had originally appeared almost as soon as it appeared in Umtali, 143 head had died, in spite of which the total number of cattle had increased. In the Umtali district "the natives have been comparatively lucky . . . a good number of Kraals in Umtassa's vicinity have not lost any cattle at all. Round Zimunya's district . . . they have suffered severe losses." The Native Commissioner for the Victoria district reported that he had allowed "practically no shifting of native cattle since April last year . . . Many transport cattle have died on the commonage of Victoria, and on the road to Selukwe. Only 25 deaths have occurred amongst native cattle, and nearly all at kraals close to the Selukwe road." There were 39,155 head of African-owned cattle in Mashonaland on March 31, 1902 and 44,564 on March 31, 1903.

It was much the same in Matabeleland, where the total number of African-owned cattle had increased from 16,077 to 19,768. Overall, "the natives have lost very few head of cattle from redwater." In Bubi, all of the cases that had occurred did so in proximity to main roads and there were thirty-seven deaths. In Bulilima-Mangwe, south-west of Bulawayo, into which the Whites had stampeded with their cattle, there had been only three outbreaks, with nineteen deaths. The Commissioner added that "During the last quarter of the year, I purchased, on behalf of the government, certain young cattle required by Dr. Koch for experimental purposes in connection with his investigation of [redwater: crossed out] African coast fever." (Koch's new name for the disease had caught on, at least near Bulawayo.) In the Matobo district, due south of Bulawayo, African Coast fever had caused only fifteen deaths. In the Insiza district, sixty-five cattle had died in twelve kraals at Mzingwani, but the African-owned cattle in Filabusi and Insiza remained free of the disease, while it had played havoc among European herds. The African-owned herds had shown an increase over the year before of 817 head, to a new total of 2,617. In Belingwe, "redwater" broke out at the end of the year and quickly spread to five kraals, but no further. No deaths had occurred in the previous six weeks. In Selukwe, there were a few losses, close to the Fort Victoria road. In Gwelo, no authenticated case had appeared among African-owned cattle although "redwater" had destroyed "a high percentage of the cattle held by Europeans." The cattle in Sebungwe 'were "thriving;" no cases had been seen in Wankie; herd size had increased 10 percent in the Tuli district. In Fingo (not a "native district" but a special region that had been given to the Mfengu people who arrived in Rhodesia between 1898 and 1902, recruited by Rhodes from the Transkei), the news was bad:

The reported outbreaks of a new cattle disease . . . caused a great deal of uneasiness amongst the Fingoes as about that time a great many wagons were passing [along the Salisbury Column Road] . . . I regret to state that not many months afterwards, the disease made its appearance [on May 8, 1902] and has been on the location ever since . . . [it has] carried off 161 head [and] I am much afraid the Fingoes [will] yet lose heavily.

The message was always the same: few deaths in African-owned cattle in areas remote from the European system of ox-transport, more than a few, and often many, deaths near the ox-transport routes.

There is some direct evidence that there was no African unrest in November, 1903.[10] On November 4, the *Financial News* published another letter from Stanley Portal Hyatt, in which Hyatt predicted that "within the next nine or ten months the civilized world may once again be horrified by tales of massacre" in Rhodesia. This provoked a cable from the London office to Milton, dated November 5, 1903:

Private translate yourself. The Financial News newspaper has published letter from Stanley Hyatt written from Umtali township stating that there is serious unrest among natives and that there is great danger of immediate rising on attempt collect increased hut tax as natives cannot pay. He states that Administrator knows this but is indifferent and takes no precaution. As these reports do great harm suggest you should telegraph giving unqualified denial to rumour in form we can publish. H. Wilson Fox.

On the same day, November 5, Milton sent a coded telegram to

H. B. Hulley, the Native Commissioner in Umtali, asking him to respond to these rumors by telegram and by letter. Hulley was not in Umtali at the time, but he replied by letter on November 16 that "there is no truth in the statement made by Mr. Stanley Hyatt, that the natives are in a state of serious unrest." Hulley added that he did think that it would be very difficult to collect an increased hut tax and blamed the rumor on the Melsetter farmers who feared that an increase in the hut tax would interfere with their supply of labor. He also attached a copy of his report for August, 1903, in which he had pointed out that at the beginning of each rainy season the Africans always left town to go to their homes "to help break up the land for the coming season and for the same reason we will have rumours of a native rising, as we always have some one who thinks that as the local boys are leaving the towns it can be for no other reason than to take part in a rebellion." As to Hyatt, Hulley said:

Stanley Hyatt was a transport rider in the Victoria District. I do not know him personally. He seems a quiet and steady young man. By trade he is an engineer and is at present in charge of the Beira Cold Storage plant here. He is, I think the author of some short stories on Kafir life . . . He is probably engaged on a bigger work and this is his preliminary bid for notoriety.

A similar telegram was sent to L. C. Meredith, Native Commissioner in Melsetter, who replied by telegram on November 7 that he was unaware of any grounds for such statements. He also attributed the rumor to the Melsetter farmers and added that "the loss of native cattle has been greatly exaggerated." On November 20, 1903, the Chief Native Commissioner for Mashonaland sent a circular to all of the Native Commissioners in Mashonaland, asking if they were aware of any unrest. Almost all of the replies said that there were no signs of unrest; the replies that admitted to a "feeling of unrest" never linked that feeling to the new cattle disease.

Rather than go through the Native Commissioners' reports for the year ending March 31, 1904[11] one by one, I will give a summary of where the disease remained rare or absent, where it appeared for the first time, and where it continued to spread. The disease had, by then, appeared in every part of Mashonaland except the M'toko district; a total of 1,292 cattle had died in Mashonaland but 850 of those deaths had occurred in a single area, the Victoria district (where Gray and Koch had conducted their test of Koch's method of immunization). In most districts there were only a few deaths, partly, the Native Commissioners thought, because of restrictions on the moving of cattle and partly because the Africans had been warned to keep their cattle off all public roads. In South Mazoe (near Salisbury) African Coast fever had broken out "at various times in nearly all . . . of the district; in certain kraals the cattle have been completely exterminated; in other places they have suffered severely." The district commissioner added that "throughout the district inoculation has been instituted in strict accordance with the instructions of Professor Koch. In certain cases it appears to have had little effect . . . Most of the farmers in the district have abandoned the process, as they believe that it is quite useless and has the effect of killing the calves."

The report from Melsetter is of special interest because the European cattle in Melsetter (now Chimanimani) had been so severely affected so early. Melsetter also was the last region in which an outbreak occurred, in 1954. The head count was very small (534) and showed a decrease of 153. Nevertheless,

Coast fever has not been able to make rapid progress amongst Native cattle owing to the herds being small and far between, and because of the very strict application of the Cattle Removal Regulations . . . the cattle on the Sabi Valley have been saved from infection. During the past two months I have not had any reports of deaths from coast fever amongst Native cattle. I cannot say that it is due to the disease becoming less severe as sufficient time has not yet elapsed to clean the District of infection. It is really due to the fact that the cattle have died [or become immune] in the infected areas and that the strict enforcement of the Regulations prevents the infection being carried to new areas.

In the Salisbury district, as might have been expected, the Africans lost many cattle, as they did, as mentioned above, in the Victoria district.

African-owned cattle were also spared in Matabeleland, but the disease had appeared in regions where it had previously been absent. The overall report said that 647 head of cattle had died, "nearly all in the neighbourhood of main roads . . . inoculation has been adopted with some Native cattle on the Fingo location; other Natives have fought shy of the experiment." In Wankie, there were no cases of African Coast fever: "This is a matter for much congratulation as the safety of hundreds of transport oxen was of vital importance as regards both the railway and colliery extensions."[12]

Later annual reports reveal the same state of affairs. The disease continued its slow spread into the regions where African-owned cattle were held, yet the African-owned cattle apparently never suffered the same depredations as the European-owned cattle. In a comparatively late report[13] we learn that in the period 1915–22, there were 105 outbreaks affecting 25,997 European-owned cattle and only 28 outbreaks affecting 10,258 African-owned cattle. Moreover the death rate was 17 percent in the European-owned herds and only 10 percent in the African-owned herds. (Those figures cannot, however, be taken as evidence that the African-owned cattle had a higher degree of immunity. For one thing, since the usual mortality rate is 95 percent, the figures of 17 percent and 10 percent must have been based on the size of the herds rather than on the number of cattle that actually fell ill. Moreover, considering the relatively unreliable nature of the figures, the difference between 17 percent and 10 percent is probably not statistically significant.)

In August, 1904, the new laws governing the movement of cattle were adopted.[14] More importantly, in spite of the expectations of Gray, Stockman and Stirling, the Africans seem to have cooperated. They presumably saw for themselves the risk of keeping their cattle too close to the main roads, and acted accordingly. Another factor that may have played a role in protecting the African-owned cattle was that those cattle tended to stay near the villages where their owners lived. Apart from cattle raids, which had died out by 1902, African-owned cattle were not ordinarily moved over distances comparable to those covered by the transport riders.

I see no reason not to believe these reports. No Native Commissioner could have expected to advance his career by reporting that there were no deaths of cattle in his district if, in fact, there were many such deaths. Any falsification would have been exposed, within another year or two. Each commissioner did, to be sure, have the responsibility for a very large territory and the Native Commissioners undoubtedly varied in their skill and diligence. Stanley Portal Hyatt certainly did not have a high opinion of most of them.[15] Speaking of a Native Commissioner whom he admired, Hyatt said that he was

quite the most efficient Native Commissioner in Mashonaland. Unlike most of his kind, he was not South African born, he had never been accused of using his office for his own private profit, of fining natives so many cattle and entering up the fine as having been so many sovereigns.

... Other Native Commissioners – most of them were Natal men, suffering from 'Natal Fever', chronic tiredness – remained all the year in their camp, surrounded by a crowd of native parasites, female and male, and allowed their black police to do much as they liked, to assess the hut tax, to levy blackmail from the whole countryside.

Whatever the merits of any individual Native Commissioner, the overall conclusion is probably correct: not only did East Coast fever affect the African-owned cattle less than it affected the European-owned cattle but the Africans cooperated with the Europeans in preventing the spread of the disease. In addition, the relatively small size of the African-owned herds and the relative remoteness of those herds from the transport routes may have shielded them for just long enough to allow them to be further protected by the even more stringent controls on the movement of cattle that were imposed in August, 1904.

That the African-owned cattle may have been spared the worst effects of East Coast fever is a somewhat unexpected conclusion. My own reading of Gray, Stockman and Stirling, and of their expectations, originally led me to the opposite assumption, namely that the Africans would move cattle when and where they chose, and that such movements played an essential role in the spread of East Coast fever. An exchange concerning "Samwiro's cattle" confirms the opposite view. On August 24, 1905, the Native Commissioner for the Marondella District wrote to the Chief Veterinary Surgeon to say that there had recently been an outbreak on "Samwiro's location" but that there was clean veld nearby.[16]

Samwiro is willing to have all the cattle in his location moved onto clean veldt but it is doubtful whether he would agree to have infected cattle destroyed without compensation of some sort. I have not questioned him on the subject of compensation but he informed me he was perfectly willing to do any thing the Government told him to do. I am certain he would not mind his own infected cattle being destroyed provided he got the meat.

There can be little doubt that an African chief would willingly deceive a Native Commissioner, but there is other evidence that the Africans were willing to cooperate with the European authorities. According to Gray's article "Inoculation for African Coast Fever,"[17] "The principles of inoculation as laid down by Dr. Koch were explained to the natives by the Native Commissioners, and a majority of them expressed their willingness to allow their animals to be treated." The Africans were, obviously, well aware of the threat that East Coast fever posed to their cattle and were willing to take part in an effort designed to ward off that danger.

Cattle were the main store of the wealth of the Africans; the main "bank account" for their owners. The land was held in common, but the cattle were owned by individuals. Both as a store of wealth and for deep symbolic reasons, cattle played an essential role in the marriage of daughters. In addition, the years spent herding cattle were a rite of passage for young boys. Joseph B. Loudon has told me that, when he studied the Zulu culture in the 1950s, old men could estimate their age by remembering that they had been herd boys in the time when the cattle died, that is during the years of rinderpest.[18] As late as the 1980s, in the remote and isolated van Niekerk ruins, a friend of mine gathered some twigs and berries of a kind that he had known when he was a herd boy. Partly, I suppose, for sentimental reasons, but partly, as he told me, to show them to his children, who had never had that experience or seen those twigs and berries.

As to the marriage of daughters, the dowry, "bride price," or "lobolo" was of profound importance to the fabric of the culture and its social structure. As Joseph B. Loudon has put it to me, it was both a symbol and a proof of descent. The cattle given to her father by his daughter's husband were provided by that husband, his father and his brothers. Their presence in her father's kraal was living proof that the familial rights and obligations of her children were those of her husband's patrilineal descent group. That could be confirmed by pointing to the cattle that the wife's father had received in return for his daughter's marriage. The cattle had belonged to the husband's family; now they belonged to the family of the wife's father. The wife had been part of her father's family but her children were now part of her husband's family. The genealogy of the cattle and their descendants became a living proof of the genealogy of the children of the new marriage.[19]

It is thus no wonder that the Africans continued to move cattle about.[20] What is more impressive is that they refrained from doing so, even for a time. When the disease appeared to have relaxed its grip, the Native Commissioner for Belingwe wrote in his annual report for the year ending March 31, 1906 that[21] "the relaxation of restrictions on stock removal have been keenly appreciated by the natives, who are once more settling down to the natural order of things and buying, selling, bartering and exchanging cattle to their hearts' content."

The Africans were a pastoral and crop-growing community. As Hulley wrote to Milton,[22] the Africans always left the towns as the rainy season approached, "to help break up the land for the coming season." And, as Stanley Portal Hyatt said,[23] the African, as a "small cultivator, whose main interests in life are his home, his family and his crops . . . wants to be home, at least during seed time and harvest . . . he is painfully human, and, knowing him well, I cannot foresee the day when the dividend of a mining company will be more important to him than the filling of a grain bin, in which the food of his wife and children is stored." Hyatt wrote to condemn his favorite enemy, the Chartered Company, and to condemn its demand that the hut tax be paid in gold, but what he said seems persuasive. Later writers certainly confirmed his view. Beach[24] characterized the earlier Shona economy as having "an agricultural base, with supporting branches of production based on herding, hunting/gathering, manufacturing and mining . . . by the late 19th century . . . the agricultural base remained of paramount importance." The paramount importance of the sowing and reaping of crops may well have brought the 1896–7 uprising to an end. Beach suggests that the "the Shona rulers were committed to the defence of their fields, without which Shona society could not continue . . . the war ended in late 1897 not so much because of the fighting but because it was vital for the people to start the 1897–8 summer crop." Keppel-Jones, in discussing Rhodes' famous *indaba* in the Matopos which led to the end of the 1896 war, says much the same.[25]

There was still food in the hills, but there were more mouths to feed. And how would the stock be replenished? That depended on the next crop, but most of the crop had to be grown in the plains, not among the rocks and impenetrable thickets of the Matopos, and the sowing season was at hand. This is the kind of problem that responsible leaders face, but that ardent young soldiers tend to brush aside.

In the event, as both Beach and Keppel-Jones argue, the choice was for peace and for crops. (One of the great successes of independent Zimbabwe has been to produce a many-fold increase in the productivity of the small farms and their farmers, who now make a very important contribution to the nation's food supply. The second annual Alan Shawm Feinstein World Hunger Award was conferred, in 1988, upon "Zimbabwe's communal farmers in honor of their efforts to alleviate world hunger." In September, 1988, the Hunger Project conferred its Africa Prize for Leadership on the President of Zimbabwe, Robert Mugabe, in recognition of the same achievement.)[26]

In summary: As far as I can determine, East Coast fever did not affect the African-owned cattle in Rhodesia as severely as it affected the European cattle, nor as soon. The African-owned cattle did not become the major focus of infection nor the chief means of spreading it. The disease did not provoke African unrest and the Africans appear to have cooperated in its control. There is nothing to suggest that East Coast fever disrupted the social fabric of African life to a degree even faintly resembling the disruption caused by rinderpest.

Many of my conclusions about the effect of East Coast fever on the African-owned cattle are at great variance with the predictions of the white settlers and of their veterinarians. The evidence for my conclusions is necessarily fragmentary and inadequate, gathered as it is from the reports of the Chartered Company's Native Commissioners and cattle inspectors. Nevertheless, these conclusions are plausible. No epidemiologist would question the conclusion that the disease spread only slowly to cattle remote from the transport roads.

As one reads the various reports of the veterinarians, one finds repeated predictions that the Africans would not cooperate. Yet those predictions are often coupled with examples of such cooperation. Statements that the Africans "will move about with the cattle no matter what is done to stop them" appear in the same report as the statement that the chiefs were cooperating to prevent cattle from moving into Bechuanaland. Statements that the Africans would have nothing to do with dipping cattle are contradicted by later reports that they did cooperate in dipping. Even Stirling, who spoke of the Africans fleeing from the first sign of disease and from the cattle inspectors, admitted that they would cooperate when they understood that it was to their advantage to do so. The early assumption that the Africans would refuse all help and would spread the disease when and if they chose to move cattle seems to be unfounded. That assumption is, I suppose, just one more piece of evidence for the success of the colonial myth that the Africans were incapable of behaving rationally even when their own social and economic interests were at stake. Not only were they capable of behaving rationally, they had well organized social and political structures and they had leaders who were willing to cooperate in measures designed to protect the cattle, measures such as the restriction of movement and, much later, regular dipping. (There is ample evidence that the chiefs cooperated willingly in the widespread killing of dogs to suppress the outbreak of rabies, presumably because of their past experience with that disease. Mad dogs had long been recognized and feared throughout the world.)[27]

Because East Coast fever spread only slowly into the African-owned herds, those herds were still relatively free from the disease in late 1904, when stringent controls were finally imposed. Those controls came too late to save the European cattle but they may have come just in time to give some protection to the African-owned cattle.[28]

10

Two more parasites and another new disease

The rod-shaped parasite that causes East Coast fever is not the juvenile form of the pear-shaped parasite that causes Texas fever. That much had been established by 1904. But a good deal of confusion remained about some rod-shaped and ring-shaped parasites, often seen in the blood of animals that had been inoculated in an attempt to immunize them against East Coast fever. Moreover, the tiny cocci that Smith and Kilborne had seen in mild cases of Texas fever also remained unexplained as of 1904: unexplained in the sense that no one had questioned the original conclusion of Smith and Kilborne that those tiny cocci were the juvenile form of the pear-shaped parasite.

The second new parasite: Theileria mutans

Koch, in his efforts to devise a vaccine, had injected blood into non-immune animals. A few weeks after such injections he regularly found what he called "ring forms" in the "immunized" animals. He took the presence of those ring forms to indicate that the animals had indeed been immunized against East Coast fever.[1] At the Bloemfontein conference of December, 1903, Theiler, apparently referring to the ring form, said that[2] "He believed it to be a new species of piroplasma and that it had nothing to do with East Coast Fever." In 1904 Theiler returned to the problem in his article "The *Piroplasma bigeminum* of the immune ox."[3] He noted that in East Coast fever the parasite can be rod-shaped or ring-shaped or can show intermediate forms. On the other hand, any animal that has recovered from Texas fever still contains the pear-shaped parasite in its blood. That can be shown by injecting its blood into a non-immune animal, which will then develop Texas fever. That is true even though the pear-shaped parasites may be so rare in cattle that have recovered from Texas fever that they escape microscopical examination.

But when young calves were injected with blood from an animal immune to Texas fever, there was commonly an initial reaction and then, after some time, a second reaction. During the second reaction, "one often sees a peculiar phenomenon, namely the occurrence of endoglobular parasites which correspond to the description of *Piroplasma parvum*." Rings and rods are seen in as many as 10 percent of the red cells. They are, Theiler said, probably the same as the rings that Koch thought were a sign of immunity to East Coast fever, but they are merely a form of the pear-shaped parasite, *Piroplasma bigeminum*. They are a form of the Texas fever parasite, a form that appears when infective blood is injected into an animal that is already immune to Texas fever. They have nothing to do with the *Piroplasma parvum* that causes East Coast fever, even though they resemble it: they are the "immune form" of *Piroplasma bigeminum*. In one experiment Theiler took an ox obtained from a district where ordinary redwater had never existed and induced redwater by injection of blood from an animal that was infected with the Texas fever parasite. Both the pear-shaped parasite and the small parasites that resemble *Piroplasma parvum* appeared, but when that ox was later exposed to infective brown ticks it contracted a fatal case of East Coast fever. Theiler concluded that "the presence of rings does not indicate that an animal is immune against East Coast Fever" and that "the rings and rods represent a phase in the life-history of *Piroplasma bigeminum* in the immune ox." The former conclusion was correct; the latter conclusion was completely wrong.

Theiler returned to the problem in his annual report for 1905–6, and in a series of articles published in 1906, 1907 and 1909 in which he showed that he had been wrong in concluding that the rings and rods are a form of *Piroplasma bigeminum*.[4] In those later studies Theiler showed that the small rings and rods that can appear in an animal inoculated with blood are neither the East Coast fever parasite nor an immune form of the Texas fever parasite. They are a distinct new species, which Theiler called *Piroplasma mutans*. Under microscopic examination *Piroplasma mutans* is very similar to the East Coast fever parasite, but it differs from it in two ways. Firstly, of course, it does not cause East Coast fever. Secondly, it can easily be transferred from one animal to another by inoculation with blood in which it is present, which is not true of the East Coast fever parasite.

In his article of 1906, Theiler concluded that

an animal which is born in the Transvaal contains as a rule piroplasma bigeminum but not piroplasma mutans. We can successively infect an animal with piroplasma bigeminum and piroplasma mutans. We have not yet been able to do the reverse, because we have not as yet met with an animal which was only infected with piroplasma mutans.

Thus, Theiler said,

My former conception of the immune form of piroplasma bigeminum has become obsolete ... the fact that the injection of blood of a redwater immune animal into susceptible cattle is followed occasionally by rings and rod-shaped parasites must now be interpreted as has been done in this paper [i.e. as the simultaneous infection of the animal with two distinct parasites].

Theiler had gone a little farther than that in his annual report by saying that "piroplasma mutans has all the characteristics of the piroplasma of the type of ordinary redwater, since it remains in the immune animal, and can be transmitted with the blood. Indeed, when we inoculate against redwater, we usually inoculate against this latter parasite." (Actually, one inoculates the latter parasite, but since no immunity develops the word "against" seems wrong.)

In his article of 1907, Theiler showed that the blue tick, which transmits *Piroplasma bigeminum* does *not* transmit *Piroplasma mutans*. The progeny of blue ticks that had fed on animals infected with both parasites caused only redwater when they fed on non-immune animals. But those animals, after they had recovered from red-water, could be infected with *Piroplasma mutans* by injecting blood that contained both parasites. Theiler added that there is, under the microscope, hardly any difference in the appearance of *Piroplasma mutans* and the parasite that causes East Coast fever. In 1909 Theiler had what he called a "stroke of luck." He had exposed two cattle to infection and one of them contracted only an infection with *Piroplasma mutans* (although it later contracted a fatal case of redwater). Theiler thus had, for a time, a supply of blood infected only with *Piroplasma mutans*, and he infected four animals with it. Three of them were later exposed to infective blue ticks and only then did they develop redwater and show *Piroplasma bigeminum* in their blood (another, Theiler said, was infected with redwater by the brown tick: "this is an exception to the general rule, but the experiments were undertaken in such a way that no other explanation is possible." He was surely wrong.)

Later work was to show that *Piroplasma mutans* is indeed a distinct species, that it can be transmitted by inoculation, and that it rarely causes serious disease. In addition, it was long thought to be transmitted in nature by the brown tick. Thus both *Piroplasma parvum* and *Piroplasma mutans* appeared to be transmitted by the brown tick, whereas both *Piroplasma bigeminum* and *Piroplasma mutans* can be transmitted by inoculation. This explains much of the confusion that resulted, in early studies, from diagnoses based only on the microscopic appearance of the parasites in the red blood cells.[5]

In 1904 both Koch and Theiler[6] assumed that a disease called tropical piroplasmosis by Dschunkowsky and Luhs[7] was identical with East Coast fever, but that disease was soon shown to be a distinct one, transferable by inoculation and transmitted in nature by a tick that belongs to the *Hyalomma* genus. The parasite that causes "tropical piroplasmosis" is now known as *Theileria annulata*. Apart from the brief period in which "tropical piroplasmosis" was confused with East Coast fever, it has little to do with our story, although the parasite that causes it has figured prominently in the experimental studies discussed in chapter 11. In 1907 the "piroplasms" were reclassified and divided into two genera. The parasite that causes Texas fever became known as *Babesia bigemina*, the parasite that causes East Coast fever became *Theileria parva*, the parasite that causes tropical piroplasmosis became *Theileria annulata*, and *Piroplasma mutans* became *Theileria mutans*.

Nor has *Theileria parva* remained a single entity. The parasite that causes classic East Coast fever is now called *Theileria parva parva* to distinguish it from two other parasites. One, *Theileria parva lawrencei*, is as lethal as *Theileria parva parva* but it does not cause widespread outbreaks because, although it is transmitted to cattle from buffalo, it is rarely transmitted from one animal to another within a herd of cattle. The other parasite, *Theileria parva bovis*, which is morphologically identical to *Theileria parva parva*, causes a disease which is less severe than East Coast fever;[8] as of 1989 it has been seen only in Zimbabwe. The three "strains" of *Theileria parva* are morphologically and serologically indistinguishable, so that, in an interesting echo of 1903, their classification is "principally based on clinical and epidemiological parameters."[9]

The third new parasite and the second new disease: Anaplasma marginale *and anaplasmosis*

One more parasite remained to be identified, and it was a very important parasite indeed, both for our story and for cattle raisers. As Henning put it,[10] throughout the studies that led to the isolation of *Theileria mutans*, Theiler "repeatedly referred to the presence of 'marginal points' in the blood of his experimental animals, but, as he was unable to explain their significance, he did not pay much attention to them at first." In his annual report for 1905–6, dated November 12, 1906, Theiler actually thought that[11] "*Piroplasma mutans, n. spec.*" might be the cause of gall sickness. But "Attention has also been drawn to a certain phenomenon which is frequently observed in connection with redwater inoculations, viz. the occurrence of marginal or peripheral points, which, although their nature is not yet clear, undoubtedly have a protozooic character." I believe that this is Theiler's first mention of the "marginal points." He again connected gall sickness with *Piroplasma mutans* in his 1907 article[12] in which he also referred to "marginal points." In his 1909 article[12] he no longer regarded *Piroplasma mutans* as pathogenic; he also said "In some animals the presence of marginal points has been noted. I am not yet in a position to explain the nature of these 'points' or to state the relation in which they stand to piroplasma mutans."

In late 1908, Theiler found funds to purchase some cattle in England and to have them sent to South Africa for experimental purposes. According to Gutsche, F. B. Smith was in London, staying at the Savile Club,[13] and Theiler asked him to approach Stewart Stockman, who selected heifers in Sussex. Stockman inoculated those cattle against redwater in London and Smith arranged for them to be sent to South Africa, where they arrived in January, 1909. After they arrived in Pretoria, as a further precaution, Theiler again inoculated them against redwater, five with blood from one animal and five with blood from another. As expected, none of them developed redwater, but about a month later nine of them developed fever, and their red cells showed "marginal points." The cattle became severely anemic and five of them actually died. Theiler managed to transmit this illness to three more cattle, and concluded that "these marginal points are the cause of a typical disease – a grave anemia . . . that they stand in no relation to piroplasma bigeminum, and that they represent a new genus of protozoon."[14] Those "marginal points" stained intensely blue and appeared to consist only of a cell nucleus without any surrounding cytoplasm. Since they had no cytoplasm, Theiler called them *Anaplasma*; and, since they were seen at the edge or margin of the cell, *Anaplasma marginale*.

Theiler had discovered another new parasite *and* another new disease. That disease, anaplasmosis, became a specific, well-defined entity which replaced part of a group of "diseases" previously known by the vague term "gall sickness." Anaplasmosis causes severe and even fatal anemia but it does not cause hemoglobinuria.

Theiler's discovery of this new parasite and of the disease that it causes, and his creation not only of a new species but of a new genus, aroused considerable skepticism and was not fully accepted for many years. But it was eventually validated, as was Theiler's suggestion that the same parasite had been the cause of the mild form of Texas fever that Smith and Kilborne had described in 1893.[15] Since Koch relied on Smith and Kilborne in interpreting the findings that he made in Dar-es-Salaam in 1897 and 1898, we must return to their study.

The original small parasite

What had Smith and Kilborne said about parasites and diseases in 1893, in their classic study of Texas fever?[16] To begin with, they said there are two types of Texas fever, an acute type and a "mild," nonfatal or chronic type. In the acute type the victims are obviously and severely ill. There is a high fever, death may occur within four or five days after the fever appears, and there is marked destruction of red cells and marked hemoglobinuria. In the mild type, red cells are destroyed, but not rapidly enough to produce hemoglobinuria. The animals are anemic and listless but not, at least to the unaided eye, obviously ill. The acute form is at its worst in mid-summer; the mild form is "largely a disease of autumn."

Moreover, in the acute form we see characteristic parasites in some of the red blood cells: two pear-shaped parasites, their tapered ends often close together. They are seen in perhaps only 5 percent of the red cells, but they are very distinctive and "there is a very rapid multiplication of the microparasite in the blood vessels corresponding to an equally rapid disappearance of the red corpuscles." Smith and Kilborne called these parasites *Pyrosoma bigeminum*; they later became *Piroplasma bigeminum* and are now called *Babesia bigemina*.

In the mild type of Texas fever as many as 50 percent of the red blood cells contain parasites. Those parasites are not large, pear-shaped and twinned; they are tiny, round and single. They are "round coccus like bodies from 0.2 to 0.5 microns in diameter and situated within the corpuscle on its border." (They were, in fact, Theiler's *Anaplasma marginale*.) Having argued that these cocci were indeed parasites and not some sort of granule or artefact, Smith and Kilborne said:

> If we admit their parasitic nature as highly probable, we have still the question of whether they are stages of the Texas fever parasite *or of another parasite transmitted with it* [emphasis added]. This question cannot be positively answered until, by methods akin to those of bacteriology, we shall be enabled to isolate the Texas fever organism and observe the transformation of one stage into the other.

Lacking that positive proof, Smith and Kilborne nevertheless concluded that the two parasites were stages of the same parasite, since both types of parasite and both types of disease were seen in every outbreak, "though at different periods of the same season." For Smith and Kilborne, the best evidence for the identity of the diseases and of the parasites came from two cattle that developed acute Texas fever in early July, complete with the pear-shaped parasites. They recovered, only to fall ill again in late August, when their red blood cells showed coccus-like bodies. Since the cattle had been kept in tick-free fields, reinfection could not have caused the relapse. But what Smith and Kilborne saw is exactly what one would expect if cattle were simultaneously infected with Texas fever and anaplasmosis, since Texas fever has an incubation period of five to ten days and anaplasmosis has an incubation period of three to six weeks. (Smith and Kilborne always emphasized that the acute form of Texas fever is at its worst in the summer whereas the mild form is seen in the fall. One thus might wonder why they thought that the juvenile form of the parasite should be seen later in the season than the adult form, but they seem to have thought that the juvenile forms seen in the fall were the offspring of the adult forms seen in the summer, since they referred to the relapse, or delayed appearance of the mild disease, as resulting from the "periodical multiplication of the micro-parasite.")

Smith and Kilborne were wrong about the tiny parasites, but their error was to have little influence on the subsequent study of Texas fever. Their three great discoveries were that Texas fever is transmitted by a tick, that it is caused by the pear-shaped parasite that they were the first to describe, and that the parasite is passed on via the tick's eggs. But, by lumping two diseases and two parasites together, Smith and Kilborne provided a model, the casual adoption of which was to mislead Robert Koch very badly indeed.

The three small parasites

At last we can solve the curious case of the small parasites:
1. In 1893 Smith and Kilborne lumped together Texas fever and anaplasmosis, and, by deciding that the small parasite was the juvenile form of the large one, lumped together the parasites that cause those diseases, namely *Anaplasma marginale* and *Piroplasma bigeminum* (now *Babesia bigemina*).
2. In 1897 and 1898, Koch, following the model provided by Smith and Kilborne, lumped together East Coast fever and Texas fever, lumped together the parasites that cause those diseases, namely *Theileria parva* and *Babesia bigemina*, and again took the small parasite to be the juvenile form of the large one.
3. In 1902 Gray and Robertson adopted Koch's interpretation of the significance of the small parasite, regarding it as the juvenile form of *Babesia bigemina*.
4. Although Laveran, in 1902 and 1903, dismissed the idea that the small parasite seen by Smith and Kilborne was the same as that described by Koch in 1898, he advised Theiler that the small *Theileria parva* was indeed the juvenile form of *Babesia bigemina*. In an article published in 1903, Laveran actually described all three parasites: tiny cocci, small bacilliform parasites and the large pear-shaped parasite (see figure 2, chapter 7). He seems to have regarded both of the small parasites as being atypical forms of the large one, although he emphasized the bacilliform parasites by saying that "in the preparations of blood that are richest in bacilliform parasites, one always finds typical *P. bigeminum*."
5. In 1903, Koch corrected himself and came to regard the small parasite as a new species, one that causes the severe disease that he called African Coast fever. But he often saw small parasites appear following inoculation. He regarded the appearance of those para-

sites as a sign that the animal had become immunized against East Coast fever, i.e. he thought that they were a (non-existent) immune form of the East Coast fever parasite, *Theileria parva*. Koch was probably looking at two simultaneous infections and two different parasites, the large *Babesia bigemina* and the small *Theileria mutans* (or, possibly, in some cases at least, the very small *Anaplasma marginale*).

6. In 1904, Theiler claimed that the small parasites seen by Koch in inoculated animals were not a sign of immunity to East Coast fever but were a sign of immunity to Texas fever. For Theiler, that small parasite now became a (non-existent) immune form of the Texas fever parasite.

7. Between 1906 and 1909, Theiler showed that some of the small parasites were neither a sign of immunity to East Coast fever nor an "immune form" of the parasite that causes Texas fever, but were a new parasite, today called *Theileria mutans*. He then discarded the idea that there is an immune form of the Texas fever parasite. He also regularly referred to the presence of "marginal points."

8. In 1909 and 1910 Theiler finally showed that the "marginal points" were a distinct parasite which he called *Anaplasma marginale*. He called the disease that they cause anaplasmosis. And he argued, correctly, that Smith and Kilborne had made two mistakes. The tiny cocci that Smith and Kilborne had described and regarded as the juvenile form of *Babesia bigemina* were *Anaplasma marginale* and what those investigators had called the "mild form" of Texas fever was anaplasmosis. Which brings us back to where the case of the small parasites began in 1893.

In principle, although I do not know that it has ever been done, one could take a healthy ox and give it Texas fever either by inoculation or by the bite of a blue tick. Having fallen ill and then recovered, the ox could then be given anaplasmosis, either by inoculation or by the bite of a blue tick. Having survived anaplasmosis the ox would then have both the pear-shaped parasite of Texas fever and the small parasite of anaplasmosis in at least some of its red cells. One could then infect it with *Theileria mutans*, at which point its blood would contain the large Texas fever parasite and *two* small parasites, *Anaplasma marginale* and *Theileria mutans*. And, if the ox were then bitten by an infected brown tick, it could contract East Coast fever and, just before it died three weeks later, its blood would contain the large Texas fever parasite and *three* kinds of small parasites: *Theileria parva*, *Theileria mutans* and *Anaplasma marginale*. Thus both a large parasite (*Babesia bigemina*) and a small parasite (*Anaplasma marginale*), can cause fever and anemia, are transmissible by inoculation, and can be transmitted by the blue tick and onward via its eggs. And there are two small parasites, indistinguishable by light microscopy, both long thought to be transmissible by the brown tick, one of which (*Theileria parva*) causes lethal East Coast fever and the other of which (*Theileria mutans*) rarely causes any serious disease. To add to the confusion, *Theileria parva* cannot ordinarily be transmitted by inoculation whereas *Theileria mutans* can easily be transmitted in that way. By 1910, the list of "small" parasites that can be found in the red blood cells of cattle included *Theileria parva*, *Theileria mutans* and *Anaplasma marginale*. Since any or even all of those parasites can appear in the red cells of animals along with the classic pear-shaped parasite that causes Texas fever, it is not surprising that the early investigators found it so difficult to assess the importance of the "small forms" characteristic of East Coast fever.

Nor is it surprising that, as a result, many mistakes were made in 1902, 1903 and 1904. What is remarkable is that Texas fever and East Coast fever were distinguished from one another within 18 months of East Coast fever appearing in Rhodesia in October, 1901, that the brown tick was incriminated as the vector of East Coast fever as early as December, 1902, and that the three small parasites had been differentiated by 1910. It does seem worth emphasizing that *all* of the small parasites that had misled not only Koch but also Theiler himself were, in fact, eventually identified as new species and named by Theiler and that his identifications have stood the test of time (very nearly, at any rate).[17]

East Coast fever and Koch's postulates

In October, 1903, Lounsbury remarked that he had suspected that the "Rhodesian disease was quite different to Redwater" as soon as he had produced the new disease by a brown tick in late 1902.[18] Theiler had said that the problem would be solved through the study of the tick. And, in retrospect, it may seem that that is how the problem was solved. Yet none of the fifteen results that Theiler cited as showing that the diseases are different and that, therefore, the causal parasites are different, made any mention of his experiments on ticks. Only in the third section of his annual report for 1904 did he turn to "Transmission of East Coast fever by ticks." Even then he did not use the fact that one kind of tick transmits one disease and another kind of tick transmits the other disease as proof that the diseases are different.[19]

It had seemed to me that Theiler had so much success and was able to correct so many of Koch's errors exactly because Koch could not transmit East Coast fever from one animal to another whereas Theiler could. Lounsbury had identified the right tick and Theiler and Lounsbury had identified the stages in the life cycle of that tick during which it is infective. Theiler could test for immunity because he could evoke a case of East Coast fever at will. Theiler could show that animals whose blood contained the "ring forms" that Koch took to be a sign of immunity were not immune, because he could infect them with East Coast fever, using an infected nymph or mature tick. And Theiler could separate the organisms that cause Texas fever and East Coast fever because the brown tick transmits only the parasite that causes East Coast fever, whereas the blue tick transmits only the parasite that causes Texas fever. To identify the causal organism, to induce the disease in a new animal by transferring that organism, to recover the organism from the animal thus infected, to infect another animal with the organism thus recovered, to show that the organism is always present when the disease is present and that the disease is always present when the organism is present – that is how one shows that an organism causes a disease. That is how one fulfills Koch's postulates. In East Coast fever it was Theiler rather than Koch who fulfilled Koch's postulates, because Theiler could transmit the parasite from a sick animal to a healthy animal and Koch could not. That, for me at least, was how Theiler identified the parasite with certainty and that is why Theiler was entitled to name it, which he did: "*Piroplasma parvum.*" (When the piroplasms were later reclassified, the East Coast fever parasite was appropriately renamed *Theileria parva*. Stephens and Christophers had, as early as November, 1903, suggested the name *Piroplasma kochi*[20] for the parasite Koch had seen in "African Coast fever" but they still referred to the occasional presence of pear-shaped forms; moreover, Theiler's priority in "isolating" the parasite by transmitting it seems clear. That is probably why Wenyon's suggestion[21] that "*Theileria kochi* may be the correct name" never caught on.)

What has all this to do with Koch's postulates? What, indeed, are Koch's postulates? Koch never gave an explicit list of those postulates, but Carter has reconstructed them in two interesting articles on the concept of causality in late nineteenth century medicine.[22] Carter's reconstruction of Koch's postulates is this:

1. An alien structure must be exhibited in all cases of the disease.
2. The structure must be shown to be a living organism and must be distinguishable from all other organisms.
3. The distribution of micro-organisms must correlate with and explain the disease phenomenon.
4. The micro-organisms must be cultivated outside the diseased animal and isolated from all disease products which could be causally significant.
5. The pure isolated micro-organism must be inoculated into test animals and these animals must then display the same symptoms as the original diseased animal.

Strictly speaking, Koch's postulates have nothing to do with proving that a new disease is in fact new. They provide criteria for showing that a particular organism is the cause of a disease that has already been identified. But a claim that a disease is new and previously unidentified obviously can be greatly strengthened if the organism that causes it can be identified and shown to fulfill Koch's postulates.

It might be noted that the question of immunity does not figure in these postulates. Moreover it is not easy (and in 1903 or 1904 it was not possible) to cultivate parasites outside a diseased animal and then induce the disease by inoculating their infectious stage into a healthy animal. In my opinion, Theiler did the equivalent of that by the use of the brown tick. He "isolated" the organism by feeding uninfected ticks on sick animals, he caused the disease by placing ticks infected in that way on a healthy animal, by microscopic examination he identified the organism in the blood of the newly infected animal, and he again recovered it, in infectious form, by allowing uninfected ticks to feed on the newly infected animal and then, after moulting, to infect a new animal. But there is no evidence that Theiler saw it that way.

Koch announced, in his interim report, that both the disease and the parasite that causes it were new. As evidence that "African

Coast fever" differs from Texas fever, he adduced the different clinical signs and clinical course of the diseases; the absence of anemia, hemolysis and hemoglobinuria in African Coast fever; the different microscopic appearance of the parasites; the fact that in African Coast fever the parasites are seen in far more red cells than the pear-shaped parasites usually are seen in Texas fever; the distinctive post-mortem findings in the two diseases; and the absence of cross-immunity. He said nothing whatever about the transmission of the causal organism which he was, in any event, never able to transmit.

As to the fifteen points that Theiler listed to prove that the new disease was not Texas fever, they were:[23]

1. Cattle which are immune against redwater . . . contracted the disease and died.
2. . . . cattle which had been hyper-immunised against rinderpest . . . and then against ordinary redwater . . . contracted the disease and died.
3. Cattle . . . immune against redwater showed, on *post mortem*, lesions of redwater and, in their blood, the *Piroplasma bigeminum*, together with the bacillary piroplasma.
4. A certain amount of cattle did not show *Piroplasma bigeminum* in their blood.
5. The average incubation period after exposure to natural infection was about 12 days; the average course of the temperature reaction was 13 days. . .
6. . . . animals which had *Piroplasma bigeminum* in their blood showed . . . haemoglobinuria . . . animals which only had the bacillary form of piroplasma present did not show this symptom.
7. . . . in the majority of cases, there was no decrease of red corpuscles, or only a very slight one.
8. The susceptibility of cattle to the disease was 100 per cent, and the mortality averaged 95 per cent.
9. . . . healthy cattle placed in stables alongside sick cattle did not contract the disease.
10. The *post-mortem* lesions . . . differed from those of ordinary redwater. . .
11. The inoculation of blood . . . which contained the bacillary piroplasma . . . did, in no instance . . . produce the disease.
12. Cattle which had thus been treated acquired no immunity; they contracted the disease after they were exposed to natural infection.
13. Cattle which were injected with blood of immune oxen did not show any reaction due to the injection of such blood, neither did they acquire any immunity therefrom.

14. Cattle which were injected with serum of immune oxen did not acquire any passive immunity when exposed to natural infection; they died as rapidly as did the controls.
15. Animals which have recovered from East Coast fever have acquired a permanent immunity.

Only one of those results had anything to do with how the disease is transmitted. Even that one had nothing to do with ticks and offered an essentially negative argument, namely that East Coast fever cannot be transmitted by inoculation of blood whereas Texas fever can. My argument that Theiler had fulfilled Koch's postulates must thus be dismissed as being purely retrospective. When Theiler said that the problem would be solved by the study of the tick he was not thinking of the tick as a device to replace the culture medium as a method for isolating the causal organism, he was thinking of it, just as he said, as "the agency by which the disease is produced." To use Carter's terms, the tick is a *necessary* cause of East Coast fever: in nature, no brown ticks, no East Coast fever. The parasite is also necessary. No parasite, no East Coast fever. In naturally occurring infections, only when the tick is infected with the parasite does it become a *sufficient* cause, invariably able to cause East Coast fever in a non-immune animal. To induce East Coast fever under natural conditions, the *infected tick* is both necessary *and* sufficient. Lounsbury and Theiler did, in fact, establish that. Since the East Coast fever parasite is not passed on via the egg of the brown tick, they were able to experiment both with uninfected ticks and with ticks that they infected by feeding them on sick animals, and to show that an infected tick feeding on a non-immune animal suffices to cause East Coast fever.

It seems obvious (but only in retrospect) that Theiler *must* have identified the parasite and induced the disease with it, thus proving that the parasite was a new one and that the disease was therefore a new one. But the record is perfectly clear. Koch and Theiler did nothing of the kind. They instead decided that the disease was not Texas fever. And from the conclusion that the diseases were different, they concluded that the causal parasites were different.

What is a new disease?

As we have seen, both Koch and Theiler, and for that matter, Duncan Hutcheon, were impressed by the same facts. Texas fever and East Coast fever have different clinical signs and a different clinical course. The post-mortem findings are different. And, finally, animals undoubtedly immune to Texas fever have no immunity at all to East Coast fever. Duncan Hutcheon made those points: he said that an organism might increase in virulence, and that, as a result, animals previously immune to it might become susceptible to it. But, he said, one would hardly expect the disease to *alter in character*. Unfortunately for Hutcheon, he was forced to back down and to conclude that the diseases were the same because expert bacteriologists had insisted that the causal parasites were merely varieties of the same parasite. At that time those expert bacteriologists were, apart from Robertson, rightly regarded throughout the world as experts: they were Koch, Laveran and Nocard. But how does one decide that a new disease *is* new?

The concept of a specific disease is somewhat elusive. The fact that two diseases differ in their signs, symptoms, clinical course and post-mortem findings does *not* prove that they are caused by different organisms. Syphilis, leprosy, tuberculosis and the diseases caused by the streptococci provide examples of that. Nor is cross-immunity an absolute guide. A solid immunity to one Lancefield type of streptococcus produces no immunity whatever to another Lancefield type, even though the types are morphologically identical and can be distinguished only serologically. The cross-immunity argument was nevertheless a strong one, almost as persuasive to latter-day microbiologists as it was to Koch, Theiler and, indeed, to Hutcheon. If animals solidly immune to one disease readily fall prey to another, the disease to which they fall ill is not the one from which they have already recovered. (That is, in fact, virtually a definition of "solid immunity.") Unfortunately, protozoan parasites are particularly gifted at changing their antigenicity, so the cross-immunity argument is less persuasive for diseases caused by parasites than it is for diseases caused by bacteria. But even if a parasite alters its antigenicity, it ordinarily produces the same disease. Hutcheon was right: one does not expect the same organism to increase in virulence, attack animals supposedly immune to it *and* produce a disease that is altered in character. One does not *expect* that, but it can happen. Influenza, caused by a virus that is notorious for its skill at antigenic variation, can change from being "typical flu" to being a disease that affects the central nervous system: more virulent, an absence of immunity *and* an alteration in character.

Ironically enough, then, the most solid single argument was that the parasite looked so different under the microscope – at least to those who were not convinced that it was only the juvenile form of an already well-known parasite! But the case rested on a set of arguments which, taken all in all, are very persuasive. And, after all, the diseases are different.

Many of the diseases with which we are familiar were described, and correctly described, long before their cause was known. Diseases were, and still are, defined by their signs and symptoms, by their clinical course, and by post-mortem findings. Diseases caused by infectious organisms are now often further defined by demonstrating the presence of those organisms. But the mere demonstration of the presence of the causal organism is a far cry from fulfilling Koch's postulates. There are many infectious diseases for which Koch's postulates have not been fulfilled, yet few serious students of those diseases have any doubts about the presence of the organism being a necessary condition for the appearance of the disease.[24]

But one cannot avoid a final question. If neither Theiler nor Koch himself had "Koch's postulates" in mind while they were investigating East Coast fever, were those postulates ever as influential as they are now thought to have been?

The stumbling blocks

In 1897 and 1898, when Koch studied seriously ill cattle at Dar-es-Salaam, he quickly reached the conclusion that they had Texas fever (some of them presumably did; most of the severely ill ones certainly had East Coast fever as well).[25] Koch saw the typical pear-shaped parasites and he also saw small parasites, just as Smith and Kilborne had done. Koch's description of the small parasites was, however, quite different from that of Smith and Kilborne. The parasites that Koch saw were not tiny, they were not round and they were not found at the margins of the red blood cells. They were "miniature staves," sometimes so strongly curved that they formed rings. Koch adopted the suggestion of Smith and Kilborne that the small parasites were the juvenile forms of the typical pear-shaped parasite. The small parasites did not look at all like those described by Smith and Kilborne; moreover they were found in severe cases, not in mild cases. For that difference, Koch offered no explanation. Instead he said

Only with regard to the early forms of the *Pyrosoma* and the relation of both it and the full-grown parasite to mild and severe Texas fever, have I come to different conclusions from the American investigators. I found namely . . . in the red blood corpuscles of cases which took a *severe form* [emphasis added] strange forms resembling miniature staves so that one might take them to be small bacilli.

But Smith and Kilborne had, after all, been wrong. The small parasite they had seen was not a juvenile form of the Texas fever parasite. Koch nevertheless persuaded himself that the small parasites that he had seen were the same as the small parasites that Smith and Kilborne had seen and he adopted their incorrect hypothesis that the small parasites are the juvenile forms of the large pear-shaped parasites, thus creating what Gray later called "a stumbling block to future investigators."

Had Laveran not persuaded Theiler that the bacilliform parasite was only an atypical form of the pear-shaped parasite, there is little reason to doubt that Theiler would have announced that both the disease and its causal parasite were new as early as October, 1902. That would have left nothing for Koch to do except identify the wrong tick as the carrier and fail to discover a vaccine. We do not know exactly what Laveran wrote to Theiler but what he later published[26] provides a fascinating counterpoint to Koch's report of 1898. Laveran did not base his conclusion on the suggestion made by Smith and Kilborne that the "small parasites" were the juvenile form of the large parasite. Quite the contrary, he explicitly refuted that suggestion. Laveran cited Koch's 1898 report, the report of Gray and Robertson, and Theiler's letters as evidence that the "atypical" form of the parasite is found in severe cases of the disease. But, Laveran said, Smith and Kilborne saw very small parasites only in the mild autumnal form of Texas fever. And that, Laveran said, suffices to prove that those very small parasites have nothing to do with the bacilliform parasites, which are seen in Africa only in very grave cases of the disease.

For Laveran, the fact that the small parasites seen by Smith and Kilborne were found in mild cases whereas those seen in Africa were found in severe cases proved that the two kinds of small parasites had nothing in common. For Koch, the same fact represented only a difference between his observations and those of the

"American investigators," caused "by inequality of season, of climate, of breed of cattle, or perhaps by dissimilarity in the method."
Koch made several mistakes in 1897 and 1898, Laveran made only
one in 1902 and 1903. Koch persuaded himself that the animals he
saw at Dar-es-Salaam had hemoglobinuria. Koch decided that the
small parasites he saw in 1897 and 1898 were the same as the small
parasites that Smith and Kilborne had described, even though they
looked quite different. Koch dismissed as an unanswered question
the fact that the small parasites that he saw were found in fatal cases,
whereas those that Smith and Kilborne had seen were found in mild
cases. And finally, accepting Smith and Kilborne's hypothesis,
Koch concluded that the small parasites were juvenile forms of the
large parasites. Laveran made none of those mistakes, but he did
conclude, for no very good reason, that the bacilliform parasites
were an "atypical" form of the large parasites. As far as influencing
other investigators, that was the only mistake that mattered. Koch
provided a stumbling block for Gray, Robertson, Hutcheon and
Watkins-Pitchford; Laveran provided another one for Theiler.
Since "plain matters of fact are terrible stubborn things,"[27] the
answer eventually emerged.

Even though we can analyze these events only in retrospect, and
in the light of knowledge acquired at a later date, they show how
hypotheses affect not only what people conclude but what they *see*.
Smith and Kilborne,[28] having decided that the small parasites were
the juvenile form of the large parasite, went on to say that they had
seen intermediate forms, and published a figure of a parasite in
transition from the coccus stage to the pear-shaped stage (see figure
4). Koch[29] said that the little staves can assume the form of a willow
leaf and that "between such forms and the pear-shaped form of the
fully-grown *Pyrosoma* there are a number of intermediate stages."
Koch also persuaded himself that the bacilliform parasites that he
had seen were somehow equivalent to the tiny cocci that Smith and
Kilborne had described *and* illustrated.

Since facts are stubborn things, to force an observation to conform with a theory with which it is not *quite* consistent can be very
misleading. A feeling for whether observations are or not consistent with one another or with a theory by which they are interpreted is an important part of the intuitive side of science. If Smith
and Kilborne had not arrived at their erroneous conjecture and, far
more importantly, if Koch had not forced his observations to

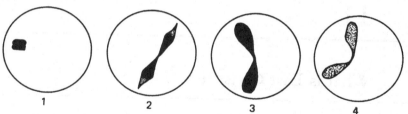

Fig. 4   An illustration supposedly showing (2) a form transitional between the "coccus" of the mild form of Texas fever (1) and the twinned, pear-shaped parasite of the acute form (3 and 4). From fig. 3 of Smith and Kilborne (see chapter 10, n. 16). In their text Smith and Kilborne said the coccus undergoes division but "the two resulting bodies are as a rule still attached to each other . . . as they continue to enlarge, the two members of the pair remaining always of the same size, a more elongated, pear-shaped outline is assumed." There is, of course, no such stage intermediate between those two unrelated parasites. Smith and Kilborne themselves said that the "enormous multiplication of the parasite in the blood shows . . . how ephemeral these intermediate stages must be."

conform with that conjecture, the entire story of East Coast fever might have been different. Different even to the point of the disease being recognized in 1897 and thereafter contained within the countries in which it long had been, and still is, endemic. From that point of view, what Koch did in 1903 and 1904 did not matter very much, but what he did and did not do in 1897 and 1898 may have mattered a great deal.

11

What is East Coast fever?

The study of East Coast fever and of other diseases caused by theilerial parasites has continued without interruption since 1910 and is very active today. I have touched very briefly on immunity and the efforts to produce a vaccine in chapter 7. Other areas of research have involved the study of the life cycle of the parasite in the tick and in the infected animal, the cultivation of the parasite *in vitro*, the taxonomic classification of the parasite[1] and the study of the way in which the parasite actually causes the disease. Each of these studies has overlapped with and involved the others but I have separated from them, somewhat artificially, a series of results that has led to the present-day view of how *Theileria parva* kills an infected animal.

Since the material reviewed in this chapter is unavoidably technical, for the reader who does not care to struggle through it, here is the bottom line: cattle suffering from East Coast fever develop what amounts to an acute leukemia[2] combined with tumors called lymphomas and, because of the destruction of the normal lymphocytes, develop immune deficiency and become susceptible to bacterial infection. Although I must use many technical terms, I often try to define them; even when I do not I hope that the gist of the argument can be grasped anyway. There is, however, no getting around three terms, lymphocyte, lymphoblast and lymphoid. Most of the cells in the blood are red blood cells, the cells that transport oxygen. For every thousand red cells in the blood there are one or two "white" blood cells (called white mostly because they are not red). Speaking very roughly indeed, one kind of white blood cell devours bacteria, bits of dead tissue and other particles that do not belong where it finds them. Another major class of white blood cells is largely concerned with producing "antibodies" to various foreign substances. That class of white blood cells is made up chiefly of lymphocytes. Some of those lymphocytes (the B cells) recognize "foreign" substances and manufacture antibodies against them; others (the T cells) also detect foreign substances but they manufacture either certain chemical messengers or chemicals that actually kill "foreign" cells.

As to the lymphoblast, it is simply a cell that divides to give rise to lymphocytes. It is the parent cell: its normal offspring, the lymphocytes, do not ordinarily divide. But they become lymphoblasts every time that they respond to a foreign substance (an "antigen"). They also become lymphoblasts if they are exposed to any substance that causes cell division (a "mitogen"). Such lymphoblasts resemble those cells in the bone marrow or the thymus that give rise to normal lymphocytes. They also resemble, more ominously, the lymphoblasts that are seen in acute lymphocytic leukemia. The word "lymphoid," often used to mean "having to do with or resembling lymphocytes" is also used to describe "lymphoid organs," such as the spleen, that are largely made up of lymphocytes.

A word of caution: although part of this chapter deals with material that belongs to the historical period, much of it deals with research done between 1960 and 1988, and does so in a field in which I have no special expert knowledge. Although I am deeply indebted to David W. Brocklesby, C. G. D. Brown, D. W. Fawcett, Maclyn McCarty, Ralph Steinman and William Trager for advice and for reading parts or all of this chapter, none of them is responsible for any omissions or misinterpretations in what is necessarily a sketchy and imperfect review of a complex series of scientific articles.

The parasite and the lymphocyte

A naive answer to the question "What is East Coast fever?" is that it is a usually fatal disease of cattle caused by a parasite that is now known as *Theileria parva parva*. But what is the nature of the disease? What part of the body is affected and why is the disease so serious?

East Coast fever does not cause hemolysis, hemoglobinuria or anemia, but all of the early students of that disease discussed it in terms of the parasites that appear in the red blood cells. The figures in Koch's article of 1898, in the joint report of Gray and Robertson, and in Laveran's article show red blood cells infested by the parasites. And the earliest debate concerned the question of whether East Coast fever was merely a variety of Texas fever, in which the parasites that occur in the red blood cells do cause hemolysis, hemoglobinuria and anemia.

But, as early as 1902, both Gray and Gray and Robertson emphasized the presence, in animals suffering from East Coast fever, of swollen lymph nodes, and pale "infarcts" in the kidneys.[3] In his interim report of March 26, 1903,[4] Koch called attention to "local lesions in certain organs which indicate that the parasites accumulate in these parts in enormous numbers." Among the lesions Koch called attention to were "the swollen and haemorrhagic condition of the different groups of lymphatic glands." Moreover, "that this is caused by the action of the parasites is proved on microscopic examination as we find in all these different parts the organisms are unusually abundant, and there we have observed a peculiar form which up to now has not been described, a form which leads to the conclusion *that here an increase of the parasites takes place* [emphasis added]." Those "peculiar forms" were presumably what we now call "Koch's blue bodies," which Koch described again in 1905.[5]

Koch's blue bodies soon came to be regarded as being sufficiently characteristic of East Coast fever to have diagnostic significance, but the fact that they are regularly seen does not prove that they are a stage in the life cycle of the parasite. K. F. Meyer, who was the first to succeed in transmitting East Coast fever by implants of spleen,[6] was convinced that they were a form of the parasite and he compared the small lymphoma-like lesions in the gut, liver, lung and kidneys to metastases. He admitted that the appearance of Koch's blue bodies in all those places could be a response to some unknown toxin but he was inclined to think that they represented the proliferation of the parasite,[6] and he remarked that "the morbid anatomy of East Coast fever resembles to a great extent the lesions found in leucaemic diseases."[7]

In a series of articles published in 1910 and 1911,[8] Richard Gonder also argued that those "peculiar forms," Koch's blue bodies, "represent a stage in the development of *P. parvum*." Gonder pointed out that the parasites undergo development in the lymphatic and "haemolymphatic" glands, in the bone marrow and in the spleen. In the blood, he added, they are seen in the large mononuclear lymphocytes. The parasite in the red blood cell, on the other hand, does not develop or divide, and can do so only "after it has entered into the tick."[9] Many of Gonder's theories of how the parasite multiplies were eventually discredited but he was correct on one crucial point: Koch's blue bodies are a stage in the life cycle of the parasite and the parasite does multiply within lymphoid cells. East Coast fever is not a disease of the red blood cells, it is a disease that affects one kind of white blood cell, the lymphocyte, and affects similar cells seen in other parts of the body. The stage of the parasite that appears in those cells is called the schizont which, to the parasitologist, means a stage that multiplies asexually, by direct splitting (schizogony). As Barnett put it in 1968:[10] "after an incubation period when no parasites can be found, schizonts are found in the lymphoid tissues of the lymph node nearest to the site of tick feeding; 1 to 3 days later, schizonts can be found in lymphoid tissues throughout the body . . . the number of schizonts increases progressively until death or recovery of the host."

The parasite thus does invade lymphocytes and, as Koch, Meyer and Gonder argued, it multiplies within them. But there are at least two possible interpretations of that fact. One is that the parasite multiplies within the lymphocytes, kills them and escapes to infect other lymphocytes. The other is that the parasites and lymphocytes multiply together, so that parasite-infected lymphocytes give rise to new lymphocytes, complete with new parasites. Gonder favored the first possibility, as did Cowdry and Danks[11] who said, in 1932, "The parasite multiplies within [the lymphocytes] without quickly killing them [but] our observations do not support the current view that the parasite acts as a powerful stimulus to the multiplication of lymphocytes." As Hulliger and her colleagues put it, much later,[12] "It was assumed by the early workers, particularly by Gonder, that the parasite, after infecting lymphocytes, multiplied by schizogony, the particles of the schizonts breaking up . . . [and then infecting] other lymphocytes."

A much more interesting possibility appeared in 1940, when Reichenow[13] claimed that "the parasites are seen in lymphocytes undergoing mitosis and the schizont can be seen to be dividing into two equal or unequal parts among the daughter cells." Normal lymphocytes do not reproduce themselves by division, either in the body or in cell culture. But Reichenow showed that, in infected cattle, at least some lymphocytes that are infected with a parasite can divide into two daughter cells and that, when they do, the parasite appears in both cells. The lymphocytes and the parasites thus multiply together.

Reichenow's finding was by no means universally accepted, but in 1945, Tsur[14] found that *Theileria annulata* will multiply in tissue culture that contains cells from the spleen. That result was confirmed by Tsur, Neitz and Pols[15] who succeeded in causing *Theileria parva* to multiply under the same conditions, as did Brocklesby and Hawking.[16] By 1962 Tsur and Adler[17] were able to carry out mass cultivation of *Theileria annulata*. (The object of such studies was, in general, to provide a supply of parasites on which the effects of drugs could be tested, or for use in experiments designed to produce vaccines.)

Reichenow's discovery came into its own in 1964, when Hulliger, Wilde, Brown and Turner published a short article in *Nature*.[18] They reported that infection of bovine lymphocytes with either *Theileria parva* or *Theileria annulata* causes those lymphocytes to divide and to proliferate. Normal lymphocytes maintained outside the animal (in "culture") do not divide; lymphocytes infected with the parasite do divide, and the parasite divides with the lymphocyte, so that each "new" lymphocyte contains a "new" parasite. And each "new" lymphocyte and its "new" parasite can and do divide again (*ad infinitum*, or at any rate for three or four months). To put the matter in simple terms, the theilerial parasite converts the normal lymphocyte into a perpetually dividing lymphoblast that resembles the cell that is seen in leukemia. Later work by Hulliger[19] and by others,[20] in particular Malmquist, Nyindo and Brown, confirmed those findings and it is now generally accepted that, as Trager put it in 1986,[21]

If a suspension of [bovine lymphocytes] from an uninfected cow is exposed to infection *in vitro* by sporozoites of *Theileria parva* . . . only those cells that become infected are capable of continuous growth *in vitro*. Similarly, in cell cultures prepared from infected cows, the already infected lymphoblasts show continuous growth *in vitro*. Each infected cell normally contains a macroschizont of the parasite with 10–17 nuclei. When the host cell divides, the parasite is also divided in two so that each daughter host cell is infected with a parasite that again grows to have 10–17 nuclei. If the parasites are killed [by use of a drug that kills the parasites but not the lymphocytes], the host cells soon stop growing. On the other hand, if the division of the lymphoblast was inhibited without inhibition of the parasites, as with colchicine or with a minimal concentration of actinomycin D, a great increase in number of parasite nuclei per cell occurred. With colchicine there were up to 100 theilerias [schizont nuclei] per lymphoblast, and the host cells showed a cytopathogenic effect . . . The association between *Theileria* and the bovine lymphoblast as it exists in tissue culture can be regarded as a symbiotic or mutualistic one even though *T. parva* is highly pathogenic to the intact bovine host. It would be of great interest to know the biochemical nature of the mitogenic effect.

The parasite and the infected animal

As Trager says, the parasite and the transformed lymphocyte develop a mutually helpful or symbiotic relationship when kept alive outside the animal, each, so to speak, causing the other to become immortal. Why *Theileria parva* is so lethal when it infects cattle thus becomes the next question. *Theileria parva* infection does produce transformed lymphocytes in infected cattle and those transformed lymphocytes do divide together with the parasites, as Reichenow showed in 1940, but there is much more to the story.

In 1960[22] Barnett found that "the production and reproduction of lymphocytes in certain tissues always accompanied the pathological changes during infection." He also found that the lesions in the kidney contained "lymphocytic masses" in which mitotic figures were common. But he regarded those "lymphocytic masses" as being "an ill-organized regenerative response to produce lymphocytes" in an animal in which the normal production of lymphocytes had been severely compromised. Barnett noted that in lymph nodes too, the early result of infection was enlargement of the node by the proliferation of lymphocytes: "many dividing forms were seen." But, in the end stage of the disease, lymphocytes disappeared from the spleen, from the lymph nodes and from the blood itself. Thus death seemed to occur not as the immediate result of a great proliferation of lymphocytes but as a result of their later disappearance.

In 1966, Jarrett and Brocklesby[23] reported that "The salient feature of the primary reaction to *T. parva* is lymph node enlargement. This is caused by replacement of the normal node architecture by massive lymphoblastic hyperplasia; examination of smears in the light microscope at this stage usually fails to reveal the presence of the parasites. The cause of this hyperplasia is unknown." Even examination with the electron microscope failed to reveal parasites in this early stage of lymph node enlargement. Only at a later stage were the macroschizonts (Koch's blue bodies) seen. Unable to explain the early proliferation of lymphocytes in which no parasites were seen, Jarrett and Brocklesby suggested that perhaps "some factor associated with the parasites causes this hyperplasia in preparation for later invasion by the parasite itself" and cited Barnett's idea that "a diffusible factor is liberated by the parasite which may be initially stimulating to [the tissues that produce lymphocytes]."

In short, a considerable gap remained between the observation that the parasite and the transformed lymphocyte divide together in tissue culture and the observation that in the infected animal no parasites are seen in the lymphocytes at the time when they begin to proliferate. Nor was the finding that infected lymphocytes and their parasites divide together universally accepted.[24] But, as we have seen, by 1970, Malmquist, Nyindo and Brown[25] had definitively confirmed that finding and had introduced a procedure for cultivating *Theileria parva* infected lymphocytes that is still in use. In 1971, Moulton, Krauss and Malmquist said that "the outstanding features of [East Coast fever] are the presence of Theileria in lymphoblasts, hyperplasia of almost neoplastic proportions, and metastasis of lymphoblasts throughout the body." They added that, at a later stage, "lymphoblasts undergo simultaneous degeneration and the parasites enter the erythrocytes."[26] In the discussion section of their article they referred to the "unlimited growth of parasitized lymphoblasts" in tissue culture and said that "it is reasonable to assume that the same process occurs *in vivo*, thus providing a means for propagation and dissemination of the parasite in large numbers." But that was still only a "reasonable assumption."

In 1973, DeMartini and Moulton[27] returned to the question in a study of the microscopic changes in lymph nodes in calves infected with East Coast fever. They published their article in our old friend, the *Journal of Comparative Pathology and Therapeutics*, its name now modernized to the *Journal of Comparative Pathology*. DeMartini and Moulton noted that "Lack of information concerning the cell type first entered by the parasite, the mechanism of spread of parasitized lymphoblasts throughout the lymphoid tissues of the body, and the ultrastructural features of affected lymph nodes and parasitized cells provided the impetus for the present study." They confirmed earlier findings of the initial proliferation and subsequent destruction of lymphocytes in the lymph nodes. And, once again, they found early proliferation of lymphocytes that did not appear to be parasitized. They also found, at a later stage, parasite-containing lymphoblasts "often in mitosis." They were unable to "elucidate the mechanism of destruction of lymphoid cells in affected nodes" but they suggested that that phenomenon might have "an immunological basis." Overall, at least implicitly, they agreed with the notion that the "immortalization" of parasite-infected lymphocytes in tissue culture must find its counterpart in the disease itself.

In 1974, Radley and his colleagues[28] studied the development of East Coast fever in cattle infected by a carefully controlled dose of material obtained from infected ticks. With larger doses of infectious material, the interval before the appearance of signs of disease (the prepatent period) was shorter, the interval before the appearance of fever was shorter, and time to death was shorter. But macroschizonts (Koch's blue bodies) were never seen, no matter how large the dose, before the fifth day. *However*, since "the relationship between prepatent period and infectious dose was otherwise linear . . . our results . . . suggest that there is another stage in the life cycle of *T. parva* . . . between the infective particle and the uninuclear primary macroschizont in a lymphoid cell." In other words, Radley and his colleagues suggested that the infectious stage of the parasite enters the lymphoid cells almost immediately and then requires a few days to "mature" into its next stage, the macroschizont. At that point, as earlier work had shown, the macroschizont and the transformed lymphocyte begin to multiply together.

In 1981, Morrison and his colleagues[29] studied the development of East Coast fever from initial infection through to the death of the animal. In particular, they examined the changes in the number of parasites and the changes in the number of lymphocytes in the various organs. A standard dose of material obtained from infected ticks was used to infect calves. Two injections were given, the lymph node nearest one injection being biopsied at regular intervals, the node near the other injection being left for study at postmortem. The infected cattle were killed at different times after being infected, apart from one that died of the disease nineteen days after being infected. Similar studies were made on nineteen other cattle.

As in earlier studies, several days elapsed before parasites were detected in any of the lymph nodes, even the node closest to the site of injection. In this study the "prepatent" period was 7.3 days on average. Once they first appeared the number of parasitized cells increased steadily. The number of lymphocytes in the nodes also showed an initial rise, but eventually fell again, to below normal, until the animal died or was sacrificed. The number of lymphocytes in the nodes, blood and spleen also increased, but eventually fell again, sometimes to levels well below normal. Overall, the findings confirmed those of Barnett: first a rise and eventually a fall in the number of lymphocytes. Morrison and his colleagues[30] reviewed these and other studies in 1986 and drew a picture of the course of the disease which, as oversimplified by me, follows.

When an infected tick bites an animal, a tiny parasite carried in its saliva enters some of the lymphocytes. After about three days, that parasite becomes closely involved with the system that causes those cells to divide. As a result it turns a normal lymphocyte into a lymphoblast. Normal lymphoblasts divide and proliferate, in a controlled way, into normal lymphocytes. But if all of the lymphocytes become lymphoblasts and divide in an uncontrolled way, leukemia is the result. Immature cells, unable to function as producers of antibodies, but able to divide, replace all of the normal cells. Instead of dividing into two normal lymphocytes, the lymphoblast divides into two more lymphoblasts, which go right on dividing. And, since normal cells become thus abnormal when invaded by the parasite, and since the parasite not only forces the cell to divide but divides with it, the body becomes pervaded by ceaselessly dividing lymphoblasts. Those cells spread throughout the body, creating small tumors such as the "white infarcts" in the kidney. And they drive out, replace, and even kill the normal lymphocytes. As Morrison *et al.* say, "These cells behave essentially like tumor cells; they multiply in an uncontrolled manner and eventually replace much of the normal lymphoid tissue in a wide variety of organs." But, as the end approaches, the abnormal lymphoid cells die. At the end, the normal lymphocytes have vanished, and, along with them, their ability to produce the antibodies that protect the animal against infection. Deprived of its lymphocytes, the animal is immune deficient. If the many tumors that spread throughout its body do not kill it, infection by other organisms will kill it. The small tumors that Barnett thought might be new centers of production of normal lymphocytes are, in fact, metastases, caused by the spread of lymphoblasts, converted to a malignant state by their embrace with the parasite. In cell culture, the embrace of the cell and the parasite causes each to become immortal. In the animal, where the lymphocyte has a vital role to play, that embrace is fatal: the host dies, and with the host, the lymphocytes and their parasites also die.

The host, its lymphoblasts and most of their parasites die, but not quite soon enough to protect future generations of cattle. Some of the "macroschizonts" or Koch's blue bodies, live long enough to give rise to "microschizonts" which leave the dying white cell and change into another form of the parasite, which in turn enters the red cells. There the parasite becomes our old friend the "bacilliform" parasite. And when a brown tick feeds on an already doomed animal, it ingests, along with its meal of blood, those bacilliform parasites. After few more transformations within the tick, some of which require the tick to moult, those parasites enter the saliva of the tick, ready to kill more cattle. The cattle die but the ticks and the parasites survive, as does East Coast fever.

Infection by inoculation

If the parasite is contained within the lymphocytes in the blood, inoculation of healthy animals with blood or with infected cells from the spleen might be expected to transmit East Coast fever. Yet, as we saw in chapter 7, early investigators failed to transmit the disease by inoculation of blood, spleen or lymph nodes. And when later investigators did succeed in transmitting the disease in that way, the success rate was variable and never reached anything like 100 percent. In 1971, Brown and his colleagues[31] returned to this problem using infected lymphocytes grown outside the animal. Injection of 10 million (10^7) lymphocytes usually transmitted the disease; in two cattle fatal cases were induced by the injection of a 1,000 million (10^9) lymphocytes. But the majority of the cattle that were injected with between 100,000 and 1,000 million cells showed only "minor or inapparent reactions." In an interesting sequel to that study, published in 1978, Brown and his colleagues showed that if blood was taken from a healthy animal and its lymphocytes were infected by allowing ticks to feed on the blood, reinjection of those lymphocytes into the donor animal *invariably* caused patent East Coast fever.[32] But the same number of infected lymphocytes, injected into other animals, never caused either East Coast fever or any sign of immunity to East Coast fever (except in the special case in which the blood was injected into an identical twin of the original donor). The injection of as few as 4 million infected cells into the animal from which they had been obtained caused East Coast fever, but had no effect on animals unrelated to the donor. Brown *et al.* suggested that when the infected cells were injected into the animal from which they came, they were easily able to multiply, and to cause the parasite to multiply with them, thus causing frank East Coast fever. But when the infected cells were injected into an animal unrelated to the donor, they were "rejected," much as an organ transplant can be rejected, and the parasites were rejected with them. Brown *et al.* thus explained why so many of the early efforts to transmit East Coast fever by inoculation failed. Such experiments succeed if the white cells are able to survive in the donor animal and fail if they are rejected. (In the earlier study infection could be transmitted, but only by the injection of some 1,000 million infected cells compared with the far smaller number of infected cells that sufficed if they had come from the same animal into which they were again injected. Presumably when many millions of cells are injected some of the parasites escape and succeed in infecting the animals even though the injected lymphocytes are themselves rejected. In later studies,[33] it has been found that the injection of as few as 100 infected lymphocytes into the animal from which they were obtained can cause East Coast fever.)

The transformed lymphocyte

As we saw earlier, infected cells obtained from the spleen can be grown in tissue culture and can continue to divide for many generations of cell and parasite. But those cells were already infected when they were removed from the animal. It was not until 1973 that Brown and his colleagues[34] succeeded in infecting normal lymphoid cells outside of the donor animal. Lymphoid cells were exposed to parasites derived from infected ticks, and some cultured cells, taken from mesenteric lymph nodes, became infected and transformed into "immortalized" lymphoblasts. But the same procedure failed to infect cultured cells taken from the spleen or from the blood. This posed a problem for the assumption that the natural infection is caused by the parasite entering the lymphocytes that circulate in the animal's blood or by entering lymphocytes attracted to the area bitten by the tick.

In 1980, Stagg and his colleagues,[35] using the electron microscope, obtained further proof for the ideas of Reichenow and of Hulliger and her colleagues by showing that the macroschizont (Koch's blue body) becomes intimately associated with the chromosomes of the lymphocyte that, once infected, divides along with its parasite. In the next year, 1981, Stagg and his colleagues[36] succeeded in the *in vitro* infection of lymphocytes obtained from bovine blood. Infectious material derived from ticks was added to lymphocytes obtained from the blood of healthy cattle; after the cells and the infective material were mixed and allowed to stand for 20 minutes, the mixture was introduced into a flask containing cultured spleen cells. Although spleen cells were present, sophisticated light microscopy showed that, within one hour, the infectious particles (the "sporozoites") attached themselves to the lymphocytes that came from the blood. By 20 hours the sporozoites were regularly detected *within* the white blood cells, where they became associated with a structure associated with protein synthesis, the Golgi apparatus. By the third day, Koch's blue bodies (macroschizonts) were seen. This study thus made a major step towards filling the gap in time between the initial infection of the lymphocyte and the later appearance of the form of the parasite that "transforms" and "immortalizes" the white blood cells and divides along with them. A *single* infectious particle (a *single* sporozoite) was enough to infect and transform a white blood cell.

In the same year, Musisi and his colleagues[37] also showed increased activity of the Golgi apparatus in cells that had not yet developed macroschizonts. They suggested that once the parasite became involved with the Golgi complex "The parasite is then treated as a chromosome and is drawn with the spindle contraction into the respective daughter cells prior to cytoplasmic division." They referred to the earlier findings of Reichenow[13] and of Hulliger *et al.*[12] as evidence that the parasite is ordinarily split between the two daughter cells. They added that "It is also not known whether these lymphoblasts are T or B lymphocyte precursors," a question that would soon be answered. Near the end of their article they asked "Could there be a relationship between what is happening here and the unexplained proliferative behavior of neoplastic cells and those having oncogenic [cancer-causing] viruses?"

Also in 1981, Kurtti and his colleagues[38] compared cultures of cells that had been parasitized for a long time (and were thus transformed into "immortalized" lymphoblasts) with cells freshly infected with the parasite. They concluded, among other things, that after some generations the newly parasitized cells increasingly resembled the cells that had been parasitized for a long time. As early workers had argued, Kurtti and his colleagues found that, after two or three days, small parasites could be found near the nucleus of newly infected cells and that cell division began around the third day.

In 1982, Fawcett and his colleagues[39] showed that the parasite can enter lymphoid cells within minutes. They pointed out that Stagg *et al.*[35] had detected very early stages of the invasion of lymphocytes by the parasite and they presented their own observations, made with the electron microscope. Fawcett and his colleagues showed that the tick-transmitted forms of the parasite, the "sporozoites," "do attach to bovine lymphoid cells *in vitro*, are rapidly interiorized, and subsequently become localized in the Golgi region." Fawcett and his colleagues expressed surprise at how quickly this happened: "somewhat unexpected was the rapidity of the entry process. Previous studies had suggested that bovine cells might be infected within an hour or two. In the present . . . study, sporozoites were frequently found within lymphoid cells within 10 min. It is likely that considerably less time is required."

The mature macroschizont (Koch's blue body) usually contains eight nuclei, whereas the form of the parasite that invades the lymphocyte (the sporozoite) contains only one nucleus, as does its successor, the trophozoite. In 1983, Jura, Brown and Kelly[40] showed that within 24 hours from a lymphocyte being infected by *Theileria annulata* the trophozoite changes into a form that has two nuclei, those two nuclei divide into four, and those four into eight. Thus within 24 hours the lymphocyte contains what might be regarded as an immature macroschizont, containing two nuclei. When the mature macroschizont, with eight nuclei, has been formed, the parasite and the lymphocyte begin to divide. Earlier studies, beginning with those of Reichenow and of Hulliger and her colleagues had shown that the parasite then splits into two parts, one of which appears in each new lymphocyte. More than that, as Jura, Brown and Rowland[41] showed in 1983, just before the earliest signs of division of the lymphocyte, the eight nuclei of the parasite divide into sixteen nuclei, so that each new lymphocyte is infected with a fully developed parasite complete with eight nuclei. Thus from the moment the parasite enters the lymphocyte, the process of mitosis begins. Initially the nuclei of the parasite multiply until a multinucleated parasite results. Just before the lymphocyte itself divides, the nuclei of the parasite undergo a final doubling in number, so that when the lymphocyte divides each new lymphocyte contains a parasite with as many nuclei as the parasite in the parent lymphocyte.

In 1984, Fawcett and his colleagues[42] pushed the moment of entry of the parasite into the cell a little earlier. They exposed bovine lymphocytes to the infectious parasite and, with the electron microscope, obtained photographs of the parasite adhering to the cell wall and then entering the cell. Although their earliest photographs were obtained 10 minutes after exposure of the cell to the parasites, they suggested that "It seems likely . . . that the actual entry process requires 5 min or less." They added that "In the intracellular environment the sporozoite rapidly begins its differentiation into [its next stage] the trophozoite." And, within 48 to 72 hours, that next stage "has usually undergone nuclear division to form a multinucleate early schizont." That "multinucleate early schizont" is of course, Koch's blue body, which goes on to cause the transformation of the lymphocyte into an endlessly dividing lymphoblast.

One part of the picture thus seemed to be reasonably complete by 1984. The form of the parasite that enters the animal via the saliva of the tick invades lymphocytes almost immediately, within at most a few minutes. It soon changes to its next stage, the "trophozoite." The trophozoites divide and provide the nuclei of the macroschizont or Koch's blue body. From then on the infected lymphocyte becomes a lymphoblast. That transformed cell and its parasite and their offspring divide repeatedly. In the infected animal, those transformed cells spread throughout the body causing small tumors and destroying normal lymphocytes, a process that ends some two to three weeks later with the death of the animal.

The T cell

But other questions arise: What kind of lymphocyte is transformed into being a malignant lymphoblast? How does the parasite convert a healthy lymphocyte into a cell that resembles a malignant tumor cell? And why are normal lymphocytes killed?

According to a recent review,[29] the parasite can even infect cells that are very different from the white blood cell, namely fibroblasts. It can also invade one kind of "scavenger" white blood cell, the macrophage.[43] But the only cell lines that perpetuate themselves in cell culture are those made up of lymphocytes and it is all but certain that the sole natural target of the parasite is the lymphocyte. There are two kinds of lymphocyte, the B cell and the T cell. They look the same under the microscope and they both "recognize" foreign substances, but the B cell produces antibodies whereas the T cell is more concerned with producing substances which act as a signal or stimulus to other white blood cells. Some T cells are also "killer" cells, producing substances that can kill cells of the body that have become abnormal.[44]

In 1965, a year after the first report by Hulliger and her colleagues, two articles appeared in *Nature*[45] reporting the discovery that human lymphocytes produce a soluble substance that promotes division of other human lymphocytes. That soluble substance soon came to be known as T cell growth factor (TCGF); in 1979 it received a new name, interleukin 2 (IL-2). By 1980[46] it had been shown both that certain kinds of T cells produce this "soluble substance" and that certain kinds of T cells multiply if, and only if, that substance is present.

Two studies appeared in 1981, one of which[47] showed that T cell growth factor can "support the long term growth of T cells ... from patients with various [malignant tumors made up of T cells]." The other study[48] showed the same thing and, in addition, showed that cells grown from such tumors can *produce* T cell growth factor. Thus[48] "It is possible that a major abnormality in these disorders is the capacity of the same malignant cell to produce and respond to its own growth factor." Later the same year one particular kind of malignant T cell was found to produce T cell growth factor in large quantities, which held out the hope that enough TCGF (IL-2) could be produced to allow its chemical structure to be determined.[49]

Meanwhile evidence had begun to suggest that the lymphocytes that become infected in East Coast fever, or at any rate the infected lymphocytes that can be maintained in cell culture, might be T cells and, in 1981, Pinder and her associates[50] announced their conclusion that "All Theileria-infected lymphoblastoid cells derived from infected cattle" appeared to be T cells and said "We submit that only lymphocytes ... [that come from] a discrete subpopulation of T lymphocytes are susceptible to transformation by the *T. parva* infective particle."

In 1985 Brown and Grab[51] developed a pure line of bovine T cells, "cloned" from a single cell. That strain of T cells was strictly dependent for its growth on the presence in the culture medium of T cell growth factor. In 1986 Brown and Logan[52] reported the results of infecting that strain of bovine T cells with *Theileria parva*. They found that infected cells in cell culture do produce a growth factor: when the solution in which those cells had been growing was added to a culture of cells that grow only in the presence of T cell growth factor some growth occurred in that second culture. Thus infected cells can produce a growth factor that resembles T cell growth factor, although Brown and Logan were not able, in 1986, to say with certainty what that factor was and referred to it only as having "TCGF-like activity." Brown and Logan also showed that infected cells proliferate more rapidly if they are exposed to externally produced T cell growth factor.

In introducing and in discussing their findings, Brown and Logan pointed out that "The schizont and the lymphocyte divide synchronously, but the mechanism by which the parasite effects lymphoproliferation is unknown." But if the cells were exposed to drugs that kill the parasite, "the resulting uninfected cells continued through only a few cell divisions before death ensued." And "Thus, the mechanism of lymphocyte transformation by *Theileria* parasites does not appear to be by permanent alteration of the host genome, but is more likely due to a reversible parasite-mediated induction of host growth regulating mechanisms." Their fundamental conclusion was that the parasite-infected lymphocytes do produce a "growth factor" that promotes multiplication of lymphocytes.

In 1988 Dobbelaere and his colleagues[53] summarized the situation by saying that Brown and Logan had shown that clones of bovine T cells do not require an outside source of growth factor to grow, once they have been infected with *Theileria parva*, and had shown that *Theileria*-infected T cells produce a growth factor. But, Dobbelaere *et al.* asked, is the growth factor that is produced by infected T cells necessary for their own growth? In their words, "no evidence has been presented that Theileria-infected lymphocytes are themselves dependent on the presence of such a growth factor." In other words, such cells might be "immortalized" for some other reason, and just incidentally happen also to produce a growth factor. Alternatively, their growth might depend on the growth factor that they themselves produce.

Dobbelaere and his colleagues concluded that when T cells are infected with *Theileria parva* they do start producing a growth factor (as Brown and Logan had shown) and it is that self-produced growth factor that leads to the continuous multiplication of the cells. The growth factor is produced inside the cell but in order to act it must bind to the outside of the cell. If there is a large number of cells in a small volume of fluid, the growth factor that diffuses out of each cell into that fluid will accumulate there in a high concentration and growth will be rapid. If there are only a few cells in a large volume of fluid, the growth factor will be diluted in that large volume and growth will be slowed. And that is what Dobbelaere *et al.* did find: if cells growing at a certain rate in a small volume of fluid were placed in a larger volume of fluid, thus diluting the growth factor, the rate of growth slowed. Moreover, the addition of growth factor to the fluid restored the growth rate.

But the presence of growth factor does not lead to proliferation of lymphoblasts unless those cells have, on their outer surface, "receptors" to which the growth factor can bind. Dobbelaere *et al.* showed that infection of the lymphocyte by *Theileria parva* has another important result: not only does it cause the cells to produce a growth factor, it causes them to develop receptors for that growth factor. Additional proof of the importance of the receptors was obtained from experiments on cells that were exposed to a drug that kills the parasite but does not harm the cell itself. The cells then stop dividing, after a time, partly because they no longer produce growth factor. But only partly for that reason. If growth factor from an outside source is added, the cells will continue to proliferate for a little while longer, but not forever. Without their parasites they stop producing the surface receptors to which the growth factor can bind and they gradually lose the receptors that they already had. Thus the parasite changes the cell in two crucial ways: its presence causes the cell to produce a growth factor *and* it causes it to create, on its outer surface, the receptors to which that growth factor must bind in order to promote cell division.

What next?

By mid-July, 1902, only four months after Lionel Cripps noted that "large numbers of cattle are dying . . . in Melsetter the disease is spreading and it is now bad in Salisbury," all of the eight cattle that had been brought from Natal to Rhodesia to see if they were immune to "Rhodesian Redwater" had died. Taking note of the death of those cattle Marshall Clarke and Alfred Milner decided that it would be prudent to have an expert come out from England to study what might, after all, prove to be a new disease. Eighty-six years later, July, 1988 saw the publication of the article by Dobbelaere and his colleagues that went some way towards explaining why animals infected with East Coast fever develop tumor-like masses made up of proliferating lymphoblasts.

But many questions remain. It is not known exactly how T cell growth factor acts to promote cell division; it is not known exactly how the parasite causes the cell to produce growth factor; it is not known how the parasite causes the cell to produce surface receptors; and it is not known why the parasite divides along with the cell. After all, the growth factor that is produced by the parasite-infected cells can promote growth in any T cell that has surface receptors for that growth factor, and those cells divide just as rapidly as parasite-infected cells. What is, in a sense, the single most distinctive feature of East Coast fever, the fact that the parasites and the cells divide together, remains wholly unexplained.

As Trager said in 1986,[21] "It would be of great interest to know the biochemical nature of the mitogenic effect." It would also be of great interest to know whether the parasite-infected lymphocyte is a realistic model of human leukemia and lymphoma. Morrison *et al.* remarked, in 1986,[30] that "the infected cells are similar in their behavior to lymphoid tumor cells" even though there is no permanent change in their genetic structure. But the very fact that the change is not necessarily permanent is one of the intriguing facts about this parasite-induced malignant tumor. As Dobbelaere and his colleagues said[53]

Most systems used to study transformation and tumorigenesis ... are irreversible because they involve permanent alterations in the genóme ... *Theileria*-infected lymphoblastoid cells are exceptional in that immortalization is caused by a parasite present in the cytoplasm of the infected cell ... the unlimited growth potential *can readily be reversed* [emphasis added] by elimination of the parasite by specific antitheilerial drugs.

Dobbelaere and his colleagues added that "The way in which the parasite effects host-cell transformation is still unresolved." The question of whether the parasite-transformed cells have something fundamental in common with the cells of lymphatic leukemia or whether the differences are more important than the interesting similarities is also still unanswered.

The possibility that the study of theileriosis might provide clues to the understanding of leukemia and lymphoma is interesting enough. Just as provocative is the fact that the cells that are infected by the theilerial parasite appear to be T cells. And once the cells have become so leukemia-like that only immature cells are left to multiply and no mature cells are left to function normally, the victim develops an immune-deficient state and may even succumb to overwhelming bacterial infection.

These facts are well known to those who study the parasite that causes East Coast fever. I do not know to what extent they have influenced those scientists who study lymphocytic leukemia and lymphoma or those scientists who study another condition caused by a failure of normal T-cell function, AIDS. If the ability of the theilerial parasite to induce leukemia, lymphomas and immune deficiency contributes in any important way to an understanding of any of those conditions, we may have to give Koch a better grade for his study of East Coast fever, simply because he said, on March 26, 1903, that the finding of "peculiar forms" in certain lesions shows "that here an increase of the parasites takes place."

12

Epilogue

An anti-heroic history of East Coast fever might go something like this: in 1901 East Coast fever invaded Rhodesia. Well-trained veterinarians failed to recognize that it was a new disease. That failure did not really matter because before anyone could have identified it as being new, the disease had entrenched itself so thoroughly that it was eradicated only after fifty years of intensive work. Robert Koch did recognize that the disease was new, and Charles Lounsbury and Arnold Theiler did identify the tick that transmits the parasite, and did characterize the parasite. None of that mattered very much, because, without a treatment or a vaccine, the fifty years devoted to controlling the disease had to rely largely on long-established techniques such as quarantine, fencing and slaughter of infected animals. Since the search for an expert was badly handled, Koch missed a whole season in which to study the disease, but that did not really matter, because Arnold Theiler and Charles Lounsbury were already at work. Koch might have reached Rhodesia sooner than he did and identified the disease as being new sooner than he did, but that did not matter because the disease had become entrenched long before any expert was invited and because Lounsbury, Theiler and Hutcheon were becoming increasingly convinced that the disease was a new one. Bruce might have been a better choice than Koch but even Bruce could not have discovered a cure or a vaccine or reversed the spread of the disease. It might have made a difference if Koch had actually identified the disease in 1897 and warned the countries of southern Africa not to import cattle from the coast of East Africa, but he did not.

What mattered most about the East Coast fever episode was that it did happen and that it caused serious social and economic problems. Both Rhodesia and the Transvaal recovered fairly quickly from what proved to be a temporary setback, but it was not obvious at the time that they would recover – a deep social unease was a major cost of the new plague. And the center did not hold. London did not provide an expert; the expert who came from Berlin provided neither cure nor immunization.

Even a determinedly anti-heroic historian might concede that there were a few other things that mattered, and some that might yet matter. The development of a relatively safe dip for cattle and the widespread introduction of its use may not seem like a glamorous breakthrough, but without it cattle-raising in Africa on the scale now practiced would be impossible. Koch did observe that the parasite that causes East Coast fever multiplies in lymphatic tissues and, as we saw in chapter 11, the pursuit of that observation has led to many exciting discoveries and may well lead to more. On an immediately practical level, the disease was discovered, its vector and its causal parasite were discovered, and, as a result, the chances of its being once again accidentally introduced somewhere in the world have been much reduced. Of equal importance, we can be all but certain that the disease would be quickly diagnosed and, one hopes, its spread quickly brought under control.

It is curious to think that if Theobald Smith had not made an error in 1893, Koch might have discovered East Coast fever in 1897. It is even more curious to think that if phylloxera had not appeared in the Cape, the government of the Cape might not have decided, in 1893, to employ an entomologist. No phylloxera, no Lounsbury?[1] Since the center did not hold, it was fortunate that there were local institutions that did work. Without the support of the Department of Agriculture of the Cape Colony and without the support of the newly-created and well-funded Department of Agriculture of the Transvaal (funded from the center, to be sure), Lounsbury and Theiler could hardly have done what they did. They did almost everything except publicly assert that the disease was a new one. Were they too cautious?

Scientific caution and rationalization

I have repeatedly suggested that Gray, Robertson, Hutcheon and Theiler held back from recognizing that "Rhodesian redwater" was a new disease because they relied too heavily on the great authority of Robert Koch, and, to a lesser degree, on the advice of Lignières, Laveran and Nocard. I have even argued that to force an observation to conform to a theory can be very misleading. But there is another side to the story: scientists, perhaps more than most people, hesitate to invoke radically new explanations or to admit that a new observation demands that all their assumptions be reinterpreted. If one does not admit that a new observation requires a radically new explanation one must find a way to fit that observation into the existing framework. One must either do that or rationalize it, i.e. explain it away. The East Coast fever episode provides many examples of rationalization.

When Smith and Kilborne noted that there were two clinically distinct forms of Texas fever and two parasites of very different appearance, they were uneasy in their conclusion that they were dealing with a single disease and with the juvenile and adult forms of a single kind of parasite. They carefully discussed and ruled out the possibility that the small 'coccus-like bodies" might be arte-facts. They added that "If we admit their parasitic nature as highly probable we have still the question before us whether they are stages of the Texas fever parasite or of another parasite transmitted with it." They said that that question could not be answered with certainty until the transformation of one stage of the parasite into the other could be seen in culture or in the blood of infected animals. But, they said, both forms were seen in every infected animal. Moreover, two animals that had recovered from the acute form of Texas fever, and in whom the number of red cells was returning towards normal, suddenly suffered a relapse; the small form of the parasite appeared and the destruction of red cells resumed. This happened at a time when the field was free of ticks, so a new infection could be ruled out. (They did not consider the possibility that simultaneous infection with two diseases might lead to the appearance of one of those diseases in a few days and to the appear-ance of the other disease only after a few weeks.) And they per-suaded themselves that they had actually seen the tiny parasites divide, elongate, and transform into the pear-shaped parasites. They even argued that the coccus-like bodies were seen most readily when their development into the pear-shaped parasite was retarded because of "a low temperature of the air . . . [or] partial immunity."

That reasoning may seem labored, but consider how improbable the correct explanation was: two distinct parasites, both seen in red blood cells and sometimes in the same red blood cell, each capable of destroying red blood cells; two distinct parasites transmitted by the same tick, each capable of passing forward via the egg of that tick; each parasite capable of being transmitted from one animal to another by the inoculation of blood; two diseases caused by the bite of a single tick, one disease arising in a few days and the other only after some weeks; and every animal always suffering from both of those diseases. The true state of affairs was indeed almost as improbable as the discovery of a new continent!

When Robert Koch studied what we now know was East Coast fever in German East Africa he had to make a number of "adjustments" to persuade himself that he was dealing only with a virulent form of Texas fever. He persuaded himself that the clinical findings and post-mortem findings were identical with those described by Smith and Kilborne, although it does not seem possible that they could have been. But his major rationalization had to do with the bacilliform parasites, which did not look like the tiny cocci described by Smith and Kilborne and were, in any event, seen only in severe and fatal cases rather than in mild cases. I am not sure whether Koch's comment on that deserves to be dignified as a rationalization: he merely said that it might be due to differences in the climate, the breed of cattle, the time of year or the experimental method.

Almost as soon as Gray saw cases of "Rhodesian redwater" he knew that it differed from ordinary redwater. It attacked supposedly immune animals, it did not produce hemoglobinuria and it caused severe pulmonary edema. Gray attributed the pulmonary edema to the altitude and he searched the literature for descriptions of disorders of the lung in Texas fever. Finding no such descriptions even in Lignières, he nevertheless "assumed" from a remark of Lignières that someone had in fact mentioned such disorders. And he did find one article that indicated that hemoglobinuria is not necessarily characteristic of redwater. As to the lack of immunity, he argued that that was only to be expected because the animals were infested with an unusually large number of ticks and because the disease had apparently increased in virulence when it was transmitted through a series of susceptible animals.

When Robertson undertook a systematic study of the blood of cattle infected with "Rhodesian redwater" he found that it almost always contained the small bacilliform parasites and almost never contained the large pear-shaped parasites typically found in Texas fever. He accepted Koch's view that the small parasite was the juvenile form of the large one, but he added a new rationalization to the growing list: the disease was so virulent that the animals died before the small parasites had time to mature into the large pear-shaped form.

Duncan Hutcheon, whose articles of early 1903 give all of the reasons why "Rhodesian redwater" must have been a new disease, backed away because of the views of "eminent bacteriologists" and because of the views on immunity that Lignières had sent to Theiler. But Hutcheon found another rationalization: the increased virulence and altered character of the disease were caused by simultaneous infection of the animal by two species of ticks. And Arnold Theiler, as convinced as Hutcheon was that the disease was a new one, and dissuaded from saying so by the same reasons that dissuaded Hutcheon, provided one final rationalization for the differences between "Rhodesian redwater" and ordinary redwater, namely "that it is principally from the location of the parasite [in the tissues] that the cause of the difference in the symptoms arises."

The interplay between the slow and tedious accumulation of experimental evidence and the acquiring of sudden insights into the meaning of the evidence thus accumulated is a well-known feature of the scientific method. The attempt to fit new facts into old interpretations may delay the process of forming new insights but it also guards against the proliferation of arbitrary hypotheses. Nor are scientific advances caused by public demands that something be done – not, at any rate, unless competent scientists, well trained and capable of solving problems, are already at work in well-administered and well-funded institutions. Theiler and Lounsbury were not the first to announce that a new disease had appeared in Rhodesia and the Transvaal, but the meticulous way in which they gathered evidence and tested their findings seems to me to provide a textbook example of the power of self-critical, systematic and methodical investigation of a complex problem.[2]

The center and the periphery

Recent studies of science in the British empire have drawn attention to the interactions between Great Britain as the center or metropolis and the colonies as the frontier or periphery. It has also been suggested that the notion of a single center be replaced by that of a "moving metropolis."[3] In the East Coast fever episode there were, in fact, several centers and several peripheral areas. We might imagine a map of the world, with small disks to identify peripheral areas, large disks to identify centers, and thick or thin arrows between the disks to show how much information flowed, and of what quality, and in what direction. But every network thus defined will differ in its elements and their relative weight from every other network. Are we to look at the map of the center–periphery relationships of the British empire as a social or political or economic phenomenon? Or should we examine the center–periphery relationships of "science," or of agricultural science, or veterinary practice, or veterinary research, or bacteriology, or parasitology, or the study of ticks, or the network of experts on Texas fever?[4] (In 1901 there was no network of experts on East Coast fever.) In addition, no single network persisted unchanged throughout the East Coast fever episode. Many centers, many peripheral areas, many networks interacting, all in flux – what can one do except look at some specific examples?

Great Britain was the place where most of the veterinarians who coped with East Coast fever had been trained: Hutcheon, Gray, Stockman, Watkins-Pitchford and all of Gray's veterinary staff.[5] Apart from that, it was one of the least important centers of the East Coast fever story, ill-equipped as it was to supply either experts or expert advice suited to a study of a parasitic disease of cattle in southern Africa. The East Coast fever episode cannot serve as an example of the relationship between the center and the periphery within the British empire proper, except as an example of what happens when the center is called upon for help and cannot produce it. Only three men in Great Britain were qualified to do veterinary research; two of them were otherwise committed and one was serving with the Army in the Boer War. And the Royal Society was able to produce one and only one additional candidate, David Bruce.

Great Britain was a center for practical veterinary education, and in 1902 it was certainly a center for science at large, with more Nobel prizes in physics in the offing than any other country in the world. Although Great Britain was a late arrival to the field of the study of parasitic diseases of human beings in 1902 it was emerging as an important center, with Ross's Nobel prize in the offing. But, unless one looks on David Bruce as a one-man center, it was not a center for research into parasitic diseases of animals in subtropical countries. Nor did the Cape Town–Edinburgh–London network of skillful practical and academic veterinarians include Bruce. Bruce's merits were recognized by a self-perpetuating Royal Society meritocracy that did not include a single Fellow who was also a Fellow of the Royal College of Veterinary Surgeons (even John McFadyean never became a Fellow of the Royal Society). The apparent absence of cross-links between the veterinary network, which did not include Bruce, and the Royal Society network, which did, is a striking feature of the search for an expert. It is equally striking that both the veterinary network and the Royal Society were unaware of the merits of Arnold Theiler, whereas Bruce asked for Theiler's services. Bruce and Theiler had formed a high opinion of each other while they were working in the periphery, i.e. in South Africa.

It might be argued that Chamberlain tried to confine the East Coast fever problem to the single center–periphery relationship of Great Britain and Rhodesia, or to that of Great Britain and the southern African colonies, whereas the Chartered Company was perfectly willing to turn to other centers for help. But the initial approaches to Texas and Baton Rouge were made by Gray, acting on his own knowledge, and the initial requests for advice directed to Lignières, Laveran and Nocard were made by Theiler, also acting on his own. They acted on their own, but they acted in terms of their professional training, skills, knowledge and traditions, i.e. as members of the network of trained veterinarians. One must not, as MacLeod[3] has reminded us, neglect the traditions "of different *corps d'élite* – the professional motivations and abilities . . . of which the stuff of history is made."

Although Lignières did not play a decisive role in the study of East Coast fever, he was a prominent member of the Texas fever network, and the role he did play provides a striking example of the existence of many centers and many peripheral areas. He began at an undoubted and major center, the long-established veterinary faculty of Alfort. He went from there to the Argentine, where his book on Texas fever, written in French, was published in Buenos Aires. Buenos Aires was surely "peripheral" at that time, but Lignières' findings were also published, in French and in France, in a major periodical. Lignières' report was translated into English in Australia and published in an agricultural journal in Queensland.

Four peripheral areas were linked when a request from Salisbury to Johannesburg was passed on to Australia and resulted in the English version of Lignières' article, written in the Argentine, being received in Salisbury without the intervention of any center.

What about the requests for advice from the United States? In terms of scientific agriculture, the United States was certainly a center in 1902, and the letters sent to Baton Rouge and to the famous Texas cattle ranch, the King Ranch, were sent from periphery to center. But the structure of scientific agriculture in the United States provides a unique example of center and periphery, since the system of land-grant agricultural colleges, Hatch Act experimental stations and extension programs had been created to deliver information from the center to newly settled and still developing areas across the country and to create new information to benefit both center and periphery. Some of those areas were not yet even states but were federal territories, colonies if you will. This was the system of the internal linking of the center to the periphery of the same country that F. B. Smith introduced, first to the Transvaal, then to the Union of South Africa, and finally to Great Britain.[6]

L. O. Howard's Division of Entomology supplied to South Africa many American economic entomologists, trained at land-grant agricultural colleges and Hatch Act experimental stations. The first of them, Charles Lounsbury, reached South Africa in 1895, eighteen years before there was a single government economic entomologist in Great Britain and at a time when he believed himself to be the only government-employed economic entomologist in all of Africa. As Worboys points out in his thesis, economic entomology provides a clear-cut example of a flow of knowledge from the periphery to the center, i.e. from the empire to Great Britain. Worboys also points out that not only South Africa but other parts of the British empire had employed economic entomologists trained in the United States. In the English-speaking world, economic entomology flowed, in the 1890s and later, from the U.S. center to various peripheral parts of the British empire and finally flowed back to the British center. But in 1902, Lounsbury, working in Cape Town with only one assistant, had to turn to another center, in Toulouse, for identification of the brown tick.

If the Cape Colony was part of the periphery it was a very special part. It had a well-developed department of agriculture and an important agricultural journal. It also had a Chief Veterinary Officer, Duncan Hutcheon, who was distinguished enough to become an Honorary Associate of the Royal College of Veterinary Surgeons and it had an active and well-equipped division of veterinary bacteriology. Australia also had a well-developed system of support for scientific agriculture.

Rhodesia was certainly part of the periphery, but its Chief Veterinarian's original reaction to the new disease was to turn for help and advice not to Great Britain but to the Cape Colony and to Texas and Louisiana. On the other hand, when Gray decided that he needed to take a refresher course he went to London to take McFadyean's course. Even that does not show that London was more than a nascent center: McFadyean's course had begun only in 1904. Yet the studies by Koch and by Theiler were quickly reprinted in British journals, the most important of which was McFadyean's *Journal of Comparative Pathology and Therapeutics.* (The British were quick to republish Koch's reports, which were written in English. The Germans translated Koch's reports and published them; they did not pay Theiler the same compliment.)

What about Arnold Theiler? Educated in a center, he was by no means an expert of the center: he reached South Africa simply as a practical veterinarian with no special qualifications as an expert. Self-taught as a bacteriologist and parasitologist, he was working alone and largely unrecognized in Pretoria when East Coast fever appeared in the Transvaal in 1902. And yet, with the backing of the Transvaal and of the Union of South Africa, Theiler's institute at Onderstepoort became a major center. By the 1920s, in terms of veterinary research, the Union of South Africa was far ahead of the United Kingdom. But in 1902 and 1903, however close he was to knowing that the new disease was a new disease, Theiler certainly deferred to the experts of the center: Lignières (ex-Alfort), Laveran, Nocard, and above all, Koch. They were wrong and he was right: but they were what Hutcheon, also misled by them, called the "expert bacteriologists": the experts of the center. By the 1920s, if an expert opinion on a disease of animals was needed anywhere in the world, it might well have been Theiler who was consulted.

There was another empire involved: the German empire. It has long been known that Koch was deeply involved with the German government, the German army, and German imperial ambitions. I have not consulted the archival sources in Germany that might shed light on Koch's role in the East Coast fever episode, but that episode was only one of Koch's many tours of duty in foreign parts, all of which deserve further study in the context of science and the German empire. Nor should such a study be limited to Koch: in Africa alone it might examine the role of Gonder, Kleine, Reichenow and many others. I would, however, surmise that the use of science as an agent of imperial power was more conscious, systematic and deliberate in the German empire than it was in the British empire.

One final, very important factor deserves attention, that of language. The only person involved in the study of East Coast fever who could speak, read and write English, French, German and Afrikaans was Arnold Theiler. On the most elementary practical level, both in Rhodesia and the Transvaal, the conflicts between the veterinarians and the Afrikaner farmers were exacerbated by the fact that many of those farmers spoke little or no English and many of the veterinarians spoke little or no Afrikaans. On another level, translations were important: Hutcheon and Gray read translations of Lignières' articles and of Koch's 1898 report.[7] On still another level, the role of the three major languages of science, English, French and German, may be relevant to the question of science and empire. The factors determining the choice of what language to use for publication when the author's first language was not English, French or German were manifold, but a judgment as to the international power and prestige of the country whose language was chosen was surely one of them.[8]

Thus there were many networks of quite different sorts of components, many centers, many peripheral areas, and a few places such as the Cape Colony and Australia that were in transition, and there was a flow of information not only from center to periphery or periphery to center, but between peripheral areas. MacLeod's concept of the role of the "moving metropolis" in what he calls the "architecture of imperial science" draws on examples taken from science in the British empire, but by "metropolitan science" he means "not just the science of Edinburgh or London or Paris or Berlin, but a way of *doing* science" that developed in eighteenth-century Europe. MacLeod emphasizes the role of multiple developments that have "reverberating effects" and argues that "the idea of a fixed metropolis radiating light from a single point source is inadequate" to explain the relationship between center and periphery. The East Coast fever episode certainly cannot be interpreted in terms of a "single point source" of knowledge even if all of the European centers are treated as one. To understand it we must examine the role of many loyalties, commitments and special interests: imperial, national, economic, political, scientific, professional and personal. An explanation that emphasizes the role of only one or two of those networks is necessarily partial and risks being tendentious. On the other hand, a full analysis of the role and interaction of all of the networks must inevitably be as intricate and complex as the very history that it is intended to illuminate.[9]

Economic causes and consequences of East Coast fever

In the late 1890s rinderpest produced a profound disruption of the economy of Rhodesia and South Africa, as well as creating widespread social tension and impoverishing many Africans. Transport was disrupted, shortages of food developed, and, in South Africa, many Africans were driven from the land and forced into the labor market.[10] But cattle that survived rinderpest became more valuable because they were then immune to the disease, and an effective vaccine was soon developed. By the time rinderpest began to come under control, the Boer War was about to break out. The cost of fighting rinderpest, the losses caused by rinderpest and the effects of the war combined to produce severe economic problems in both South Africa and Rhodesia. And the treaty that ended the Boer War was not signed until May 31, 1902, when East Coast fever had already invaded both Rhodesia and the Transvaal. Neither country could afford the cost of an all-out attack on the new disease. The slaughter of herds and the compulsory fencing of fields were ruled out in both places as being too expensive. Quite apart from the general economic depression, Rhodesia had lost its principal backer, Rhodes, who died on March 22, 1902. Rhodesia could no longer look to Rhodes as a source of funds or as an advocate of investment; it could look only to the financially troubled Chartered Company itself. Because East Coast fever was not quickly brought under control, the economic situation worsened, and, as we saw in chapter 8, European settlers began to leave, just as they began to leave Natal after East Coast fever swept through that country. Nor were the Africans spared: East Coast fever may have spared the

African-owned cattle in Rhodesia, at least to some degree, but it did not do so in the Transkei or in Natal. A fence was built to protect the Cape Colony, but East Coast fever appears to have entered the Transkei from the coast, just as it entered Rhodesia, the Transvaal and, presumably, Natal. The need to restock herds depleted by rinderpest led to cattle being brought from Dar-es-Salaam to Beira and Umtali; some of the cattle imported into the Transvaal were presumably "repatriation cattle," intended to restock herds depleted during the Boer War. It probably became steadily easier and cheaper to move cattle by sea; if so, that was an unfortunate form of "progress" as far as spreading East Coast fever.

On the other hand, in line with the British government's policies of promoting development in the colonies and the Commonwealth, the European-oriented parts of the economies of both South Africa and Rhodesia continued to develop.[11] South Africa remained a successful farming country, the gold and diamond mines survived, ox-transport gave way to the internal combustion engine, and industrialization went ahead. Southern Rhodesia, which saw some degree of industrialization after 1946 and more after the formation of the Federation of Rhodesia and Nyasaland in 1953, remained heavily dependent on mining and agriculture. Its mines, never as rich as those of South Africa, did contain immense deposits of coal as well as gold, asbestos and chromium. The raising of cattle and of tobacco also became very successful activities.[12] Nor did all of the early settlers flee to England, to the Argentine, to South Africa or to Australia.[13] East Coast fever was thus, for South Africa and Rhodesia, a serious but temporary setback. In the parts of Africa where East Coast fever was endemic before it invaded Rhodesia and where it remains endemic, there is a far larger cattle industry than there was in 1900. For that reason the absolute economic burden of East Coast fever is much greater than it was in 1900.[14] Were East Coast fever again to be introduced into any part of the world that contains ticks capable of transmitting it, and not swiftly brought under control, the economic consequences for cattle-raising could be serious. The equally serious effects of widespread disruption of transport would, of course, not be comparable to those experienced in 1902.[15]

L'envoi

No one who fought East Coast fever between 1901 and 1910 survives to tell the tale. Duncan Hutcheon died in 1907. Robert Koch, awarded the Nobel Prize in 1905, died in 1910. Arnold Theiler died in 1936; fifteen years later, his son Max Theiler was awarded the Nobel Prize for developing the yellow fever vaccine. Charles Gray died in 1937 and Fred Neufeld in 1945. Kleine and Watkins-Pitchford died in 1951, leaving only Charles Lounsbury, who died in 1955.

The appearance of East Coast fever in Umtali in October, 1901 is thus beyond living memory, but its immediate after-effects are not. On March 18, 1902, Lionel Cripps mentioned the new cattle disease in his diary. An earlier entry in that diary reads "26 Dec. 1900, Baby (Hereward) born at 12:15 AM." On August 22, 1987 I spent a pleasant afternoon at the Cripps homestead, Cloudlands, in the hills above Umtali, with Hereward Cripps, his sister Angela Cripps, and his brother's widow, Mrs. Derek Cripps. They recalled the days when leopards and lions were often seen on the home farm and they recalled talk about the death of cattle at their father's "new" farm (Ferndale). They all remembered the years in which draft oxen had been replaced by mules and donkeys brought up from South Africa and they spoke of the lost cattle being replaced by stock brought from the north (across the Zambezi), "hump-backed" cattle that seemed more resistant to disease. Hereward Cripps also recalled that, when he was a cattle inspector at Chipinga in 1925, he saw cattle that had been in quarantine for seven years, cattle by then too fat to fit into the dipping tank. Perhaps because we had been talking of a time of deprivation and trouble, he also recalled the English version of the Shona rendering of the cry of the Namaqua dove: "Oh, my father! My father is dead, my mother is dead, my relatives are all dead. [I am] alone, alone, alone."[16]

Notes and references

In citing material from the National Archives of Zimbabwe I prefix the citation by *NAZ*; in citing material from the Public Record Office of the United Kingdom, I prefix the citation by *PRO*. In citing PRO material, the group, class and piece number are followed by the number of the file or despatch. For example, in the citation *PRO* CO 417/344/31876, *PRO* means that the material is at the Public Record Office, CO 417/344 identifies the volume in which it is found and 31876 identifies a file or despatch within that volume. *CAD, TAD* and *SAW* identify material in the Cape Archives Depot (Cape Town), the Transvaal Archives Depot (Pretoria) and the State Archives Windhoek (Windhoek, Namibia). Since *TAD* also identifies the Transvaal Agricultural Department, some citations begin *TAD* TAD.

PREFACE

1 H. Barty-King, *Girdle Round the Earth*, London, Heinemann, 1979. The Indian Ocean cable linking South Africa to Australia went into service on November 1, 1902. The search for an expert, described in chapter 4, was conducted by telegrams and cables. The speed with which telegraphic messages could be sent and received did not speed up that search, but the inadequacies of "compressed" messages often had a bad effect. Matters were dealt with in "telegraphic" style, not always to the advantage of the reaching of sensible conclusions. Barty-King (p. 125), discussing the outbreak of the Boer War, refers to the telegraphy system's "not entirely satisfactory nature as a medium for conveying the subtleties of diplomatic thinking on which lives can depend."

2 H. Butterfield, *The Origins of Modern Science 1300–1800*, London, Bell, 1949, pp. viii–ix.

3 K. S. Warren, The Great Neglected Diseases of Mankind, in J. P. Kreier (ed.), *Malaria: Immunology and Immunization*, New York, Academic Press, 1980, pp. 335–338.

4 J. Pino, The Neglected Diseases of Livestock, in M. Ristic and J. P. Kreier (eds.), *Babesiosis*, New York, Academic Press, 1981, pp. 545–554.

5 That theme is dealt with in a broader context by Worboys (M. Worboys, Science and British Colonial Imperialism 1895–1940, unpublished D.Phil. thesis, University of Sussex, 1979. I am indebted to Dr. Worboys for lending me a copy of his thesis.) See also R. MacLeod, On Visiting the 'Moving metropolis': Reflections on the Architecture of Imperial Science, *Historical Records of Australian Science* 5: 1–16, 1982.

6 P. F. Cranefield, Public Health Education, Philately and Medical History: The 1982 Zimbabwe Stamps Commemorating the Discovery of the Tubercle Bacillus, *Bulletin of the New York Academy of Medicine* 62: 206–208, 1986.

7 D. Dwork, Koch and the Colonial Office, 1902–1904: The Second South African Expedition, *N.T.M. Schriftenreihe für Geschichte der Naturwissenschaften, Technik und Medizin* 20: 67–74, 1983.

8 D. N. Beach, *War and Politics in Zimbabwe, 1840–1900*, Gweru, Mambo Press, 1986.

9 T. W. Baxter, *Guide to the Public Archives of Rhodesia*, vol. I (1890–1923), Salisbury, National Archives of Rhodesia, 1969.

10 B. A. Matson, *Theileriosis due to Theileria parva, T. Lawrencei and T. Mutans: Bibliography 1897–1966*, Weybridge, England, Commonwealth Bureau of Animal Health, n.d. [1967?]. R. Uskavitch, *East Coast Fever: A Bibliography 1925–1972*, United States Department of Agriculture, Agricultural Research Service, Plum Island Animal Disease Laboratory, Post Office Box 848, Greenport, Long Island, New York, 1972. Extensive bibliographies are found in many reviews, among them J. K. H. Wilde, East Coast Fever, in C. A. Brandley and C. Cornelius (eds.), *Advances in Veterinary Science* 11: 207–259, New York, Academic Press, 1967; W. O. Neitz, Theileriosis, gonderioses and cytauxzoonoses: a review, *Onderstepoort Journal of Veterinary Research* 27: 275–430, 1957; and W. O. Neitz, Theileriosis, in C. A. Brandley and E. C. Jungherr (eds.), *Advances in Veterinary Science* 5: 241–297, New York, Academic Press, 1959. A particularly useful source for the earlier work is M. W. Henning, *Animal Diseases in South Africa*, South Africa, Central News Agency Ltd., 1949.

11 P. J. Posthumus, *An Index of Veterinarians in South Africa*, 4th edition, vol. I, A–L, vol. II, M–Z, Pietermaritzburg, privately printed, 1982. I am indebted to Mr. Posthumus for sending me a copy of this work.

1 PROLOGUE

1 Earl Grey was Administrator of Rhodesia in 1896 and 1897. His letters are in *NAZ* Historical Manuscripts GR 1/1/1; the passage about the dead cattle has been cited before, e.g. by R. A. Blake, *A History of Rhodesia*, London, Eyre and Methuen, 1973.

   The name "Rhodesia" was adopted for postal purposes in December, 1895, but Joseph Chamberlain did not approve it as the official name of the country until April 2, 1897 (in a letter to Lord Rosmead, *NAZ* LO 5/10/5).

Rhodesia was, of course, named after Cecil John Rhodes, who died on March 26, 1902, probably unaware of the new plague that had struck his beloved Rhodesia. Rhodes not only haunts the early part of the story of East Coast fever, he haunts historians and biographers. Until recently the standard (and official) biography of Rhodes was that by J. G. Lockhart and C. M. Woodhouse (*Cecil Rhodes: The Colossus of South Africa*, New York, Macmillan, 1963). But 1987 saw another biography (B. Roberts, *Cecil Rhodes: The Flawed Colossus*, London, Hamish Hamilton, 1987). And, in 1988, a biography first published in Russian in 1984, appeared in English translation (A. Davidson, *Cecil Rhodes and His Time*, Moscow, Progress Publishers, 1988). It was soon followed by another important study: R. I. Rotberg, *The Founder: Cecil Rhodes and the Pursuit of Power*, New York, Oxford University Press, 1988. Rotberg cites twenty-three earlier biographies of Rhodes; his and Davidson's bring the total to twenty-five. Rotberg's preface cites many earlier calls for a definitive biography and remarks that "Rhodes cannot be encompassed or revealed in one dimension." Near the end of their biography, Lockhart and Woodhouse said "There can be no final judgement, and Rhodes would have been pleased that it should be so." Writing in Moscow, Apollon Davidson noted that Maxim Gorky once expressed his regret that no really talented novel had been written about Rhodes. A haunting figure indeed! Davidson, who draws with great effectiveness on the poetry of Kipling, says that scholars in Europe, South Africa, Zambia, Zimbabwe and Russia continue "to return to the figure of Cecil Rhodes." I agree with Davidson that "it is highly unlikely that they have said their final word on the subject."

2 S. P. Hyatt, *The Old Transport Road*, London, Andrew Melrose, 1914; reprint: Bulawayo, Books of Rhodesia, 1969. For a biographical note on Hyatt see chapter 8, n. 33.

3 *NAZ* A 1/5/4.

4 Although enzootic and epizootic are the correct terms to describe diseases that affect animals, almost all of the early writers used the terms endemic and epidemic and I have usually done the same.

5 The major newspapers in Rhodesia in 1902 were the (Salisbury) *Rhodesia Herald*, the *Bulawayo Chronicle* and the (Umtali) *Rhodesia Advertiser*. They were owned by the Rhodesia Printing and Publishing Company, which was controlled by the Argus Printing and Publishing Company of Cape Town, which had worked closely with Rhodes ever since he invested in it in 1881. The Argus Company also printed and published the Rhodesian *Government Gazette* and other official publications of the British South Africa Company. ([W. D. Gale], *The Rhodesian Press*, Salisbury, Rhodesian Printing and Publishing Company, n.d. [1962?]). Although these newspapers were controlled by the British South Africa Company, they were quite uninhibited in their reporting of local problems and of protests against the Company and its policies.

6 *NAZ* Historical Manuscripts CR 1/4/2. Lionel Cripps (1863–1950) was born in India, emigrated to South Africa in 1879, and later became a successful farmer in Rhodesia. After Rhodesia attained "responsible government", i.e. became a self-governing colony, Cripps was the first elected Speaker of the Legislative Assembly (T. W. Baxter and E. E. Burke, *Guide to the Historical Manuscripts in the National Archives of Rhodesia*, Salisbury, National Archives of Rhodesia, 1970, pp. 130–131).

7 Report of the Native Commissioner for Bulilima-Mangwe for the year ending March 31, 1903 (*NAZ* LO 4/1/14). By the time that report was written the term African Coast fever had been introduced by Koch.

8 Government Notice No. 178 of 1902; see *NAZ* EC 4/4/7.

9 *NAZ* EC 4/4/7; *NAZ* LO 1/2/16.

10 *PRO* CO 417/345/44055. See chapter 4 for the context of this note.

2   THE PLACES AND THE PLAYERS

1 The early history of what is now Zimbabwe is presently the subject of active investigation and re-assessment. Two convenient sources for information on specific topics are R. K. Rasmussen, *Historical Dictionary of Zimbabwe/Rhodesia*, Metuchen, N.J. and London, Scarecrow, 1979; and D. Berens (ed.), *A Concise Encyclopaedia of Zimbabwe*, Harare and Gweru, Mambo Press, 1988.

According to Rasmussen (pp. 87–88) each "feira" contained "a market center, small fort, Dominican mission church, and a few Portuguese houses." To speak of Matabeleland and Mashonaland, or to speak of the Ndebele and Shona language groups is, of course, a simplification. But it does (however roughly) distinguish between the part of the country that came to be dominated by Mzilikaze's peoples and the rest of the country. The north-eastern part of Mashonaland was then and still is called Manicaland, a name by which I occasionally refer to it.

2 The quotation from Rudd and my description of the early years of the British South Africa Company are based on A. Keppel-Jones, *Rhodes and Rhodesia: The White Conquest of Zimbabwe 1884–1902*, Pietermaritzburg, University of Natal Press, 1983 (also Kingston and Montreal, McGill-Queen's University Press, 1983). Keppel-Jones has provided what seems likely to be a definitive work both in terms of content and in terms of citations of primary and secondary sources.

The British government took it for granted that the new "Chartered Company" owned the Rudd concession. That concession in fact remained the property of the Central Search Association and its successor, the United Concessions Company. After the Chartered Company had been formed, and had sold shares to raise capital, it made a deal with the United Concessions Company: the Chartered Company would bear all expenses of development, while the United Concessions Company would receive half of the profits and would continue to own the Rudd concession even if the Chartered Company went bankrupt, which it very nearly did in 1892.

Although this arrangement was made known to would-be purchasers of shares in the Chartered Company, it worked to the disadvantage of anyone who owned only the newly traded shares in the Chartered Company and to the advantage of Rhodes, Beit and any other "insiders" who owned shares of both the Chartered Company *and* the United Concessions Company. Although Rhodes' dream of empire was certainly real, he obviously did not neglect the chance for profit. Keppel-Jones has provided persuasive evidence that if this "insider" arrangement had been generally known before the charter was granted it never would have been granted.

3 The government of Rhodesia certainly hanged people. And the British South Africa Company did issue stamps, beginning on January 2, 1892. The combined imprint of "British South Africa Company" and "Rhodesia," which began in 1909, remained until 1923 and such stamps were not finally withdrawn until March, 1924. (See *The Rhodesian Stamp Catalogue*, Salisbury, Salisbury Stamp Company, 1982.)

4 Keppel-Jones, *Rhodes*, pp. 555–556; see also T. W. Baxter, *Guide to the Public Archives of Rhodesia*, vol. I (1890–1923) Salisbury, National Archives of Rhodesia, 1969, p. xx. The introduction to Baxter's *Guide* provides useful information on the evolution of the administrative machinery of Rhodesia between 1890 and 1923, as does L. H. Gann, *A History of Southern Rhodesia: Early Days to 1934*, London, Chatto and Windus, 1965.

5 The material on ticks in these paragraphs is based on sources cited in notes to chapters 5 and 7. For information on parasitic diseases, and on the way in which they are transmitted, see W. Trager, *Living Together: The Biology of Animal Parasitism*, New York, Plenum, 1986.

In view of the great economic importance of tick-borne diseases of animals and the serious nature of tick-borne diseases of human beings (such as Rocky Mountain spotted fever and Lyme disease) it is distressing to read that the systematic study of arthropod vectors may now be underfunded by the government of the United States (see J. H. Oliver, Jr., Crisis in Biosystematics of Arthropods, *Science* 240: 967, 1988).

6 A useful source of information on the diseases of cattle in Southern Africa is M. W. Henning, *Animal Diseases in South Africa*, 2nd edition, South Africa, Central News Agency, 1949. Henning's treatment of each disease begins with a useful historical review and ends with an excellent bibliography.

7 T. O. Ranger, *Revolt in Southern Rhodesia*, London, Heinemann, 1967.

8 C. van Onselen, Reactions to Rinderpest in Southern Africa, *Journal of African History* 13: 473–488, 1972.

9 T. Smith and F. L. Kilborne, *Investigations into the Nature, Causation, and Prevention of Southern Cattle Fever*, U.S. Department of Agricul-

ture. Bureau of Animal Industry, Bulletin no. 1, Washington, Government Printing Office, 1893; reprinted in [E. C. Kelly], *Medical Classics*, vol. I, no. 5, Baltimore, Williams and Wilkins, 1937, pp. 341–597.

10 Milton was born in Newbury, Berkshire, England on December 3, 1854 and died in Cannes on March 6, 1930; for a sketch of his career, which was spent entirely in the Cape and in Rhodesia, and for information on many other figures mentioned in the present volume, see T. W. Baxter and E. E. Burke, *Guide to the Historical Manuscripts in the National Archives of Rhodesia*, Salisbury, National Archives of Rhodesia, 1970; for Milton see also the *Dictionary of South African Biography*, vol. III, p. 618.

11 NAZ LO 1/2/15.

12 Biographical information about Kotzé and many others who figure in the story of East Coast fever can be found in *Standard Encyclopaedia of Southern Africa*, Cape Town, N.A.S.O.U., 1970–6. For Kotzé in particular, see vol. VI, 1972. See also the *Dictionary of South African Biography*, vol. I, pp. 438–441. For the Kruger episode see J. P. Fitzpatrick, *The Transvaal from Within*, New York, Stokes, 1900 and B. A. Tindall's preface to volume II of J. G. Kotzé, *Memoirs and Reminiscences*, Cape Town, Maskew Miller, 1952. The statement that the Kotzé affair convinced Milner that Kruger was "irredeemable and inaccessible to reason" is that of J. G. Lockhart and C. M. Woodhouse (*Cecil Rhodes: The Colossus of South Africa*, New York, Macmillan, 1963, p. 437). H. Rider Haggard's actual title in Kotzé's court was Master and Registrar; he later spoke with great warmth of his memories of riding the circuit with Kotzé. Kruger's dismissal of Kotzé caused a great furore. On June 20, 1898, Haggard presided over a dinner of the Anglo-African Writers Club in London, at which both he and Kotzé gave speeches about Kotzé's dismissal (see the *African Review*, June 25, 1898, pp. 516–518).

13 Orpen was born in Dublin, where his father, C. E. H. Orpen, was a physician and an early figure in the education of the deaf and dumb (see E. L. LeFanu, *Life of Dr. Orpen*, London, Charles Esterton, 1860). For Joseph Orpen see the *Standard Encyclopaedia of Southern Africa*, vol. VIII, pp. 392–393; J. J. Oberholster's introduction to J. M. Orpen, *Reminiscences of Life in South Africa*, Cape Town, Struik, 1964; Orpen's obituary in the *Rhodesia Herald*, December 23, 1923; and the *Dictionary of South African Biography*, vol. I, pp. 602–603. Orpen died in East London, South Africa on December 12, 1923. An article on bushman mythology that Orpen published in 1874 was important enough to be mentioned in 1930 in Schapera's classic study (I. Schapera, *The Khoisan Peoples of South Africa*, London, Routledge, 1930, p. 125, n. 3).

14 Orpen's connection with Rhodes seems to have been genuine, even though he may have exaggerated it in later years. Rotberg mentions Orpen eight times in his biography of Rhodes (R. I. Rotberg, *The Founder: Cecil Rhodes and the Pursuit of Power*, New York, Oxford

University Press, 1988). As to Orpen's claim to have met Rhodes in 1877, when Rhodes was only twenty-four, Rotberg (p. 103 and p. 703) cites a letter written when Orpen was nearly ninety years old. Although it may reflect a certain embellishment of the actual event, it makes interesting reading. Orpen, his brother and two other guests dined with Rhodes, who told his guests that the "object to which I intend to devote my life is the defence and extension of the British Empire." Orpen replied that he was "delighted to hear of his excellent intentions" and Orpen's brother proposed that whenever the members of the dinner party wrote to one another they should add "the symbol of a five on the dice – the pyramid of brothers." Rhodes scholars indeed!

15 The first quotation is from *NAZ* LO 2/1/16; the second from *NAZ* EC 4/4/7.

16 P. J. Posthumus, *An Index of Veterinarians in South Africa*, 4th edition, Pietermaritzburg, privately printed, 1982, vol. I, pp. 82–83.

17 L. E. W. Bevan, Autobiography, n.p., n.d., typed (*NAZ* Historical Manuscripts BE 11/7/1). The description of Gray is on pp. 63–64. Bevan adds that he introduced Gray to his father who later said: "He is quite the ugliest little man I ever saw, but I should think he is a very honorable little fellow." As the result of his father's favorable opinion of Gray, Bevan accepted Gray's invitation to join the Rhodesian Veterinary Service. (For a biographical note on Bevan see chapter 3, n. 52.)

18 *Veterinary Record* 49: 812–813, 1937. Gray died in Jersey on June 14, 1937.

19 For (Sir) Marshall James Clarke, see the *Dictionary of National Biography* (second supplement (1901–11), vol. I, pp. 368–369); Keppel-Jones, *Rhodes*, p. 556; and the *Dictionary of South African Biography*, vol. III, pp. 154–155. Born on October 18, 1841, in Shronell, County Tipperary, he died on April 1, 1909, in Enniskerry, County Wicklow. He had been Commissioner of Police of the Cape Colony and Resident Commissioner of Basutoland and Zululand. Keppel-Jones says that Clarke's appointment as Resident Commissioner in 1898 "was a measure of the importance attached to the job." Clarke remained as Resident Commissioner until 1905. Although he had a long and important career, Clarke does not stand forth with any vividness from the newspaper stories, letters and telegrams that document the story of East Coast fever. Perhaps he was not a colorful person; on the other hand most references to him are found in the documents of his "opposition," the Chartered Company. His career included remarkable episodes: according to the *Dictionary of South African Biography* he lost his left arm in India in a fight with a tiger which he killed with a carving knife and he was present at the coronation of Cetshwayo.

20 For the Jameson raid, see J. van der Poel, *The Jameson Raid*, Oxford University Press, 1951; E. Pakenham [E. Longford], *Jameson's Raid*, London, Weidenfeld and Nicolson, 1960: 2nd edition, E. Longford, *Jameson's Raid*, London, Weidenfeld and Nicolson, 1982; J. P. Fitz-

patrick, *The Transvaal from Within*, New York, Stokes, 1900; C. Headlam, The Jameson Raid, in A. P. Newton, E. A. Benians and E. A. Walker (eds.), *Cambridge History of the British Empire*, Cambridge University Press, vol. VIII, 1936, pp. 552–565 and J. H. Hofmeyr, The Results of the Raid, *ibid.*, pp. 566–567; G. Wheatcroft, *The Randlords*, New York, Atheneum, 1986; and Rotberg, *The Founder*, pp. 515–550. Both Wheatcroft (pp. 285–286) and Rotberg (pp. 737–741) cite many additional sources. A few often-overlooked and very savage comments on Rhodes, the raid and the official enquiry into the raid can be found, in the preface and elsewhere, of S. C. Cronwright-Schreiner, *The Land of Free Speech*, London, New Age Press, 1906. Cronwright-Schreiner, who was Olive Schreiner's husband, shared his wife's disillusion with Rhodes.

21 S. P. Hyatt, *The Old Transport Road*, London, Andrew Melrose, 1914; reprint: Bulawayo, Books of Rhodesia, 1969.

22 D. A. Lawrence, Southern Rhodesia (Rhodesia), in *A History of the Overseas Veterinary Services*, pt. II, London, British Veterinary Association, 1973, pp. 267–268.

23 The *Southern Rhodesia Civil Service List*, Salisbury, Argus, 1900. (The title varies: for 1900 and 1901, as cited; for 1902–1907, *Rhodesia Civil Service List*; for 1910–1922, *Civil Service List of Southern Rhodesia*.)

24 Duncan Hutcheon was a much revered figure. Born near Peterhead, Scotland on June 27, 1842, he died in Cape Town on May 5, 1907. He completed his veterinary studies in Edinburgh in 1871 and went to the Cape in 1880. He was the second Chief Veterinary Surgeon of the Cape and, eventually, Director of Agriculture. Under his direction of the Cape Veterinary Department its bacteriological services were created, with the appointment of Alexander Edington and William Robertson. He battled heroically against the rinderpest outbreak and was made an Honorary Associate of the Royal College of Veterinary Surgeons in 1902. (Miss Benita Horder, librarian of the R.C.V.S., tells me that the designation Honorary Associate of the R.C.V.S. conferred genuine distinction on its recipients.) For more details of his career see Posthumus, *Index of Veterinarians*, vol. I, pp. 101–103; *Veterinary Record*, 19: 757, 819–821, 1907; and *Veterinary Record*, 20: 90–91, 1907.

3 A NEW DISEASE?

1 C. Headlam (ed.), *The Milner Papers: South Africa*, vol. II, London, Cassell, 1933, pp. 75–76. This letter, written when Rhodes was already very rich *and* seriously ill, provides a striking example of his restless ambition.

2 *PRO* CO 417/344/28488. (I believe that most of this correspondence relating to the Australian cattle is in both *PRO* CO 417/344/28488 *and NAZ* RC 3/7/6, but since some of my photocopies are from one file and some from the other and since I do not have a complete set of copies of either file I have cited my actual source.)

3 This letter, which is in *PRO* CO 417/344/28488, is the same letter in which Milner was advised that Natal had prohibited the importation of Rhodesian cattle (see chapter 4, n. 5).
4 *PRO* CO 417/344/28488. According to Stewart's letter, the cattle were purchased in the districts of Singleton and Tenterfield.
5 The entire episode offers an interesting example of the existence, in 1902, of an international network of governmental and scientific communication. Dr. J. Lignières had been Chief of Staff of the leading veterinary college of France (Alfort); he had been selected by the Pasteur Institute to investigate infectious disease of cattle in Argentina; he published his report in French in 1900; it was translated into English in Australia, where it appeared in mid-1901. Less than a year later, when it was needed in South Africa and Rhodesia, a copy was in the hands of Milner.

Lignières' report appeared both in book form as J. Lignières, *La "Tristeza" ou Malaria Bovine dans la République Argentine*, Buenos Aires, Peuser, 1900 and as J. Lignières, La "Tristeza" dans la République Argentine, *Bulletin de la Societé Centrale de la Médecine Vétérinaire*, N.S. 18: 735–774, 1900 and Transmission expérimentale de la Tristeza, *Bulletin de la Societé Centrale de la Médecine Vétérinaire*, N.S. 18: 818–880, 1900. The two versions are substantially the same but the book has more plates. For the translations, by A. J. Boyd, see The "Tristeza" in the Argentine Republic, the *Queensland Agricultural Journal* 8: 455–475, [June] 1901; and Experimental Transmission of Bovine Malaria, the *Queensland Agricultural Journal* 9:252–275 + 16 plates, [August] 1901 and 9:339–353, [September] 1901.

The material forwarded by Hopetoun also included offprints of F. Tidswell, Report on Protective Inoculations Against Tick Fever, New South Wales Department of Public Health, Sydney, 1899 [10 pp.]; Second Report, 1900 [17 pp.]; 3 short pamphlets on the techniques of inoculation, and a plan of a dipping tank. All in *NAZ* RC 3/7/6.
6 *NAZ* RC 3/7/6.
7 J. M. Sinclair, History of African Coast Fever, in *Report of Committee of Enquiry on African Coast Fever*, Salisbury, Government Printer, 1910, appendix, pp. 15–18 [copy in *NAZ* SR Misc. Reports, 1909–1916]. An expanded version of this article is found in J. M. Sinclair, A Short History of the Infective Diseases Amongst the Domestic Animals of Southern Rhodesia Since the Occupation: African Coast Fever, *Rhodesia Agricultural Journal* 19: 10–16, 1922. The report that the cattle had been purchased in a district in which redwater had never existed shows that the Australian cattle had never been exposed to redwater and had no immunity to it. In retrospect it seems astonishing that the Australian cattle were sent to Africa without being immunized against redwater.
8 R. F. Stirling, East Coast Fever and its Control, Royal College of Veterinary Surgeons Fellowship Thesis, 1912. Typed copy in the

library of the Royal College of Veterinary Surgeons, Belgrave Square, London.

9 As late as 1908, Theiler still stated that although the Australian cattle neither introduced the disease nor contracted it at Beira, they did die of it when they reached Umtali in January, 1901. (A. Theiler, Report of the Government Veterinary Bacteriologist [dated January 13, 1908]. In *Transvaal Department of Agriculture, Annual Report. 1906–1907*, Pretoria, Government Printing and Stationery Office, 1908, pp. 87–131.) In support of that view Theiler cited an article by Orpen that appeared in the March 18, 1905, issue of *South Africa* in which Orpen claimed that *before* the arrival of the Australian cattle, some cattle from German East Africa had been imported to both the Umtali commonage and to Salisbury and that "not long after this and just in those two places, some cases occurred . . . and then spread along the various roads." But the Australian cattle died in January, 1901 and the events to which Orpen referred (the appearance of the disease in Salisbury and its spread along the roads) occurred in January, 1902.

Professor John Lawrence of the veterinary faculty of the University of Zimbabwe tells me that it is generally accepted that East Coast fever was introduced into Umtali by cattle imported from East Africa in October or November, 1901, i.e. well after all but three of the Australian cattle had died. The voyage by sea from Dar-es-Salaam to Beira took about a week. Allowing for two or three days at Beira and a day by train to Umtali, cattle could easily have reached Umtali ten days after they left Dar-es-Salaam. Since the incubation period of East Coast fever is usually ten days or longer, cattle infected just before leaving Dar-es-Salaam could have arrived in Umtali ten days later in apparent good health. Professor Lawrence has made determined but unsuccessful efforts to identify the exact shipment of cattle responsible for the introduction of the disease.

In the report of the 1910 Committee of Enquiry (*NAZ* ZAB 2/1/1), A. W. N. Strickland, an early settler in Umtali, claimed that the outbreak of 1902 was brought from Beira to Umtali and "from here it was taken by transport by Patterson's cattle."

10 The telegrams are in *NAZ* V 1/2/1/1.

According to Posthumus (P. J. Posthumus, *An Index of Veterinarians in South Africa*, 4th edition, Pietermaritzburg, privately printed, 1982, vol. I, p. 109), Edmund Mullinger Jarvis was born in England on December 14, 1873, and qualified as M.R.C.V.S. on December 14, 1894 and as F.R.C.V.S. on December 8, 1910. Posthumus says Jarvis served in Rhodesia from 1901 to 1907, then moved to South Africa, and eventually returned to farming in Umtali. The *Rhodesia Civil Service List* (Salisbury, Argus) for 1902 indicates that Jarvis joined the Rhodesian Veterinary service on January 6, 1901, but he presumably remained in that service well past 1907 since he was Acting Chief Veterinary Surgeon in 1911 (see chapter 8).

11 C. E. Gray, Annual Report 1901–1902, typed copy: *NAZ* LO 4/1/17.

Published in *The British South Africa Company: Reports on the Administration of Rhodesia, 1900–1902*, Printed for the Information of Shareholders [London, 1903]. Gray's report for 1901–1902 is on pp.
224–230.

Gray's letter to Hutcheon, dated April 11, 1902, is in *CAD* CVS
1/62; the copy sent to Edington (the Director of the bacteriological
institute in Grahamstown) is in *CAD* BIG 1/3/11. Pages 2–14 of the
letter are nearly identical with pages 225–230 of the printed report, but
the letter to Hutcheon begins by thanking him for a letter of March 25
"on the subject of our present epidemic and for the numerous opinions
quoted therein; although they are somewhat conflicting I incline to Dr.
Edington's." I have not found a copy of Hutcheon's letter to
Gray.

12 Alexander Edington (1860–1928) was a physician and bacteriologist
who was the bacteriologist at the Cape of Good Hope in 1891 and later
at Grahamstown. According to Posthumus, *Index of Veterinarians*, vol.
I, pp. 60–61, Edington had a somewhat unconventional career and
seems to have made some serious errors. He claimed to have discovered a microbe that caused rinderpest and to have produced an
attenuated form of the horse sickness virus. He believed that the new
outbreak was a mixed infection of "imapunga" (Coast gall sickness or
bossiekte, i.e. heartwater) and redwater. On April 2, 1902, Gray sent
Edington a long telegram (*CAD* BIG 1/3/11) emphasizing the pulmonary lesions, saying they resembled those of horse sickness, and asking
if Coast gall sickness could present in a similar way. Having received
Edington's reply, Gray wrote again on May 8 to say that "your
description of Imapunga hardly tallies with conditions found during
our present outbreak ... further, effusion into the pericardium is not a
feature of the present epidemic." Edington continued to press his view
(see the [Grahamstown] *Journal* for July 24, 1902), and went to Rhodesia to study the outbreak. On September 20, 1902, Kotzé sent a cable
to request that Edington be recalled "as he denies that dogs have rabies
& cattle redwater." (*TAD* PMO/276). On September 25, Hutcheon
sent Gray a telegram: "Am informed that Edington has reported that
disease of cattle not redwater & disease of dogs not rabies. I expected
this ... stick to your guns on dipping." Edington did do some important early work on heartwater, but he certainly did nothing to clarify
the nature of East Coast fever. As late as December 11, 1903 Edington
sent a sixteen-page letter to the Under Colonial Secretary in Cape
Town in which he claimed that East Coast fever was identical with
what he had long before described as "veld sickness" or "South
African fever" which, he claimed, affected horses, cattle and goats.

13 C. E. Gray, *Redwater, Tick Fever, Texas Fever or Bovine Malaria*,
[Salisbury], Argus, 1901 (unpaginated: cover plus 8 pages). Copy in
historical collection, Bulawayo Public Library.

14 *NAZ LO 1/2/16.*

15 *The Rhodesian Landowners' and Farmers' Association, Bulawayo. Sixth*

Annual Report for the Year 1902, Bulawayo, Argus Printing and Publishing Co., 1903. See p. 13. (Copy in *NAZ* LO 4/1/15.)

16 *NAZ* LO 1/2/16. (Copies of these telegrams reached the Directors of the B.S.A.C. in London after a delay of a few weeks; copies of these particular telegrams were received in London on June 30, 1902.)

17 Clippings of these articles are in *NAZ* LO 5/3/3, vol. 1; typed transcripts are in *NAZ* LO 1/2/15.

18 *NAZ* LO 1/2/15.

19 *NAZ* LO 5/3/3, vol. 1. (The *Bulawayo Chronicle* of May 8, 1902, reported that Milton "had cabled to England for a first class man to be sent out from the Veterinary College of Surgeons by the first steamer," but I can find no evidence that he had done so.)

20 *NAZ* LO 1/2/16; *NAZ* EC 4/4/7. Robertson was born in Scotland in 1872 and died in Grahamstown, South Africa, December 12, 1918. See Posthumus, *Index of Veterinarians*, vol. II, pp. 175–176. After qualifying as a veterinarian in 1893, he studied at the Pasteur Institute. In 1896 he became assistant to Alexander Edington, the bacteriologist at Grahamstown; in 1902 he was based in Cape Town, under Hutcheon.

21 Gray wrote to Edington on May 8 that Robertson was en route and "I half expected him tonight" (*CAD* BIG 1/3/11).

22 Typed, hand-corrected, signed copies of Robertson's interim report and Gray's interim report are in *NAZ* EC 4/4/7; final typed copies embodying the corrections were sent to London by Orpen on May 22, and are in *NAZ* LO 1/2/16. Robertson's subsequent letters to Hutcheon are in *CAD* CVS 1/62.

23 *NAZ* EC 4/4/7; *NAZ* LO 1/2/16.

24 [C. E. Gray and W. Robertson], *Redwater Disease in Cattle*, Salisbury, Argus, 1902. Copy in *NAZ* RC 3/7/6 and in historical collection, Bulawayo Public Library.

Orpen's letter of May 22 (see n. 22 above) and the reports by Gray and Robertson were also published in the *Government Gazette* and almost immediately reprinted in Natal under the collective title *Redwater in Rhodesia* ([Natal] *Agricultural Journal* 5: 237–248, [June 20], 1902). The reports by Gray and Robertson were also published in England, again almost as soon as they reached there (*Veterinary Record* 15: 42–48 [July 26], 1902).

25 *NAZ* LO 1/2/16; also published in the Association's annual report for 1902, see n. 15 above.

26 *NAZ* LO 1/2/16.

27 *NAZ* LO 1/1/35.

28 In late September and early October, three directors of the Chartered Company, Beit, Jameson and Michell, then in Rhodesia (A. Keppel-Jones, *Rhodes and Rhodesia: The White Conquest of Zimbabwe 1884–1902*, Pietermaritzburg, University of Natal Press, 1983, pp. 623–628), formally assured the Chamber of Mines and the Farmers and Landowners Association that E. Ross Townsend would soon take over the duties of Minister of Agriculture. On October 4, Alfred Beit

told The Mashonaland Farmers Association that: "The Company has already practically decided to divide the two Departments and to have separate heads, we were approached in Bulawayo on the same question, and we said we should recommend this to the Administration and I have no doubt that it will be carried out and that there will be a competent head appointed to it" (*NAZ* A 11/2/7/2). E. Ross Townsend soon took over the duties of Minister of Agriculture.

29 *NAZ* LO 1/2/16.
30 Keppel-Jones, *Rhodes and Rhodesia*, p. 339.
31 Orpen was still defending himself and his actions on November 18, against the mockery of the Legislative Council that, in a half-bitter, half-friendly debate, discussed a motion to reduce his salary (as Surveyor-General; he was no longer Minister of Agriculture) by £2,000 "in order to draw attention to the redwater outbreak." The motion was made by Dr. Wylie, who said that he "did not intend, as had been suggested by his colleagues, that [Orpen] should quit the service of the Government ... he moved the reduction simply as a peg upon which to base an enquiry into the very serious epidemic." (Orpen: Hear, hear!) Dr. Wylie went on

regardless of consequences, the [Australian] animals were removed from Beira to Umtali, without preventive inoculations ... [and became] the focus of the terrible scourge ... The excuse of the Government was that transport riders would not obey [quarantine regulations] but what was the use of an Agricultural Department if it could not enforce its own regulations ... No longer did they see the streets paraded by sleek teams of oxen, and the haggard face of many a man told that his occupation was gone.

Orpen responded with a vigorous defence of Gray, himself and his department, and attacked the lack of public cooperation. As to the charge of senility, "the Premier of the Cape Colony was 72; Lord Salisbury was 72; ... Mr. Chamberlain was now 66." Orpen gave as good as he got, and the debate ended amicably when "Mr. Holland moved ... to reduce the Surveyor General's salary by £250 instead of £500, as he had shown himself possessed of £250 worth more vitality than he imagined he possessed (laughter). The Surveyor General: 'Hear, hear!'" The amendment to reduce Orpen's salary was withdrawn and his budget approved. As to his physical energy, Orpen outlasted the debate by twenty-one years. Born in 1828, he lived until 1923 and seriously considered taking up golf at the age of ninety-two! Quite apart from that, the debate, which occurred late in 1902, was pervaded by remarks proving that most laymen still thought that the cattle disease had been introduced into the country by the Australian cattle. See *Southern Rhodesia. Debates in the Legislative Council during the Years 1899 to 1903*, Salisbury, Argus, 1904, pp. 136–138.

In the course of the debate Orpen read a long prepared statement (*Southern Rhodesia: Memorandum by the Surveyor General Relating to the Disease of Redwater Among Cattle*, Salisbury, Argus, 1902). In that statement Orpen continued to maintain that the disease was redwater, traced the history of redwater in Rhodesia since 1892, defended the policies of the Department of Agriculture, attacked the farmers, mining companies and transport riders for not cooperating with the government, and defended Gray. In other words he took the same position on every point that he had taken in May.

32 *NAZ* LO 1/2/16.

33 *NAZ* LO 1/2/16; *NAZ* LO 1/1/35; also in *The Rhodesian Landowners' and Farmers' Association, Bulawayo, Sixth Annual Report for the year 1902.*

34 A clipping, pasted on large sheets of paper, is in the B.S.A.C. files (*NAZ* A 11/2/2/14, vol. 1); Orpen's point-by-point refutations are written alongside the clipping.

35 See C. van Onselen, Reactions to Rinderpest in Southern Africa, *Journal of African History* 13: 473–488, 1972.

36 Cable to Kitchener and Kitchener's reply, *NAZ* A 2/8/8. Rail service was established between Mafeking and Bulawayo in October, 1897. The first train from Umtali arrived in Beira on February 4, 1898. Service between Umtali and Salisbury began on May 22, 1899. The Salisbury–Gwelo connection opened on June 1, 1902 and the Salisbury–Gwelo–Bulawayo service opened on December 1, 1902 (A. H. Croxton, *Railways of Zimbabwe*, Newton Abbot and London, David and Charles, 1982).

37 Government Notice No. 178 of 1902; copy in *NAZ* EC 4/4/7.

38 *NAZ* LO 1/2/16; *NAZ* LO 3/2/28; *NAZ* LO 3/2/29; *NAZ* A 11/2/18/64; *NAZ* EC 4/4/7.

39 *NAZ* A 11/2/2/14, vol. 2.

40 *NAZ* RC 3/7/6.

41 *NAZ* LO 1/2/16; Orpen's letter and Gray's memo were reprinted in *[Natal] Agricultural Journal*, 5: 422–424 [August 29] and 5: 437–438 [September 12], 1902.

42 *NAZ* LO 1/2/16.

43 *NAZ* EC 4/4/7.

44 *NAZ* LO 1/2/16 (cable and reply).

45 Orpen's letter is in *NAZ* A 11/2/2/14, vol. 2. A letter from Robertson to F. B. Smith dated Salisbury, August 4, 1902, refers to a letter from Smith of July 23 and states that he would be willing to serve under the Transvaal government as veterinary surgeon (*TAD* TAD 342/36511). Nothing came of the proposal; in 1905 Robertson succeeded Edington as Director of Research at Grahamstown.

46 All of the material that I have located and quote from is in *NAZ* A 11/2/2/14, vol. 1, apart from Orpen's original proposal, which is in *NAZ* A 11/2/2/14, vol. 2, and a letter from the Department of Public Works, cited below (see n. 48).

47 I do not know whom Gregory thus disparaged. It may well have been Alexander Edington, who had a somewhat unconventional career (see n. 12 above).

48 See *NAZ* W 1/1/1; the original plans are in *NAZ* A 11/2/2/14, vol. 1.

Other locations, including Bulawayo, were considered but in April, 1903, Dr. Moore, the medical officer for Salisbury, wrote,

I naturally favor the [site] that Dodgson, Gray and I selected . . . the bacteriologist should live at the institute. You will understand that bacilli, like other members of the vegetable kingdom, grow and flourish best at certain temperatures, and every endeavour is made by delicate mechanical contrivances to keep the incubators at an even temperature; a variation of a few degrees being often fatal.

A bacteriologist who has taken weeks, even months, to think out and elaborate a series of delicate experiments is not going to trust to a mechanical apparatus; he must and he will live with his 'bugs'.

Further, it is hardly an exaggeration to say that the study of bacteriology to the expert becomes a hobby, and till he reaches this stage of slavery, his labours are often futile.

I would urge that the mere fact of placing a man outside the precincts of town free from interruption may tend to success, not failure, in experimental work.

49 *NAZ* A 11/2/2/14, vol. 1.
50 The search for a bacteriologist had become entangled with the problem of finding a replacement for Loir (see chapter 4, n. 44) at the Rabies Institute. On December 30, 1902, Loir sent a cable to the London office of the B.S.A.C: "Communicate the following to Calmette Lille Government asks me to teach Antirabic treatment before departure that is within fortnight to Medical Officer who is not a bacteriologist what must we do cable LOIR." On December 31, Calmette replied to the B.S.A.C. from the Pasteur Institute in Lille saying "To give direction of a treatment of this kind to a doctor who was not a specialist in the study of bacteriology would expose the population to grave danger." Calmette offered to send a replacement for Loir. On January 4, 1903, Andrew M. Fleming wrote to the B.S.A.C. that he had consulted Professor Hunter Stewart, who thought that Loir might be able to instruct someone with some background in a month, but not in two weeks. Fleming said that since plans were already underway for establishing a bacteriological institute it would be foolish to set up a separate rabies institute. Thus, Fleming said, whoever is chosen to head the bacteriological institute should first visit the Pasteur Institute in Paris to learn their methods. Meanwhile Loir should remain in Rhodesia. The gist of this advice was forwarded to Milton on January 5, who replied to London on January 7 that arrangements had been made for a bacteriologist "to take over the Institute from Loir." He presumably meant Dodgson. See *NAZ* LO 1/2/18.
51 Robert W. Dodgson was born in 1871 and qualified in 1895 after studying at St. Mary's Hospital, London. In 1898 he obtained a gold medal for his M.D. examination. In 1899 he went to South Africa to evaluate the results of typhoid inoculation in British troops. From 1901 to 1903 he directed a government research laboratory in Cape Town.

In later years he became an expert on the transmission of typhoid by shellfish. He died on March 4, 1952. (See the *British Medical Journal*, 1952, vol. 1, p. 871 and *The Lancet*, 1952, vol. 1, pp. 676 and 931.) The *Medical Directory* for 1905 lists Dodgson as having been Director of the Pasteur Institute of Rhodesia in 1903 but it is not clear whether he actually took up the post before his illness.

52 See L. E. W. Bevan, Autobiography. n.p., n.d., typed (*NAZ* Historical Manuscripts BE 11/7/1), and see D. A. Lawrence, Southern Rhodesia (Rhodesia), in *A History of the Overseas Veterinary Services*, London, British Veterinary Association, part II, 1973, pp. 267–268.

L. E. W. Bevan was born in England in 1878, qualified as a veterinarian in 1904 and died in South Africa on March 17, 1957. In 1922 he finally became the first Director of Veterinary Research in Rhodesia. An obituary in the *Veterinary Record* (69: 421–422, 1957) implied that he was something of a controversialist, but Professor John A. Lawrence tells me that Bevan's great merit was that "he got things done." The main building of the Veterinary Research Laboratories in Harare is named Bevan House.

53 C. E. Gray and W. Robertson, *Report upon Texas Fever or Redwater in Rhodesia*, Cape Town, Argus, 1902.

54 See McFadyean's *Journal of Comparative Pathology and Therapeutics* 15: 368–378, [December 31] 1902; *Agricultural Journal of the Cape of Good Hope* 21: 435–458, [November] 1902; *Veterinary Journal* 7: 136–142 and 7: 217–222, [March and April] 1903.

55 See chapter 5 for a detailed discussion of that report.

56 W. H. Dalrymple (April 24, 1856–July 17, 1925) was born in Scotland and graduated as a veterinarian in Glasgow in 1886. He was Professor of Comparative Medicine at Louisiana State University and Director of the Louisiana Agricultural Experimental Station from 1889 to 1893 and again from 1897 to 1919, when he became Dean of the College of Agriculture. He was a major figure both in Louisiana and nationally (for an obituary see the *Veterinary Record* N.S. 5: 891–892, 1925; see also *American Men of Science*, 3rd edition, 1921, p. 162). Gray and Dalrymple corresponded for some months: two letters from Dalrymple to Gray (*NAZ* V 1/2/1/1) are dated October 12 and October 27, 1902. On October 12 Dalrymple, replying to a letter from Gray of July 25, says that the "white frothy exudate from the nostrils" is not seen in Louisiana, but that very few animals die from "tick fever" at the Experimental Station now that inoculation with blood is used to immunize cattle. Dalrymple closed this three-page letter by saying "I shall be extremely pleased to hear from you . . . at any time you care to write to me on this important subject." On October 27, Dalrymple sent some blood smears from a heifer that had been feverish even though she had been inoculated: "the films may be of interest to you in comparing the forms with those found in the disease as you have it."

57 The Santa Gertrudis is the heart of the King Ranch. Gray and Robert-

son said, in their joint report, that dipping tanks were in the process of construction, "modelled upon the plan of those erected at the Santa Gertrude Ranche, Texas, with certain modifications adopted from the plans of dipping tanks published in the Natal Agricultural Journal, in order to enable warm arsenical dips to be used." The plan of a dipping tank reproduced in the report had just appeared in the [Natal] *Agricultural Journal* 5: 301–302, [July 18], 1902; it showed the tank in use at Nel's Rust. The owner of Nel's Rust, Joseph Baynes, had long been a proponent of dipping cattle.

According to Tom Lea (T. Lea, *The King Ranch*, Boston, Little Brown, 1957, pp. 492–493), Cooper Curtice had surmised that Texas fever was tick borne even before Theobald Smith had proved that. As a result "the world's first cattle dipping vat" was invented and built at the Santa Gertrudis in 1891. For Curtice see: G. Dikmans, In Memoriam: Cooper Curtice, 1856–1939, *Journal of Parasitology* 25: 517–520, 1939.

Dikmans does not mention the dipping tank at the Santa Gertrudis but he does point out that although "the idea that cattle ticks were in some way connected with the problem of tick fever was not new ... Dr. Curtice's determination [in 1889] of the life cycle of the ticks made it possible to settle the question." Curtice urged that "experiments be undertaken to demonstrate that cattle ticks were the actual vectors of tick fever." Those were the experiments that were carried out by Smith.

58 C. E. Gray, East Coast Fever: A Historical Review, in *Report of the South African Association for the Advancement of Science. Sixth Meeting, Grahamstown, 1908*, Cape Town and Johannesburg, published by the Association, 1909, pp. 194–208. Full details and citations of Koch's work at Dar-es-Salaam are given in chapter 5.

59 The correspondence is in *NAZ* V 1/2/1/1.

60 D. E. McCausland, Rhodesia, in A. P. Newton, E. A. Benians and E. A. Walker (eds.), *Cambridge History of the British Empire*, Cambridge University Press, vol. VIII, 1936, pp. 662–670.

4   THE SEARCH FOR AN EXPERT

1 Milner was a brilliant and controversial figure, admired by supporters of the empire and despised by anti-imperialists. He was born in Giessen, Hesse-Darmstadt on March 28, 1854 and died near Canterbury on May 13, 1925. See C. Headlam (ed.), *The Milner Papers: South Africa*, 2 vols., London, Cassell, 1931–3; the *Dictionary of National Biography* (1922–30), pp. 588–602; and J. E. Wrench, *Alfred Lord Milner: The Man of No Illusions*, London, Eyre and Spottiswoode, 1958. A more recent study is that of A. M. Gollin, *Proconsul in Politics: A Study of Lord Milner in Opposition and in Power*, London, Anthony Blond, 1964. See also J. Marlowe, *Milner: Apostle of Empire*, London, Hamish Hamilton, 1976;

T. H. O'Brien, *Milner: Viscount Milner of St. James's and Cape Town*, London, Constable, 1979. Earlier biographies are cited in Basil Williams' sketch of Milner in the *Dictionary of National Biography* (*D.N.B.*).

Milner was a member of Lloyd George's small "War Cabinet" and Wrench comes close to suggesting that without his analytic and administrative abilities Great Britain might have lost the First World War. Acting on no authority but his own, Milner persuaded Clemenceau to place Foch in supreme command (over Haig and Pétain) after Amiens. After the war, according to the *D.N.B.*, Milner "was chiefly responsible for the establishment of the new Ministry of Health." Churchill's comment was made when he was a war correspondent for the *Morning Post*; I have taken the comment from Wrench, *Alfred Lord Milner*.

2 For Milner's role in reorganizing the Agricultural Department of the Transvaal, see W. B. Worsfold, *The Reconstruction of the New Colonies under Lord Milner*, London, Kegan Paul, 1913, vol. II, pp. 91–117. Worsfold remarked that "there is no part of the national life of the new colonies which was more profoundly benefited by Lord Milner's administration than agriculture."

3 My remarks about Smith are based in part on his entry in the *Dictionary of South African Biography*, vol. IV, pp. 578–580, which is by Theiler's biographer, Thelma Gutsche (see chapter 7, n. 1), and in part on information provided by John Garnett of the U.K. Ministry of Agriculture. The details of Smith's appointment as agricultural adviser are in *TAD* GOV 14/244. The documents relating to the approval of his plan and his authorization to proceed are in *TAD* CS 120/8972, which also contains the only copy of Smith's report to Milner that I have been able to locate. For the agricultural advisory service see N. F. McCann, *The Story of the National Agricultural Advisory Service – A Mainspring of Agricultural Revival 1946–1971*, Haddenham, Ely, Cambridgeshire, England, Providence Press, 1989.

4 *PRO* CO 417/344/28488.

5 All material referred to in this paragraph is in *PRO* CO 417/344/28488. The proclamation prohibited the importation into Natal of cattle from Rhodesia, Queensland, Texas and Louisiana, i.e. from places where true Texas fever was thought to exist. The proclamation appeared, among other places, in the [Natal] *Agricultural Journal* 5: 204, [June 6] 1902, as did a brief announcement, on the same page, that Watkins-Pitchford had left for Rhodesia with a number of Natal cattle to determine whether the outbreak in Rhodesia was "capable of being communicated to Natal stock."

The *Agricultural Journal and Mining Record*, to give it its full title, was an official fortnightly publication of the Department of Agriculture of Natal. It is usually cited as the *Natal Agricultural Journal* but Natal was not part of the title until 1904.

6 *PRO* CO 417/344/34191. Manuscript copy: *NAZ* RC 3/7/6. A brief

note in the [Natal] *Agricultural Journal* (5: 302 [July 18], 1902) said that the "disease is a form of redwater, but of so severe a type as to break down the immunity generally possessed by the Natal cattle. He [Watkins-Pitchford] considers, however, that there is no cause for anxiety concerning the spread of disease to this country." Two official reports soon appeared: "Redwater in Rhodesia. Report by H. Watkins-Pitchford, F.R.C.V.S. Experiments with Natal Cattle" and "Second Report," ([Natal] *Agricultural Journal* 5: 341–347, [August], 1902). The long first report, dated June 25, 1902, spoke of the great haste with which the journey was begun: in order to catch the ship Watkins-Pitchford assembled and loaded eight cattle within 36 hours since the next ship to Beira was not due to leave for three weeks. The cattle were disembarked at Beira on June 14 and taken by rail to Salisbury, reaching there on June 16. As of the first report (June 25, 1902) the cattle remained in good health. By the second report, dated July 19, 1902, all of the cattle had died, but Watkins-Pitchford said that they had died only because "redwater" had become more virulent: "This is the only explanation possible in the absence of the supposition that a strange or hitherto unknown disease exists concurrently with Redwater ... I see no reason to suppose this is the case."

These reports were reprinted as a pamphlet (H. Watkins-Pitchford, *Redwater in Rhodesia: Experiments with Natal Cattle*, Salisbury, Argus, 1902, cover plus 11 pages); the only copy of that pamphlet I have come across is in the Colonial Office library, now part of the library of the Foreign and Commonwealth Office, London.

7   PRO CO 417/344/34191; also *NAZ* RC 3/7/6.
8   *NAZ* RC 3/7/6 (Manuscript copy and typed copy).
9   See C. E. Gray and W. Robertson, *Report upon Texas Fever or Redwater in Rhodesia*, Cape Town, Argus, 1902, p. 23.
10 Some of these letters and telegrams are in the Resident Commissioner's files (*NAZ* RC 3/7/6), others are in the Administrator's files (*NAZ* A 11/2/2/14, vol. 2); some are in both.
11 Agriculture Register of Letters Received (by the Cape Department of Agriculture), *CAD* AGR 1/62: on August 13, an entry reads "Bacteriologist expert – recdg. either McFeaden, Dr. Koch or Prof Nocard" and again on August 13: "Bacteriological expert – suggesting selection be left to McFadyean if he cannot come." The letters themselves have not survived in either the Cape Archives Depot or the National Archives of Zimbabwe.
12 McFadyean (June 17, 1853 – February 1, 1941) graduated from the Royal (Dick) Veterinary College, Edinburgh in 1876. He became Professor of Pathology and Bacteriology at the Royal Veterinary College, London, in 1892 and Principal of that college in 1894. See I. Pattison, *John McFadyean*, London, J. A. Allen, 1981.
13 PRO CO 417/344/36657.
14 *NAZ* RC 3/7/6.
15 Milner and the Colonial Office had other things on their mind at the

time. On September 6, Milner, discouraged by Afrikaner influence in the Cape, asked to be allowed to resign. On August 25, Chamberlain had decided to visit South Africa; he left London for Durban on November 25 on a mission that must have required a good deal of planning both by Milner and in London.

16 D. Dwork, Koch and the Colonial Office, 1902–1904: The Second South African Expedition, *N.T.M. Schriftenreihe für Geschichte Naturwissenschaften, Technik und Medizin* 20: 67–74, 1983.

17 Manuscript draft of the letter to McFadyean is in *PRO CO* 417/344/36657; McFadyean's reply is in *PRO CO* 417/369/38001.

18 Woodhead (April 29, 1855 – December 29, 1921), Professor of Pathology at Cambridge, was the first editor of the *Journal of Pathology and Bacteriology*. For obituaries and tributes, including one from the great James Mackenzie, see *British Medical Journal*, 1922, vol. 1, pp. 39–41 and 81–82; and *The Lancet* 1922, vol. 1, p. 51.

19 Auguste Sheridan Delépine (January 1, 1855 – November 13, 1921), Professor of Pathology at Owens College, Manchester, was known for bacteriological work related to public health. For obituaries see *British Medical Journal*, 1921, vol. 2, pp. 921–922 and *The Lancet*, 1921, vol. 2, p. 1080.

20 *PRO CO* 417/344/38303.

21 *PRO CO* 417/344/38303; Delépine's replies are in *PRO CO* 417/368/39501.

22 Bruce was born in Australia on May 29, 1855 and died in England on November 27, 1931. See *Dictionary of National Biography* (1931–40), pp. 108–110 and *Obituary Notices of Fellows of the Royal Society*, vol. 1 (1932–5), pp. 79–85.

23 *PRO CO* 417/370/41566.

24 T. S. P. Strangeways (December 28, 1866 – December 23, 1927) was originally named Thomas Strangeways Pigg; he later changed his name to Thomas Strangeways-Pigg and finally to Thomas Strangeways Pigg Strangeways. The research institute that he headed from 1902 to 1926 was later named the Strangeways Research Laboratory; it was to become particularly well known under the leadership of Dame Honor Fell. In 1902 Strangeways was Woodhead's assistant; like Woodhead and Delépine he had no experience with redwater or other diseases of cattle, although he had once studied human malaria.

Strangeways was best known for his work on arthritis. For obituaries see *British Medical Journal* 1927, vol. 1, p. 28 and *The Lancet*, 1927, vol. 1, p. 56. See also E. D. Strangeways, F. G. Spear and H. B. Fell, *History of the Strangeways Research Laboratory, 1912–1962*, Privately printed, 1962; and J. A. Witkowski, Dame Honor Fell, *Trends in Biochemical Sciences* 11: 486–488, 1986.

25 *PRO CO* 417/345/42435.

26 Letter dated June 29, 1988.

27 Stewart Stockman stayed on in the Transvaal as its chief veterinarian after the end of the Boer War, and did join Arnold Theiler in in-

vestigating East Coast fever. In view of Pattison's analysis, one can hardly fault McFadyean's advice (apart, perhaps, from wondering why he overlooked David Bruce). Stockman was born in Edinburgh in 1869 and died in England in 1926. He was a pupil and friend of John McFadyean; in 1905 he became Chief Veterinary Officer of Great Britain. Stockman later married McFadyean's daughter. For an analysis of the long-time cooperation between Stockman and McFadyean, and for an evaluation of Stockman's later great importance in the veterinary profession see I. Pattison, John McFadyean and Stewart Stockman, *Veterinary History*, N.S. 1: 2–10, 1979. See also Stockman's obituary in the *Veterinary Record*, N.S. 6: 498–499, [June 12] 1926.

28 A. Keppel-Jones, *Rhodes and Rhodesia: The White Conquest of Zimbabwe 1884–1902*, Pietermaritzburg, University of Natal Press, 1983, pp. 623–628. Keppel-Jones argues that these events were the first step towards independence. That argument is confirmed in an interesting way by the resolution that The Rhodesian Farmers and Landowners Association adopted opposing abrogation of the charter (*The Rhodesian Landowners' and Farmers' Association, Bulawayo. Sixth Annual Report for the Year 1902*, Bulawayo, Argus Printing and Publishing Co., 1903, p. 26). That resolution ended with the words "industry will be best maintained and fostered under the Charter until the white community has increased to such an extent as to enable it to demand self-government."

29 *PRO* CO 417/344/38303.

30 *PRO* CO 417/345/47498.

31 Manuscript draft of cable in *PRO* CO 417/370/41566.

32 *NAZ* RC 3/7/6.

33 *PRO* CO 417/345/47498. On October 13, Gray wired to Hutcheon "I have recommended that Koch be approached at once as our observations have coincided with his . . . at Dar-es-Salaam . . . will be glad to know that you endorse my recommendation." Hutcheon was not in Cape Town. The message was forwarded to him by the Department of Agriculture on October 15 with an appended statement "What do you advise? On your recommendation we stipulated for either McFadyean or someone recommended by him" (*CAD* AGR 1/157).

34 *PRO* CO 417/345/42435.

35 *PRO* CO 417/435/47498.

36 *PRO* CO 417/435/44055.

37 *PRO* CO 417/435/44055. The first minute on that file reads "The point seems to be that the man who has made his name would refuse to go while a younger man who has not yet done so but is probably quite as good would take the appointment. The Priv. Sec. might approach Professor Koch and if he refuses, fall back on Mr. Strangeways. A.J.H." Another minute, dated October 24, reads "Private Secretary, Professor Koch must be approached through the Foreign Office, I suppose."
    The first response to Chamberlain's note was: "Mr. Chamberlain, I

understand that the F.O. [Foreign Office] will write ["are writing" crossed out] to Sir F. Lascelles to try and get Dr. Koch.

"Do you think it necessary to go to the Royal Society.

"I had sent the telegram to the F.O. before you wrote this minute."

Another plaintive note, from the Foreign Office, dated Friday, October 31, reads: "Dear Monkbretton, We have done nothing about getting Dr. Koch or any other German Bacteriologist for the cattle in Rhodesia because you wrote to me on Oct. 28 asking me to stop the proposed despatch to Lascelles as Chamberlain did not see why bacteriology should be made only in Germany. Are we to go on?"

38 Dwork, Koch and the Colonial Office, in an excellent summary of the events of September 2 – November 27, transcribed Chamberlain's all but illegible note slightly differently.

39 Minutes of the Malaria Committee, in the library of the Royal Society.

40 *PRO* 417/345/44055.

The full text of Lankester's note follows:

Unofficial
Nov. 5th.
My dear Sir,
    I have just attended a committee of the Royal Society which decided unanimously to recommend to you Surgeon Colonel Bruce F.R.S. as the right man to go to South Africa to investigate Red-water fever. You will learn this from Sir Michael Foster. But I think I may take the liberty of saying something about the remarkable qualifications of Colonel Bruce – which may not appear at once when his name is mentioned to you. Colonel Bruce is the discoverer of the cause of two most important diseases – Malta fever and (later) Tsetze [*sic*] Fly disease [of cattle] or Nagana. His work in both cases was admirable and his merit in both matters is universally recognized both at home and abroad. There is no one – not even Dr. Koch himself – who has shown so special an aptitude for the kind of investigation required. He is the one man whom we can put forward with confidence as able both from previous experience and special aptitude to carry out the investigation of Red-water fever to a successful issue.
    He holds at present a high post in the new committee for Army Medical Education. But valuable as his services must be there – it is in carrying out such a mission as that desired in South Africa – that Colonel Bruce's exceptional qualities as a discoverer & scientific man can alone be made full use of. I venture to write this unofficial note – because I am sure that you always desire to obtain the services of the right man and in this instance – if Colonel Bruce can be granted leave from the War Office – there is, I am quite confident, no possibility of doubt that he is the man whom you would wish to employ – as being really capable and one whose performance & reputation can be preferred to those of Dr. Koch.
    I am, my dear Sir, Very faithfully yours,

E. Ray Lankester.

Lankester's note was written on stationery headed "Arts Club. 40, Dover Street. Piccadilly W." The Arts Club is still on Dover Street. In 1902 the Royal Society was quartered in Burlington House, which is a two-minute walk from Dover Street. Lankester also belonged to the Savile Club, located at 107, Piccadilly. Perhaps he was so anxious to write his letter that he went to the Arts Club because it was closer to the Royal Society. The Savile Club, which was founded in 1868, quickly became a gathering place for bright young biologists. Of the five original members of the Malaria Committee, all but Lister were or had been members of the Savile; two later members of that committee, Charles Sherrington and Clifford Allbutt also were or had been members of the Savile (*The Savile Club: 1868 to 1925*, privately printed, 1923).

41 Manuscript draft in *PRO* 417/345/44055, with note: "Sent 10:35 A.M. 11/11." A copy was sent to the Foreign Office.

42 The letters are in *NAZ* A 11/2/2/14, vol. 2.

43 The full text of Orpen's letter follows:

Dear Mr. Milton

Yesterday evening after Chief Veterinary Surgeon Gray's return from Mazoe, I was for the first time able to meet him about the obtaining of an expert of high reputation from Europe to investigate the present cattle disease.

He says negotiations to obtain any of the highest class through Professor Mac Fadyen have not been successful – and that he cannot personally come? He recommends that if Mac Fadyen cannot come then *Koch* should if possible be obtained at joint expence of South African governments because he has already partially investigated similar disease at Dar es Salaam. If Koch cannot be obtained then he would advise Professor Nocard be obtained if possible.

Gray finds dipping not the success he hoped and learns from Queensland that inoculation is not giving satisfaction.

I believe that disease very similar to that so destructive here is spreading in Swaziland and may spread much further into Transvaal Natal &c and that if application is made through the High Commissioner the several South African Colonial Governments will agree and a cable could be sent to Europe to secure the services of an expert of European reputation.

Yours faithfully,

Joseph M. Orpen, S.G.

This letter, which had very important results, is a little mysterious since much of the information that it contained had already been sent by Kotzé to Milner and even by Milner to the Colonial Office. Perhaps it was written to bring Milton up to date. Or perhaps Gray and Kotzé had been consulting without bothering to tell Orpen and used Orpen as a cat's paw to attract Milton's attention.

44 The generally dismal situation in Rhodesia had become even worse when a terrifying epidemic of rabies spread throughout Matebeleland. On September 3 an appeal was made to the London office to send out an expert. On September 20, Pasteur's nephew, Dr. A. Loir, sailed from London with all necessary apparatus, having agreed to spend six months in Rhodesia for a fee of 1,000 pounds, "that is to say, five hundred pounds to be paid to me or my wife in Paris, before I start, and five hundred at the expiration of my voyage; or in case of my death, immediately to my wife or children" (*NAZ* LO 1/1/35). The rabies episode offers a remarkable contrast to the search for an East Coast fever expert, but the disease was obviously rabies, there were people in

Rhodesia able to determine that it was rabies, and the obvious place to
seek an expert was the Pasteur Institute. While still in Bulawayo, Loir
delivered a talk in which he said that he agreed that the cattle disease
was actually Texas fever although "What struck me most . . . is the
enormous quantities of the red corpuscles . . . which are infected by the
parasite, the rarity of the characteristic pyrosoma form, and the fre-
quence [*sic*] with which one finds the bacillary form."

Loir read his paper before the Rhodesia Scientific Association on
December 17, 1902 and it was published as *Notes on Rhodesia from a
Bacteriological Point of View*, Bulawayo, Argus, n.d. [1903?], 15 pp.
This pamphlet also contains a letter to Loir from Pasteur, dated June
15, 1891, in which Pasteur discusses the question of whether Australia
should suspend its six-month quarantine on imported dogs.

45 A 11/2/2/14, vol. 2; copy received by Milner in *PRO* CO
417/345/48426.
46 *PRO* CO 417/345/48426.
47 *NAZ* LO 1/1/37.
48 Milner's telegram and the various replies are in *PRO* CO
417/345/53185.
49 *NAZ* A 11/2/2/14, vol. 1.
50 Smith's letter is in *TAD* CS 178/15398; Milner's cable is in *PRO* CO
417/345/48336.
51 *NAZ* LO 1/2/18; *PRO* CO 417/365/50262 (but see n. 68 below).
52 Koch's full reply was:

In reply to your letter of the 22nd November I have the honour to inform you
respectfully that should the British South Africa Company decide to send an
Expert to Rhodesia to combat the cattle disease prevailing there, I should be
very pleased to undertake the mission. My conditions would be as follows:

(1) Two of my Assistants will accompany me.

(2) The expenses of the journey of myself and two Assistants are to be paid.

(3) I am to be paid daily £3, each of the Assistants £2, (reckoning from the
commencement of the journey until the return to Berlin) as daily allowance.

(4) There is further to be paid to me for the duration of one year (inclusive of
the outward and return journey) a fee of £6,000 and to each of the Assistants a
sum of £1,000. If the expedition should last a shorter time, then the fee will be
reckoned in proportion to the lesser time, but it is not to be less than the half of
the named sum. Should the expedition last longer than the year, then the fee
will be proportionately increased.

(5) Payment of the expenses for the scientific equipment which will amount to
about £400 to £500. (This equipment will remain the property of the British
South Africa Company and will be handed over to the Company at the close of
the expedition.)

(6) For the acquisition of the personal and scientific equipment as also for the
initial expenses of the journey the sum of £1,000 is to be paid to me immediately after the conclusion of an Agreement.

(7) It would be very agreeable to me if the services of Herr Otto Henning,

Veterinary Surgeon in Bloemfontein, who rendered me excellent service during my researches in connection with the Rinderpest in Kimberley in 1896 and 1897, could be placed at my disposal. For my part I would undertake that the British South Africa Company should derive all the advantages of the scientific and practical results of the expedition without any further conditions whatsoever. I would also undertake at the same time to make researches with a view to ascertaining the nature and the remedy of other diseases in animals, of which the British South Africa Company should desire the study.

In respect of the fee I take the liberty of stating that I cannot estimate it at a lower figure, as I lose during the period of the expedition, both my existing pay and also other revenue.

I have not found the original of Koch's reply, all copies in various archives (*NAZ LO 1/2/18; PRO 417/365/50262*) being headed "Translation."
53 *NAZ A 11/2/2/14*, vol. 1.
54 According to T. W. Baxter (*Guide to the Public Archives of Rhodesia*, Salisbury, National Archives of Rhodesia, 1969), material in the London board private files was intended "to keep Milton privately informed of the views of the London Board on all matters of importance," in other words this material was (illegally) intended to be kept secret from the Colonial Office in London, from High Commissioner Milner in Johannesburg and from the Resident Commissioner in Salisbury. L. H. Gann (*A History of Southern Rhodesia: Early Days to 1934*, London, Chatto and Windus, 1965, p. 143) says: "Colonial Office access to Company correspondence meant less in reality than on paper, for important communications which the Company wished to keep out of Imperial hands simply found their way into private letters between Directors and the Administrator on the spot." I assume that those of Milton's messages to London that were conveyed via the Company's agent in Cape Town (J. A. Stevens) were also intended to be kept "out of Imperial hands." The private files are *NAZ A 1/5/1* to *A 1/5/9*.
55 *NAZ A 1/5/4*.
56 *PRO CO 417/345/53185*.
57 *PRO CO 417/345/53185*.
58 *PRO 417/365/50262*.
59 On the same day that Milton cabled to Milner, i.e. November 28, the London office of the Chartered Company wrote to the great French bacteriologist, Edmund Nocard, who had been the second choice of both Hutcheon and Gray [*NAZ LO 1/2/18*]. Whether this was done at the instigation of Milton or because the London board was so alarmed by Koch's charges I do not know. The letter sent to Nocard on November 28 was almost identical to the letter that had been sent to Koch on November 22. Nocard declined on December 7, saying that he was totally committed to a study of foot-and-mouth disease:

I regret it all the more because during the past few years I have given a great deal of study to the piroplasmoses of cattle, dogs and sheep . . . and because from an examination of the preparations which have been sent to us by M. Theiler ... I have been able to assure myself that the cattle disease which is troubling you is only a form, though apparently a more malignant one, of Redwater...

Nocard suggested that the B.S.A.C. seek the services of "Dr. Nicolle" who had recently studied redwater in Turkey. Since Nocard described his candidate as being "the Director of the Imperial Institute of Experimental Medicine in Constantinople," the man he had in mind was not Charles Nicolle, who received the Nobel Prize in 1928, but Charles Nicolle's then better-known older brother, Maurice Nicolle.

The B.S.A.C. thanked Nocard on December 18, expressing its regret that it could not approach Nicolle. Nocard, who had discovered the causative agents of psittacosis and Nocardiosis, died less than a year later, at the age of fifty-three. Nicolle, Nocard said, "would be perfectly prepared for the study of the Rhodesian disease. I think that no other important business would prevent him from accepting this mission." Nicolle eventually became a professor at the Pasteur Institute in Paris.

60 *PRO CO* 417/435/48336. The staff of the Colonial Office did not approach the Foreign Office as soon as it heard from Milner, as a series of minutes on this file shows:

Mr. Fiddes, In view of this I presume Professor Kock [*sic*] will be approached?

Local feeling too strong to go against. G.G. [Gilbert Grindle] 22/11.

Sir M. Ommanney, See Mr. Chamberlain's minutes on note paper and my minute in consequence both attached to 44055. I suppose we can only proceed as proposed above?

Lord Onslow, I note that on the telegram 44055 [recommending Bruce] we did not call Lord Milner's attention to the feeling which was evoked here when a German subject was employed on the last occasion [rinderpest] and to the assumption which is involved that no competent British subject is available. But, meanwhile, Lord Milner has communicated with the other Govt's concerned and the result leaves us no option but to approach Prof. Koch.

Sir M. Ommanney, I gather from Mr. C's minute on 44055 that if Koch is to be approached it should be through the B.S.A.Co. Might we not let them do it? [Onslow] 23/11 [Koch had been approached by the B.S.A.C. the day before, but the Colonial Office did not know that].

Lord Onslow, It is not, at this stage, a question of his being approached by the B.S.A.Co. Lord Milner has been acting in this matter for all the S. African Govt's including Rhodesia. He has ascertained that all are willing to contribute towards the employment of Koch and asks us to approach him. I think we should ask F.O. [Foreign Office] to find out if he can go at an early date and what his terms will be. 25/11.

(Written in the margin of the above: "Then I suppose we must do it 25/11" and, finally, "Proceed as originally proposed [Onslow] 26/11.")

61 *PRO CO* 417/359/49680.

62 *PRO* CO 417/360/49829.
63 *PRO* CO 417/360/49830.
64 *PRO* CO 417/345/49654.
65 *NAZ* A 11/2/2/14, vol. 2.
66 *PRO* 417/365/50262.
67 *PRO* CO 417/435/49851.
68 *NAZ* LO 1/2/18; *PRO* CO 417/365/50262. I cited this letter in n. 51
    above, with reference to the events of November 22, but at that time
    no copy had been sent to the Colonial Office.
69 *NAZ* LO 1/2/18; manuscript draft minuted "Mr. Orpen," *NAZ* A
    11/2/2/14, vol. 1.
70 The Chargé d'Affaires learned from Dr. von Muhlberg on December 1
    that Koch had already been approached and what his terms were and
    sent that information to the Foreign Office. Presumably before he
    heard from von Muhlberg, on the same day, December 1, the Chargé
    d'Affaires launched a second, rather bizarre, approach to Koch (*PRO*
    CO 417/360/50190). As he wrote to the Foreign Secretary, the Mar-
    quess of Lansdowne,

    I today requested Mr. Collier who met Professor Koch last night at a dinner
    given by Dr. Hillier, the leader of the Deputation of Friendly Societies which
    has recently been travelling about Germany, to interview the Professor on the
    investigation of the cattle disease in Rhodesia . . . Dr. Koch stated that he had
    already received a communication from the South Africa Company in this
    sense, and handed to Mr. Collier a list of the conditions on which he was
    willing to undertake the investigation, copy and translation of which I have the
    honour to enclose. He stated at the same time that he had already communi-
    cated these conditions to the South Africa Company, and said he supposed he
    might regard the proposals which he had received from the two sources as
    identical.

    Presumably even Koch was beginning to get a little muddled, since
    this was the third time in nine days that he had been asked to go to
    Rhodesia, the third time he had agreed to do so, and the third time he
    had given identical terms for doing so. (The list that Koch handed Mr.
    Collier on December 1 contained the same terms that he had sent to the
    B.S.A.C. on November 24 but is somewhat differently worded; he
    did not simply hand Mr. Collier a copy of his letter to the B.S.A.C.)
    The proposals that Koch handed Mr. Collier are dated December 1. It
    took the embassy three days to get them translated and sent, via the
    Foreign Office, to the Colonial Office, where they arrived on Decem-
    ber 5.
71 *PRO* CO 417/345/49851.
72 *PRO* CO 417/365/50262. Bruce's detailed terms were as follows:

    (1) Time. Six months to one year;

    (2) Salary . . . Present military pay of £865:15:4 plus five guineas per diem for
    travelling and out of pocket expenses;

    (3) Free passage to Cape Town and back, for self, Mrs. Bruce and a Lab-

oratory Assistant; Mrs. Bruce acts as unpaid Secretary and Laboratory Assistant. Could go by Government Transport if available.

(4) Pay for second Laboratory Assistant probably about £80 to £100 per annum;

(5) Free transport over Government Railways or by wagon, &c.

(6) Use of Laboratory, materials, experimental animals, &c. I would bring out apparatus which might form nucleus ["e" in "neucleus" crossed out: Bruce or his wife surely typed this letter] of Government Laboratory when left behind. It is possible that there is a Laboratory established in Rhodesia already. The cost of apparatus would be between £150 to £200;

(7) I would require, especially at first, the assistance of a Veterinary Surgeon accustomed to handle cattle.

[Signed] David Bruce, Lt. Colonel R.A.M.C.

73 *PRO CO* 417/368/50603.
74 I have taken the wording of Onslow's cable to Milner from a copy that the Colonial Office sent to the London office of the B.S.A.C. (*NAZ LO* 1/2/18). The rest of Milner's telegram to the colonies I have taken from Milner's confirming letter to the Colonial Office, which did not include the text of Onslow's cable to Milner, presumably because the Colonial Office already had that text (*PRO* 417/371/13474). A third copy, hand written, which included all of Milner's telegram to the colonies and all of Onslow's cable to Milner, is found in *NAZ A* 11/2/2/14, vol. 1. It is presumably the version that Milton saw.

No two of these three versions are identical. It makes one wonder about the influence of copyists, typists and telegraphists on the course of events. None of the minor variations in these versions could have affected what happened, but it is interesting to realize that no two people read exactly the same message.
75 *PRO CO* 417/371/13474.
76 *NAZ LO* 1/2/18.
77 *PRO CO* 417/345/51830.
78 *NAZ LO* 1/2/18.
79 *NAZ V* 1/2/1/1.
80 *NAZ LO* 1/2/18.
81 *NAZ LO* 1/2/18; *PRO CO* 417/365/52902.
82 *PRO CO* 417/345/51830.
83 *PRO CO* 545/12, South Africa Register, alphabetical section, entry for December 24, 1902.
84 Castellani, who originally believed that a streptococcus was the cause of sleeping sickness, had seen trypanosomes in the spinal fluid before Bruce reached Uganda and called them to Bruce's attention when Bruce arrived in Uganda. Castellani did publish his finding and his surmise that the trypanosomes might be the cause of sleeping sickness. Davies argues that since the presence of the trypanosomes in the spinal fluid and the existence of tsetse flies in Uganda were made known to Bruce as soon as he arrived, Bruce's role was to some extent only to

confirm the importance of those observations (see J. N. P. Davies, The Cause of Sleeping Sickness? Entebbe 1902–1903, Part I, *East African Medical Journal* 39: 81–99, 1962; J. N. P. Davies, The Cause of Sleeping Sickness? Part II, *East African Medical Journal* 39: 145–160, 1962; J. N. P. Davies, Informed Speculation on the Cause of Sleeping Sickness, 1898–1903, *Medical History* 12: 200–204, 1968). Boyd argues that Castellani was not aware of the significance of his finding until Bruce pointed it out to him. (See J. Boyd, Sleeping Sickness: The Castellani–Bruce Controversy, *Notes and Records of the Royal Society* 28: 93–110, 1973). It seems to me that Bruce's further work, in particular his work on the role of the tsetse fly, justifies the statement that he *established* both the role of the trypanosome and the role of the tsetse fly. S. R. Christophers, in his sketch of Bruce in the *Dictionary of National Biography* (1931–40, pp. 108–110), used the same word to characterize Bruce's contribution: "it was Bruce who, with his extraordinary power of systematic research, first established the nature and cause of this disease." In the course of that research Bruce daily exposed both himself and his wife to the risk of contracting the disease and did so for some six months, which suggests that he, at any rate, was not persuaded that the problem had been solved even before he began to study it.

5 ROBERT KOCH IN BULAWAYO

1 *NAZ* LO 1/2/18.
2 *PRO* CO 417/365/52902.
3 Robert Koch was born on December 11, 1843 and died on May 27, 1910. He was one of the greatest medical scientists of the nineteenth century and his work, with that of Pasteur, created modern bacteriology. He was awarded the Nobel Prize for Physiology or Medicine in 1905, chiefly for his work on tuberculosis. C. E. Dolman's excellent and thoroughly documented article on Koch does not go into the East Coast fever episode in any detail (see *Dictionary of Scientific Biography*, vol. VII, New York, Scribner, 1973, pp. 420–435). Heymann's unfinished biography of Koch covers only the years 1843–1882 (B. Heymann, *Robert Koch, I. Teil 1843–1882*, Leipzig, Akademische Verlagsgesellschaft, 1932). Möllers provides many useful letters and much background material concerning Koch's work in Rhodesia (B. Möllers, *Robert Koch: Persönlichkeit und Lebenswerk, 1843–1910*, Hannover, Schmorl und Seefeld, 1950). Brock, in his recent biography of Koch (T. D. Brock, *Robert Koch*, Madison, Science Tech Publishers; Berlin, Springer, 1988), bases his account of the East Coast fever episode largely on Dwork's article (D. Dwork, Koch and the Colonial Office, 1902–1904: The Second South African Expedition, *N.T.M. Schriftenreihe für Geschichte der Naturwissenschaften, Technik und Medizin* 20: 67–74, 1983). Brock barely touches upon the German East Africa episode of 1897 and 1898, claiming, probably correctly, that Koch's

report of the work he did in that period contains "really little of enduring interest."

4 Koch spent more than a year in German East Africa. His first letter concerning "Texas fever" is dated November 15, 1897, his last is dated March 6, 1898. I do not know if his official reports, in the form of letters to various government officials, were modified before being published in book form in 1898 as R. Koch, *Reise-Berichte über Rinderpest, Bubonenpest in Indien und Afrika, Tsetse- oder Surrakrankheit, Texasfieber, Tropische Malaria, Schwarzwasserfieber*, Berlin, Julius Springer, 1898. Reprinted in J. Schwalbe (ed.), *Gesammelte Werke von Robert Koch*, Leipzig, Thieme, 1912, vol. II, pt. 2, pp. 688–747. I usually quote from the reasonably but not entirely accurate English translation of the section on Texas fever that was so often quoted by Hutcheon, Gray, Robertson and others. It appeared in the *Agricultural Journal of the Cape of Good Hope* 14: 658–667, 1899.

5 T. Smith and F. L. Kilborne *Investigations into the Nature, Causation, and Prevention of Southern Cattle Fever*, U.S. Department of Agriculture. Bureau of Animal Industry, Bulletin No. 1. Washington, Government Printing Office, 1893: reprinted in [E. C. Kelly], *Medical Classics*, vol. I, no. 5, Baltimore, Williams and Wilkins, 1937, pp. 341–597.

6 C. E. Gray, East Coast Fever: A Historical Review, *Report of the South African Association for the Advancement of Science. Sixth Meeting, Grahamstown, 1908*, Cape Town and Johannesburg, published by the Association, 1909, pp. 194–208.

7 According to Möllers (*Robert Koch*, p. 265), Koch wrote to his friend Arnold Libbertz on December 29, 1902 that he was about to leave for Rhodesia to investigate a disease of cattle and that he could hardly refuse because the investigation was, in a way (*gewissermassen*), a continuation of the work that he had begun in 1896. One might assume that he wrote 1896 in error for 1897 and that he had in mind his work on Texas fever. But, on the same day, he wrote to Georg Gaffky (Möllers, *Robert Koch*, p. 264) that the work was a continuation of the work he had begun in the Cape Province (Kaplande) six years before. Thus he seems to have had his study of rinderpest in mind when he wrote to Libbertz and to Gaffky. Yet he had already suggested to the B.S.A.C. that he travel via Mombasa, Dar-es-Salaam and Beira. Of course the entire earlier journey (to South Africa, India and German East Africa) was a single journey and it did begin in 1896.

8 *NAZ* A 11/2/2/14, vol. 1.

9 As far as I can determine, G. Stanley Bruce was not related to David Bruce: all of the letters are addressed in a formal and respectful way. According to the records of the Royal College of Veterinary Surgeons, George Stanley Bruce qualified in London on July 16, 1901, became F.R.C.V.S. on May 16, 1908, and died on March 19, 1946. His R.C.V.S. fellowship thesis on East Coast fever is less interesting than his letters to David Bruce.

The letters from G. Stanley Bruce to David Bruce were deposited in the Wellcome Tropical Institute Archive by the Royal Society of Tropical Medicine and are reproduced by permission of Miss Sue Bramley of the Wellcome Tropical Institute Archive. (The Wellcome Tropical Institute Archive has been amalgamated with the Wellcome Institute for the History of Medicine Contemporary Medical Archive Centre, which now has custody of these letters.)

10 Koch's reports were submitted to the British South Africa Company and were published in Salisbury by the Argus Printing and Publishing Company on behalf of the Legislative Council: (1) *Interim Report on Rhodesian Redwater, or "African Coast Fever"*, title page + 8 pages, dated March 26, 1903; (2) *Second Report on African Coast Fever*, title page + 5 pages, dated May 28, 1903; (3) *Third Report on African Coast Fever*, title page + 9 pages, dated September 25, 1903; (4) *Fourth Report on African Coast Fever*, title page + 7 pages + charts on pp. 8–13, dated February 29, 1904. They appear to have been written in English; a carbon copy of the typed version of the *Interim Report* (*NAZ LO 4/1/14*) has corrections in English in Koch's hand and is signed by him. The reports also appeared, in full or in part, in the *Bulawayo Chronicle*, the *Rhodesia Herald* and the *Rhodesian Agricultural Journal*, as well as in various veterinary journals. For example, the *Interim Report* can be found in the *Transvaal Agricultural Journal* (1, pt. 4: 112–117, 1903); the *Veterinary Record* (16: 72–76, 1903); the *Agricultural Journal of the Cape of Good Hope* (23: 33–39, 1903); the [Natal] *Agricultural Journal* (6: 313–320, 1903); the *Journal of Pathology and Experimental Therapeutics* (16: 273–280, 1903); and, in German, as Vorläufiger Bericht über das Rhodesische Rotwasser oder "Afrikanische Küstenfieber," (aus dem Englischen übertragen), *Archiv für wissenschaftliche und praktische Tierheilkunde* 30: 281–295, 1904. It was even excerpted at some length in the popular magazine *South Africa* (July 25, 1903, p. 284). Koch's work on the new disease thus attracted widespread attention, as did the disease itself.

The other reports were also widely republished. The most convenient place to find them is in the *Journal of Comparative Pathology and Therapeutics* (Second report, 16: 280–284, 1903; Third report, 16: 390–398, 1903; Fourth report [without all of the tables summarizing the immunization studies] 17: 175–181, 1904). The reports, and the reports on horse sickness, which Koch also studied in Rhodesia, can also be found in German translation in Schwalbe, *Gesammelte Werke von Robert Koch*, vol. II, pt. 2, pp. 749–798. (In *Gesammelte Werke*, the fourth report (pp. 787–798) is, for some reason, in English; it does include the tables.)

A frequently cited report of Koch's work was a summary written by Kleine and approved by Koch: F. K. Kleine, Die Ergebnisse der Forschungen Robert Koch's über das Küstenfieber der Rinder und über der Pferdesterbe gelegentlich seiner letzten Expedition nach Südafrika, *Deutsche medizinische Wochenschrift* 31: 912–915, 1905. This article was also reprinted in *Gesammelte Werke* (vol. II, pt. 2, pp. 799–805), where an editor's footnote states that it contains modifications of Koch's original reports. As far as I can see it neither mentions nor corrects any of Koch's errors and certainly does not mention Theiler or Lounsbury.

11 Because they stain blue in slides exposed to certain then commonly used stains, in particular the Giemsa stain and the Romanowsky stain.

12 Möllers, *Robert Koch*, pp. 265–266.

13 *NAZ* LO 4/1/14 (typed copy). Published in *The British South Africa Company: Reports on the Administration of Rhodesia, 1900–1902*, Printed for the Information of Shareholders [London, 1903], pp. 224–230.

14 *PRO* 417/371/16877.

15 *PRO* CO 417/371/15226.

16 See chapter 7.

17 Möllers, *Robert Koch*, pp. 266–269.

18 Stanley Portal Hyatt, *The Old Transport Road*, London, Andrew Melrose, 1914, p. 299; reprint: Bulawayo, Books of Rhodesia, 1969.

19 Möllers, *Robert Koch*, pp. 267–268.

20 Koch's assistants were Fred Neufeld (born in Neuteich, January 17, 1869; died in Berlin, April 18, 1945) and Friederich Karl Kleine (born in Stralsund May 14, 1869; died in Johannesburg, March 22, 1951). For more details on their lives and careers see n. 30 below.

21 F. K. Kleine, Mit Koch in Afrika, *Fortschritte der Medizin* 50: 959–966, 1932. See also F. K. Kleine, Mit Robert Koch in Afrika und in der Heimat, *Zeitschrift für Hygiene und Infektionskrankheiten* 125: 265–286, 1943, which is reprinted, along with other articles by Kleine, a biographical sketch of Kleine by Herbert Kunert, and a bibliography of Kleine's publications, in F. K. Kleine, *Ein deutscher Tropenarzt* (Einführung von Herbert Kunert), Hannover, Schmorl and von Seefeld, 1949.

The second article is longer and more detailed than "Mit Koch in Afrika." In it, Kleine identifies the Rhodesian side of the staff at Hillside Camp as being Gray, Sinclair, "Kerney" (presumably P. X. Kearney, a cattle inspector who sent Gray several detailed reports from Hillside Camp in November and December, 1902, reports which are in *NAZ* V 1/2/1/1), a green (*blutjunger*) lad named Hinds (C. F. Hinds, later an important administrator at Theiler's laboratory in Onderstepoort) and a "Mr. F.," who loved whisky and thought that the two greatest men in the world were Buffalo Bill and Robert Koch! Kleine also speaks of the garden parties and polo games of Bulawayo; as to polo "our Sinclair was Chief Matador."

22 Koch, *Second Report on African Coast Fever*. See n. 10 above.

23 See n. 9 above.

24 Koch, *Third Report on African Coast Fever*. See n. 10 above.

25 Theiler and Robertson made the same point. (For Theiler, see *Transvaal Department of Agriculture. Report of the Government Veterinary Bacteriologist, 1906–1907*, Pretoria, Government Printing and Stationery

Office, 1908; see pp. 8–9.) Two German writers, Luhe and Schilling, had challenged Theiler's assertion that the blue tick does not transmit East Coast fever, citing as evidence Koch's experiment in which he sowed a field with larvae to cause it to become infective. In rebuttal, Theiler quotes Koch at some length and italicizes the words "*previously only occasional cases of African Coast fever had occurred.*" Theiler added that this means that "*The larval ticks were distributed on an already infested area,*" as was surely the case. As early as 1904, Robertson commented "Professor Koch claims to have produced the disease through the agency of the blue tick ... but, as the Professor's experiments consisted in sowing these ticks on the veldt (and in an infected area), the chances of natural infection were not excluded." (W. Robertson, African Coast Fever, *Journal of Comparative Pathology and Bacteriology* 17: 214–221, 1904).

26 *Rhodesian Agricultural Journal* 2: 73–78, [February] 1904.
27 *Report of the Proceedings of the Conference on Diseases Among Cattle and other Animals in South Africa held on the 3rd, 4th and 5th December, 1903*, Bloemfontein, Argus, 1904.
28 Möllers, *Robert Koch*, pp. 276–277.
29 Koch, *Fourth Report on African Coast Fever*. See n. 10 above.
30 Fred Neufeld, Erinnerungen aus meiner 50 Jährigen Tätigkeit als Bakteriologe, *Ärztliche Wochenschrift* 1: 146–150 and 186–189, 1946.

Since Neufeld says that he began as a bacteriologist in 1894, the fifty years covered by his reminiscences were 1894–1944. According to an editor's note, the published version of the reminiscences was based on a shortened version of a manuscript found in Neufeld's effects after his death. If the unedited version still exists, it might repay study.

Among Neufeld's many notable achievements was his work on pneumococci. He "obtained the first solid evidence for the diversity of pneumococcal strains," discovered the capsular swelling phenomenon that occurs in the presence of type-specific antiserum, and confirmed the finding that the R (rough) and S (smooth) forms of pneumococci are interconvertible *in vitro*. All of that work played an important role in setting the stage for the later proof that the pneumococcal transforming principle is DNA (see M. McCarty, *The Transforming Principle*, New York, Norton, 1985, pp. 60, 64, 77, 78, 94).

Neufeld was President of the Robert Koch Institute from 1917 to 1933. He resigned a year before he reached 65, after a severe attack of pneumonia. He continued to work at the Institute as an honorary member until his death in Berlin in 1945. According to McCarty, Neufeld is said to have died of starvation. A brief eulogy of Neufeld by Kleine, which was probably Kleine's last published article (F. K. Kleine, Fred Neufeld, *Zeitschrift für Hygiene und Infektionskrankheiten* 127: 185–186, 1948), also says that Neufeld died of starvation (*Entkräftung*). In his eulogy, Kleine spoke of Neufeld with great warmth and respect.

According to Kunert (Kleine, *Ein deutscher Tropenarzt*), Kleine devoted most of his career to the study of trypanosomes and
trypanosomiasis, and did the field tests of the first drug that was useful
in the treatment of trypanosomiasis, Bayer 205 or "germanine." (The
late Ernst Friedheim, himself a great figure in the development of
anti-trypanosomal drugs, told me shortly before his death that Bayer
205 remains a useful agent. He added that the Germans, resentful over
the loss of their African colonies after the First World War, deliberately
called the drug germanine to remind those who used it in the former
German colonies that it was a German invention.) Kleine succeeded
Neufeld as President of the Koch Institute, in 1933, but served only
until he retired a year later at the usual age of 65. Kleine made many
visits to Africa in connection with his work on trypanosomiasis and
became a friend of Arnold Theiler and a great admirer of Theiler's
institute at Onderstepoort. Both Kunert (Kleine, *Ein deutscher Tropenarzt*) and Fortner (see below) state that Kleine left Germany for South
Africa in July, 1947 at the invitation of his old friend Major-General
Dr. A. J. Orenstein (a German-born American citizen who had
worked with Gorgas and then moved to South Africa where he
became both chief physician to the gold mines of the Rand and a
long-time friend of Arnold Theiler; see T. Gutsche, *There was a Man:
The Life and Times of Sir Arnold Theiler*, Cape Town, Timmins, 1979,
and see the *Dictionary of South African Biography*, vol. V, pp. 555–557).
Kleine died in Johannesburg in 1951.

Fortner's biographical sketch of Kleine and Fortner's reminiscences
of his own life during the Nazi period are of considerable interest (J.
Fortner, Dem Freunde des tierärztlichen Wissenschaft Geheimrat Friedrich Karl Kleine, *Tierärztliche Umschau* 15: 336–338, 1960; J. Fortner,
Geschichtliche Notizen aus meiner Zeit bis 1945, *Tierärztliche Umschau*
19: 567–574, 1964). Fortner points out that Neufeld was not Jewish and
that his slightly premature resignation was indeed the result of his
severe attack of pneumonia. Himself a vigorous anti-Nazi, Fortner
emphatically denies that Kleine was either a Nazi or in sympathy with
the Nazis. Although Kleine was awarded the "Adlerschild des Deut-
schen Reiches" on his seventieth birthday, i.e. May 14, 1939 (see
Möllers, *Robert Koch*, p. 390), the fact that he was re-appointed to a
post at the Koch Institute in 1946 and was allowed by the Allies to
emigrate to South Africa in 1947 supports Fortner's view, as does the
fact that according to the *Dictionary of South African Biography*, Kleine's
friend and patron A. J. Orenstein was the son of Jewish immigrants to
the United States. Fortner's articles are of great interest in relation to
the effects of the Nazi period on the Koch Institute. I am indebted to
Professor F. J. Fehrenbach and Mr. Klaus Gerber of the Robert Koch-
Institut des Bundesgesundheitsamtes for some of the above information and for copies of the articles by Fortner.

31 For the proposal to extend Koch's services see *PRO CO*
417/385/38482; *PRO CO* 417/374/42379; *NAZ* A 11/2/2/14, vol. 1,

and *TAD* LTG 55/69/17. For the objections of the Transvaal authorities, see *TAD* LTG 55/69/17.

32 M. W. Henning, *Animal Diseases in South Africa*, 2nd edition, South Africa, Central News Agency.

33 C. E. Gray, Immunization against Horse-Sickness by the method recommended by Professor Koch, *Journal of Comparative Pathology and Therapeutics* 17: 344–351, 1904. In this article Gray presented the final tabular results of the experiments initiated by Koch and concluded that "the lines of treatment laid down by Dr. Koch require important modifications."

34 *NAZ* "Koch, Dr, 1902/3", negative 5852.

35 *NAZ* T 2/29/6/2.

36 K. Baedeker, *London and its Environs*, Leipzig, Karl Baedeker, 1908. A single room could be had at the Ritz or Claridge's for ten shillings and sixpence (10/6), at the Savoy for 9/6, and at the Coburg (now the Connaught) for a mere six shillings.

37 A. Conan Doyle, A Case of Identity, *The Strand Magazine*, September, 1891.

38 According to the Bank of England, the retail prices index, if extrapolated back from 1915 to 1903, indicates that the purchasing power of £1 in 1903 was comparable to that of £34.88 in 1988. It may seem arbitrary to compare prices in 1888, 1898, 1904 and 1908 with those of today, but, as Keynes pointed out, "Money is important only for what it can procure," and "for the period of close on a century from 1826 to the outbreak of war [in 1914], the maximum fluctuation in either direction was only 30 points, the index number never rising above 130 and never falling below 70." See J. M. Keynes, *A Tract on Monetary Reform*, London, Macmillan, 1923, p. 1 and pp. 11–12.

39 *Cape of Good Hope. Department of Agriculture. Report of Proceedings at Inter-Colonial Veterinary Conference (Adjourned from Bloemfontein 5th December, 1903) on Animals' Diseases in South Africa. Held at Cape Town on 25th, 26th, 27th, 28th, 30th and 31st May, 1904*, Cape Town, Cape Times Ltd., Government Printers, 1904 [G.87–1904].

40 C. E. Gray, Inoculation for African Coast Fever, *Rhodesian Agricultural Journal* 2: 8–9, 1904; *Journal of Comparative Pathology and Therapeutics* 17: 203–205, 1904.

41 *PRO* CO 417/392/30208.

42 Alexander was an important farmer in Natal. Comments by him on agricultural matters often appeared in the *Natal Witness* and in the *Natal Agricultural Journal*. The *Standard Encyclopaedia of Southern Africa* (vol. I, p. 228) says that he was the first chairman of the Intercolonial Agricultural Union of South Africa, which was formed July 25, 1904.

43 Many of the comments in Alexander's article are, of course, consistent with the attack Watkins–Pitchford later made on Koch at the Bloemfontein conference. The opinions of Watkins-Pitchford that I have quoted appeared as follows, all in the [Natal] *Agricultural Journal*, vol. 5, 1902: H. Watkins-Pitchford, Redwater, June 6, pp. 197–198; [un-

signed news report], July 18, p. 302; H. Watkins-Pitchford, Redwater in Rhodesia. Experiments with Natal Cattle, August 1, pp. 341–346 (first part), pp. 346–347 (second part); H. Watkins-Pitchford, The Rhodesian form of Redwater, November 21, pp. 597–600.

Watkins-Pitchford later made a crucially important contribution to the eventual control of East Coast fever by developing the arsenical dips that are discussed in chapter 8 below. But he seems often to have felt that he did not receive adequate credit for other contributions, among them the work he did with Theiler on rinderpest. Alexander's article is not the only place in which it is suggested that Watkins-Pitchford was deprived of well-deserved recognition. The rinderpest question is discussed by Gutsche, *There was a Man*. The claim that he was denied recognition is also made in a short pamphlet published anonymously with no date, place or publisher given: *The Past Work of Lieut. Col. H. Watkins-Pitchford C.M.G., F.R.C.V.S., F.R.S.E. Being extracts from various Official and Press Sources*, a photocopy of which is in the library of The Royal College of Veterinary Surgeons. On pp. 5–6 of that pamphlet we find that in the study of East Coast fever

The odds . . . were all against Pitchford . . . for the world-famed Koch and his assistants, specially imported from Berlin at great cost, naturally had at command the fullest modern facilities, while Theiler of the Transvaal, with his magnificently equipped laboratory and ample means and staff, 'carried all the guns' so to speak in comparison to Pitchford.

The *Dictionary of South African Biography* (vol. III, p. 833) remarks that "he devoted himself to the causes of the animal diseases rinderpest and East Coast fever, sometimes in conjunction with and sometimes in opposition to the veterinarian A. Theiler." The *Dictionary of South African Biography* also states that Watkins-Pitchford was born in Bath on June 3, 1865 and died in Natal on June 25, 1950. The same source says that he became the Principal Veterinary Surgeon of Natal in 1896, later became its first Government Bacteriologist, and was, for some years, Commandant of the veterinary school at Aldershot. P. J. Post-humus, *An Index of Veterinarians in South Africa*, 4th edition, Pietermaritzburg, privately printed, 1982, vol. II, pp. 227–229, states that his work on various animal diseases and his production of vaccines were very valuable and says "here was a man who was a Veterinarian, Soldier, Artist and Writer whose road in history was a thorny one. His treatment by the Natal Government which he so ably served was to say the least, shoddy." Latter-day experts on East Coast fever, including John A. Lawrence and C. G. D. Brown, have spoken highly to me of his perfection of methods of dipping cattle to control ticks.

44 G. D. Alexander, The Inconsistency of Dr. Koch, *Veterinary Record* 16: 268–269, [October 31] 1903.

45 L. E. W. Bevan, Autobiography, n.p., n.d., typed (*NAZ* Historical Manuscripts BE 11/7/1).

46 Gray, East Coast Fever, see n. 6 above.

6 JOSEPH CHAMBERLAIN

1 See, for example, the Dictionary of National Biography (1912–21), pp. 102–118; J. L. Garvin, The Life of Joseph Chamberlain, vols. I–III, London, Macmillan, 1932–4, continued as J. Amery, The Life of Joseph Chamberlain, vols. IV–VI, London, Macmillan, 1951–68; and D. Judd, Radical Joe, London, Hamish Hamilton, 1977. An early biography by Marris, wholly uncritical and laudatory, contains many interesting personal details about Chamberlain (N. M. Marris, Joseph Chamberlain: The Man and the Statesman, London, Hutchinson, 1900).

2 University College London was founded in 1828 to provide an institution of higher learning for students who were not members of the Church of England. In 1830 the University College School was established as a preparatory school for children of similar background. See N. Harte and J. North The World of University College London, 1828–1978, London, University College, 1978 (for the school in particular, see pp. 4, 5, 48, 49, 72, 132, 133).

3 M. Sanderson, The Universities and British Industry 1850–1970, London, Routledge and Kegan Paul, 1972.

4 Charles W. Boyd (ed.), Mr. Chamberlain's Speeches, London, Constable, 1914, vol. I, pp. 43–44.

5 Boyd, Mr. Chamberlain's Speeches, vol. I, p. 62.

6 See Garvin, Joseph Chamberlain, vol. I, pp. 549–550; and Boyd, Mr. Chamberlain's Speeches, vol. I, pp. 130–135.

7 See Garvin, Joseph Chamberlain vol. I, p. 554.

8 See Judd, Radical Joe, pp. xiii–xv.

9 W. Churchill, Great Contemporaries, New York, G. P. Putnam, 1937, p. 57.

10 Amery, Joseph Chamberlain, vol. IV, pp. 222–238.

11 W. Churchill, A Roving Commission: My Early Life, New York, Scribner, 1930, pp. 94–100. Churchill had made a similar comment a few years earlier (W. S. Churchill, The World Crisis, vol. I, New York, Scribner, 1923, pp. 20–21). In 1895, Churchill said, Sir William Harcourt told him that "the experiences of a long life have convinced me that nothing ever happens." Churchill added "Since that moment, as it seems to me, nothing has ever ceased happening ... I date the beginning of these violent times in our country from the Jameson Raid."

12 For the notorious Kruger telegram in which the Kaiser implied he would have intervened had he been asked to do so, see Garvin, Joseph Chamberlain, vol. III, p. 92.
    Germany extended a veiled offer to intervene even before the raiders were captured. Kotzé, then still on intimate terms with Kruger, tells the story in J. G. Kotzé, Memoirs and Reminiscences, Cape Town, Maskew Miller, 1952, vol. I, pp. 235–236. On the morning of December 31, 1895, Kotzé went to Kruger's office where he found Kruger, General Kock and other members of the government studying maps of

the farms near Krugersdorp (the commandos had not yet captured Jameson and his party). The German Consul-General suddenly appeared, "in full official uniform with cocked hat and sword!" Told that Kruger was busy, he insisted on delivering a message, namely "now that an armed foreign force had invaded the Republic" his Government requested permission "to move a body of fifty marines from a German warship at ... Lourenço Marques" to protect the Consulate. Kruger's reply, which evoked the laughter of his colleagues, was "Tell him that, if he is afraid, I will give him 50 of my burghers to protect him." Kotzé surmised that it was the Kaiser's resentment of this humorous rebuff of an implied offer of German intervention that twice led him to refuse to receive Kruger when Kruger was in exile during the Boer War.

13 T. Gutsche, *There Was a Man: The Life and Times of Sir Arnold Theiler*, Cape Town, Timmins, 1979, p. 79.

14 The Certificate Book of the Royal Society (1881–1895) and its ballots are preserved in the library of the Royal Society, and I have obtained these various statistics from them. Of 293 certificates between November 30, 1880 and December 12, 1895, only 22 were for members of the Privy Council. Fourteen people signed for Chamberlain, including Huxley, Stokes and Michael Foster. I may have miscounted, but it appears that of the twenty-two ballots for members of the Privy Council, Lister signed only three.

15 *Year Book of the Royal Society of London*, 1899, pp. 142–160, in particular, pp. 149–150.

16 R. J. Godlee, *Lord Lister*, London, Macmillan, 1917, p. 582.

17 See the entries on Chamberlain (pp. 102–118) and Lister (pp. 339–343) in the *Dictionary of National Biography* for 1912–21.

18 P. H. Manson-Bahr and A. Alcock, *Life and Work of Patrick Manson*, London, Cassel, 1927. For Manson and Chamberlain see also the biographical sketch of Manson in H. H. Scott, *A History of Tropical Medicine*, London, Arnold, 1939, vol. II, pp. 1068–1076; M. Worboys, Science and British Colonial Imperialism 1895–1940, unpublished D.Phil. thesis, University of Sussex, 1979, chapter 3; M. Worboys, Manson, Ross and Colonial Medical Policy: Tropical Medicine in London and Liverpool, 1899–1914, in R. MacLeod and M. Lewis (eds.), *Disease, Medicine and Empire*, London, Routledge, 1988, pp. 21–37; and M. Worboys, The Emergence of Tropical Medicine: a Study in the Establishment of a Scientific Specialty, in G. Lemaine, R. MacLeod, M. Mulkay and P. Weingart (eds.), *Perspectives on the Emergence of Scientific Disciplines*, The Hague, Mouton, 1976, pp. 75–98.

19 I have not located the letter of July 22, but its date is mentioned in the Royal Society's acknowledgment of its receipt, which is dated July 25, 1898 (New Letter Book, N.L.B. 17, library of the Royal Society). In another letter to the Royal Society dated August 8, 1898, signed C. P. Lucas, it was stated that in considering the plans for the Malaria Committee, Mr. Chamberlain "has also had the advantage of a per-

sonal conference with Lord Lister and Dr. Patrick Manson" (Malaria Committee minute book, library of the Royal Society). See also n. 29 below.

20 P. Alter, *The Reluctant Patron: Science and the State in Britain, 1850–1920*, Oxford, Berg, 1987.

21 W. T. Thiselton-Dyer, Joseph Chamberlain – In Memoriam, *The Royal Botanic Gardens Bulletin of Miscellaneous Information*, London, H.M.S.O., 1914, pp. 233–236. Chamberlain's role in supporting completion of the Temperate House was further commented on, in the same volume, by Austen Chamberlain (pp. 298–299) and by Thiselton-Dyer (pp. 393–394). I have taken Chamberlain's remark to Parliament from G. B. Masefield, *A History of the Colonial Agricultural Service*, Oxford, Clarendon Press, 1972, p. 24. Worboys, *Science and British Colonial Imperialism*, locates it in *Hansard Parliamentary Debates*, 4th. series, 63: col. 882. Worboys' comments on Chamberlain's motives for becoming Colonial Secretary are in chapter 2 of his thesis. See also Garvin, *Joseph Chamberlain*, vol. III, pp. 3–10.

In spite of the importance of Kew for colonial agriculture before and during Chamberlain's term as Colonial Secretary, it was not primarily a government center for agricultural research. E. J. Russell, who was a major figure in the development in the United Kingdom of scientific research applied to agriculture points to Lloyd George's establishment in 1910 of a development fund of £1,000,000 as "the first time that a British government had made itself responsible for scientific work in agriculture" (E. J. Russell, *The Land Called Me*, London, Allen and Unwin, 1956, p. 117).

The library at Kew still reflects the involvement of Kew with agriculture in the South African colonies: it has excellent long runs of the *Agricultural Journal of the Cape of Good Hope*, the *Natal Agricultural Journal* and the *Transvaal Agricultural Journal*.

22 [Royal Society], Minutes of Council, vol. 7, p. 285 (Meeting of July 2, 1896). See also the minute book of the Tsetse Fly Committee in the library of the Royal Society.

23 [Royal Society] Minutes of Council, vol. 7, p. 293 (Meeting of October 29, 1896).

24 *Ibid.*, p. 317. "Kanthack" was undoubtedly Alfredo Antunes Kanthack (March 4, 1863 – December 12, 1898), a brilliant young pathologist whose premature death was lamented by Virchow himself (see the *British Medical Journal* 1898, vol. 2, pp. 1941–1942; *The Lancet* 1898, vol. 2, p. 1817 and the *Journal of Pathology and Bacteriology* 6: 89–91, 1898). "Stevenson" may have been J. S. Stevenson (August 24, 1872 – July 30, 1900), an officer in the Indian Medical Service who had studied plague in India and Mauritius and had headed a sanitary commission in India (see the *British Medical Journal*, 1900, vol. 2., pp. 699–700 and *The Lancet*, 1900, vol. 2, p. 354).

The notion that the employment of Koch to investigate rinderpest was not well received in England was no fantasy. In its issue of July 31,

1901, the *North British Agriculturist,* commenting on Koch's controversial claim that bovine tuberculosis is not transmissible to human beings, asked its readers "whether he himself has established a claim for accuracy?" After commenting on Koch's claim that tuberculin was a cure for tuberculosis, it said "Then he went out to South Africa to investigate the disease of rinderpest, and in a few weeks time he discovered a cure for that disease; but that cure proved to be as fallacious as his tuberculin cure for tuberculosis." The *Veterinary Record* (14: 79–80, [August 3] 1901) reprinted a short extract from that article. On April 4, 1903, the *Veterinary Record* (15: 632) published a letter from W. Stapley of San Dimas, California, commenting on the employment of Koch to investigate rinderpest, praising Watkins-Pitchford and saying of Koch's work on rinderpest that "He blurted out a false theory – all askew with the laws of immunity." Stapley recommended "Let the [veterinary] profession lay hold with both hands to its own affairs, push the laboratory trained veterinarian into the position that should be his – fire out the foreign crowd. The profession has to so advertise itself that when the colonies want a laboratory man they will turn to *us* – and not to Berlin." The resentment aroused by the employment of Koch to investigate rinderpest obviously smoldered for a long time. Stapley's letter was reprinted in the [Natal] *Agricultural Journal* 6: 369–370, [June 26] 1903.

25 See Manson-Bahr and Alcock, *Patrick Manson.*

26 [Royal Society] Minutes of Council, vol. 7, pp. 437–438 (Meeting of July 7, 1898). Also letters of July 7, 1898, New Letter Book (N.L.B. 17), library of the Royal Society.

27 Burdon Sanderson had been a member of a commission that studied rinderpest in 1865. In 1896, when Koch was in London *en route* to the Cape, Burdon Sanderson sent him a copy of the report of that commission. Koch replied that he had long regarded that report "as the best aetiological and pathological investigation of this disease that has been made" and that he had, as soon as he had agreed to go to the Cape, obtained a copy ˙which he was taking with him. Koch's letter to Burdon Sanderson was extraordinarily warm and generous: since he already had a copy of the report "I return the copy that had kindly been placed at my disposal, as it is probably the only one in your possession, and of much value to you ... Accept my cordial thanks, and do not forget Yours most faithfully, R. Koch." See Lady Burdon Sanderson, *Sir John Burdon Sanderson: A Memoir,* Oxford, Clarendon Press, 1911, pp. 64–69. For Foster, Langley and Burdon Sanderson, see also G. Geison, *Michael Foster and the Cambridge School of Physiology,* Princeton, Princeton University Press, 1978. Foster and Chamberlain, both born in 1836, were at University College School at the same time (see Marris, *Joseph Chamberlain).* The possibility that they met at that time and remained in touch has not, as far as I know, been explored.

28 See the *Dictionary of National Biography* (1922–30), pp. 472–473 and the obituary notice of Kirk, *Proceedings of the Royal Society, Series B,* 94:

xi–xxx, 1922–3. For Kirk at Zanzibar see R. Coupland, *The Exploitation of East Africa 1856–90*, London, Faber & Faber, 1939; 2nd edition, 1968. H. Rider Haggard managed to mention Kirk in a footnote to chapter 5 of *She*.

29 A series of letters in the New Letter Books of the Royal Society (N.L.B. 17) and a series of entries in the minute book of the Malaria Committee make it clear that Manson, through Chamberlain, was trying to influence the attitude of the Malaria Committee towards the work of Ross. The Royal Society was not prepared to veto Chamberlain's suggestion that Manson and Lucas be added to the Committee (see n. 19 above), but as late as July 3, 1899, they were described in the minutes as having "attended on behalf of the Colonial Office."

On August 2, 1898, the Colonial Office wrote to agree with the Royal Society that "an observer from Bombay should be sent to study under Surgeon–Major Ross at Calcutta" but added the suggestion that "a second expert . . . should be nominated by [Chamberlain], on Dr. Manson's recommendation . . . to study under Surgeon–Major Ross." At its meeting of August 12, 1898, the Malaria Committee decided that *"if the expert appointed by Mr. Chamberlain were sent to study under Surgeon-Major Ross, he should do so under direct instructions from Mr. Chamberlain independently of the Royal Society* [emphasis added]." This message was conveyed to Chamberlain in a long letter of August 16, signed by Michael Foster; that letter is somewhat more tactfully worded than the resolution of the Malaria Committee. It nevertheless went so far as to say that

With regard to the proposal that the expert nominated by Mr. Chamberlain should be sent out 'to study under Surgeon-Major Ross' (quoting the words of Mr. Lucas's letter), I am directed to make the following observation. The Committee fully recognize the great interest attaching to Surgeon-Major Ross's observations, an account of which, through the kindness of Dr. P. Manson they have had the advantage of studying, they also recognize that the main inquiry which it is proposed to carry out cannot be considered as having been brought to a fully successful issue unless it furnishes some solution or some approach towards a solution of the problems involved in the life history of the Malarial organism outside the body . . . *whether mosquitos play a part in that life history or no* [emphasis added]. But taking even the most favourable value of Surgeon-Major Ross's researches, they are unwilling, acting on behalf of the Royal Society, to commit themselves to an expression of the opinion that that work is of such a character as to demand that an observer . . . be sent to Calcutta to study under that gentleman.

The letter went on to say, in effect, that if Chamberlain wanted such an expert he should send him himself; moreover, that the Committee "assumes" that the observers "whether they be two or more, will receive their instructions . . . from the Committee, and will report to the Committee . . . in order that the Committee may exercise a general superintendence over the whole enquiry." This seems like a strong reply for the Royal Society to send to the Colonial Secretary. The observers chosen by the Malaria Committee were the well-known malariologists, J. W. W. Stephens and S. R. Christophers, but, in the first instance, they were sent not to Ross but to West Africa. Chamberlain did eventually send an observer (C. W. Daniels) to work with Ross, entirely at the expense of the Colonial Office; the Colonial Office contributed £2,400 and the Royal Society £600 to the expenses of the other two observers (minutes of the Malaria Committee, November 12, 1898). Meanwhile, on September 3, the Malaria Committee agreed to Chamberlain's request (demand?) of August 30, that Manson and Lucas "should join the Committee whose duty it will be to superintend the proposed investigation." The Malaria Committee may have been formed at Chamberlain's request, but it obviously had no intention of agreeing to suggestions simply because they came from Chamberlain or from Manson! Nor was it prepared to accept the role of the mosquito. For more information on Manson's dedicated support of Ross, see R. Ross, *Memoirs*, London, John Murray, 1923. In his *Memoirs*, Ross spoke with great bitterness about the way he had been treated by the Royal Society and the Malaria Committee. In fact, the only support Ross did receive was that of Manson and Chamberlain, and it is indeed fortunate that Manson persuaded Chamberlain to support Ross. The source of the resistance of the Malaria Committee to Ross and his views was presumably Ray Lankester.

30 The Foulerton Committee and the Medical Research Committee of the Royal Society (formerly the Tropical Diseases Committee) were merged in 1936. The Medical Research Committee of the Royal Society should not be confused with the governmental Medical Research Committee which later became the Medical Research Council.

31 For a recent examination of that subject see Roy MacLeod's introduction to R. MacLeod (ed.), *Government and Expertise: Specialists, Administrators and Professionals, 1860–1919*, Cambridge, Cambridge University Press, 1988, pp. 1–24.

32 G. B. Masefield, *A Short History of Agriculture in the British Colonies*, Oxford, Clarendon Press, 1950, pp. 68–69.

33 When Stewart Stockman became Chief Veterinary Officer of Great Britain in 1905, the Board of Agriculture had as a "laboratory" only "a room adapted for the diagnostic examination of morbid specimens . . . a slaughter house would have served the purpose equally well." Stockman immediately created a laboratory in the modern sense at Sudbury and later at Alperton Lodge and was largely responsible for the founding of the Laboratory at Weybridge of which he became the first director in 1917. His successor at Weybridge, W. H. Andrews, had also worked with Arnold Theiler (see N.H.H. [N. H. Hole?], The Central Veterinary Laboratory Weybridge, 1917–1967, the *Veterinary Record* 81: 62–68, 1967).

The reliance on advice from agencies such as Kew was strengthened during the period when Lord Elgin was Colonial Secretary (see chapter 12 of R. Hyam, *Elgin and Churchill at the Colonial Office 1905–1908: The Watershed of the Empire-Commonwealth*, London, Macmillan, 1968). But it was Milner's experiences in Lloyd George's "War Cabinet" that provided the final impetus for "professionalization" of the Colonial Office, especially in the area of agriculture. John Garnett, of the Ministry of Agriculture, advises me that

In June, 1915, Milner was appointed to chair a Committee of the Board of Agriculture to consider the need for action to maintain and increase food production in England and Wales, on the assumption that the war continued beyond September, 1916 ... thanks to the ideas of F. B. Smith ... it was cogently argued that there was need for a system to pass on official advice on how best each area might maximize its output. This system ... had conspicuous success during the food production campaigns of 1917 and 1918.

In 1920 Milner, by then Colonial Secretary, appointed a committee that studied the availability of veterinary services in the colonies (see *Report of the Committee on the Staffing of the Veterinary Departments in the Colonies and Protectorates*, London, H.M.S.O., 1920, Cmd. 922; that report dealt with the question of salaries).

The professionalization of the resources of the Colonial Office was carried a further step by L. S. Amery while he was Colonial Secretary. See, for example, *Colonial Agricultural Service. Report of a Committee Appointed by the Secretary of State for the Colonies*, London, H.M.S.O., 1928, Cmd. 3049, and *Colonial Veterinary Service. Report of a Committee Appointed by the Secretary of State for the Colonies*, London, H.M.S.O., 1929, Cmd. 3261. Arnold Theiler served on the latter committee; the two committees jointly recommended the creation of the Colonial Advisory Council of Agriculture and Animal Health. See also *Memorandum showing the Progress and Development in the Colonial Empire and in the Machinery for Dealing with Colonial Questions for November, 1924 to November, 1928*, London, H.M.S.O., 1929, Cmd. 3268. Amery, who was a disciple and admirer of Milner, discussed Milner and the reconstruction of the Transvaal in his autobiography (L. S. Amery, *My Political Life*, London, Hutchinson, 1953, vol. I, pp. 161–168). He also discussed "Colonial Development and Research" in vol. II, pp. 335–370 of that autobiography.

Arnold Theiler's interactions with Great Britain (he was knighted in 1914) were only part of an influence that was world-wide. Until 1914, when the trustees of the Rockefeller Institute for Medical Research decided to found a division for research on animal pathology, the only institution of that kind in the world was Arnold Theiler's institute at Onderstepoort; it is still a very important center.

34   Letter from E. H. Ackerknecht to P. F. Cranefield, January 21, 1986. See also G. H. F. Nuttall, who remarked that "in Germany Koch's activities were not confined to research and teaching. He was constantly called upon by his Government in an advisory capacity ...

Many felt that the weight of Koch's authority in his domain was at times too great, especially in its influence on Government" (G. H. F. Nuttall, Biographical Notes Bearing on Koch, Ehrlich, Behring and Loeffler, with their Portraits and Letters from Three of Them, *Parasitology* 16: 214–238, 1924; the section on Koch is on pp. 214–223).

35 Amery, *Joseph Chamberlain*, vol. IV, pp. 191–195. Eckardstein [Eckhardtstein] was in active charge of the embassy, Ambassador Hartzfeld being ill. Eckardstein is said to have hoped to become Ambassador himself. See also Baron von Eckardstein, *Ten Years at the Court of St. James 1895–1905*, translated and edited by G. Young, London, Thornton Butterworth, 1921. Young says that Eckardstein was "the ally of those English statesmen who were trying to reestablish the peace of Europe on the firm foundation of an Anglo-German alliance."

36 A few remarks about the economic climate in Rhodesia in 1903 will be found in chapter 8. As far as I can make out, Chamberlain thought that the best way to restore the industrial efficiency and competitiveness of Great Britain and to relieve unemployment was to form the countries of the Empire into a "Common Market." And, also as far as I can make out, his hopes were frustrated by the inability to agree on a "Common Agricultural Policy," but my mind may have become inflamed by my reading too much about 1992 in *The Economist*.

The phrase "Made in Germany" had received wide currency as a pejorative in 1896 when it was used as the title of a book by a barrister who was an advocate of protectionism (E. E. Williams, *"Made in Germany"*, London, Heinemann, 1896). Williams' book contains a detailed and very interesting analysis of why German industry had come to produce manufactured products that were superior to those of British industry; for Williams, free trade was only part of the problem.

An interesting discussion of Chamberlain's role in the debate over the perceived decline in British power is found in A. Friedberg, *The Weary Titan: Great Britain and the Experience of Relative Decline, 1895–1905*, Princeton, Princeton University Press, 1988. On p. 33 of his book, Friedberg agrees with Worboys on the question of Chamberlain's motive for becoming Colonial Secretary: "In 1887 Chamberlain decided that, if he ever held high office again, he wanted to be Colonial Secretary. It was the empire, he felt quite certain, that held the key to England's future." Friedberg took the title of his book from yet another of Chamberlain's vivid remarks, made at the 1902 Colonial Conference: "The Weary Titan struggles under the too vast orb of its fate."

7 ARNOLD THEILER, CHARLES LOUNSBURY AND DUNCAN HUTCHEON

1 My summary of Theiler's early career is based on T. Gutsche, *There was a Man: The Life and Times of Sir Arnold Theiler*, Cape Town, Timmins, 1979. See also G. Theiler, *Arnold Theiler 1867–1936: His Life*

and Times, Publikasies van die Universiteit van Pretoria, Nuwe Reeks Nr. 61, 1971; P. J. Du Toit and C. Jackson, The Life and Work of Sir Arnold Theiler, *Journal of the South African Veterinary Medical Association* 7: 135–186, 1936; and H. H. Curson, Theiler and the Rinderpest Epidemic of 1896–1903, *Journal of the South African Veterinary Medical Association* 7: 187–203, 1936. Theiler died July 24, 1936 while on a visit to England.

2 Arnold Theiler's daughter, Gertrud Theiler says that Theiler was released, at the strong recommendation of David Bruce and the Transvaal Medical Officer, George Turner, to assist in the British army hospital, but was soon allowed to resume bacteriological research (G. Theiler, *Arnold Theiler*).

3 My remarks about Lounsbury are based on the *Dictionary of South African Biography*, vol. III, pp. 539–540; M. C. Mossop, Obituary. The late Mr. C. P. Lounsbury, *Journal of the Entomological Society of South Africa* 18: 144–148, 1955; and C. P. Lounsbury, The Pioneer Period of Economic Entomology in South Africa, *Journal of the Entomological Society of South Africa* 3: 9–29, 1940. Lounsbury mentions several other American entomologists who later came to South Africa at the recommendation of L. O. Howard; the United States was at that time a leader in the field of economic entomology and most of the people Howard recommended had studied at land-grant agricultural colleges such as Iowa, Wisconsin, Illinois, Ohio and, especially, Cornell.

M. Worboys (Science and British Colonial Imperialism, 1895–1940, unpublished D.Phil. thesis, University of Sussex, 1979, chapter 7) points to economic entomology as an excellent example of the movement of science from the periphery to the center, i.e. from the colonies to the United Kingdom. The first entomologist attached to what was to become the U.S. Department of Agriculture was appointed in 1853. According to Worboys, there was no government entomologist or entomological research organization in Great Britain until 1913; in 1911, when there was no government entomologist in Great Britain, there were "thirty such posts in the Empire; not surprisingly, most staff had been recruited from the United States or trained on the spot." Arriving as he did in the Cape in 1895, Lounsbury must have been among the earliest government economic entomologists in the Empire. By 1913 he had a large staff and an international reputation.

See also L. O. Howard, *A History of Applied Entomology (Somewhat Anecdotal)*, Smithsonian Miscellaneous Collections, vol. 84 (whole volume), Washington, Smithsonian Institution, 1930 [Publication 3065; 564 pp. + 51 plates]. Howard mentions Lounsbury several times, in particular on pp. 372–374 and pp. 523–524. Howard attributed the flourishing of applied entomology to the creation, by the Hatch Act of the 1880s, of the State Agricultural Experiment Stations; Lounsbury's earlier practical work was done with C. H. Fernald at the Massachusetts Hatch Experiment Station. The Cape Archives Depot contains an extensive collection of letters to Lounsbury from L. O. Howard and members of his staff (*CAD* ENC 1/3/1).

4 A. Theiler, The Rhodesian Tick Fever, *Transvaal Agricultural Journal* 1, no. 4: 93–110, + 1 plate facing p. 104, [July] 1903. This article was probably written in June, 1903, since the latest event discussed in it occurred on June 3, 1903, yet it makes no reference to Koch's interim report. An extract from Theiler's article appeared in the [Natal] *Agricultural Journal* 6:503–504, [August 7] 1903.

5 A. Theiler, Rhodesian Cattle Disease and Rabies, *Transvaal Agricultural Journal* 1, no. 1: 37–44, [October] 1902.

6 *TAD* CS 130/10152.

7 *TAD* CS 139/11208. According to Turner's letter the recommendation that Theiler sent to Rhodesia was made "by the Board called together for framing regulations for the prevention of diseases amongst stock."

8 I do not know when Theiler sent specimens to Nocard. In his letter to the B.S.A.C. of December 7, 1902 (see chapter 4, n. 59) Nocard spoke of having studied specimens that Theiler had sent him.

9 A. Laveran, Sur la Piroplasme bovine bacilliform, *Comptes rendus Académie des Sciences* 136: 648–653, 1903.

10 Gutsche, *There was a Man*, p. 191, describes Deixonne as having been a "subordinate of Nocard at Alfort." She adds that he and Edington had been working together in Mauritius and had gone to Bulawayo to study the new outbreak.

   Laveran cites "Deixonne, *Rapport fait au retour d'une mission dans le Sud africain*, Port-Louis, 1903." I have not been able to locate a copy of this book, which sounds like it might be interesting. I assume that it was published in Port Louis, Mauritius. Although Laveran both quotes from the book and gives a citation that is precise and persuasive, the book is indeed elusive. No copy is listed in the (U.S.) *National Union Catalogue* or in several other printed catalogues that I have consulted (including A. Toussaint and H. Adolphe, *Bibliography of Mauritius (1502–1954)*, Port-Louis, Mauritius, Esclapon, 1956). No copy is found in the British Library or in the library of the Colonial Office (now part of the library of the Foreign and Commonwealth Office, London), or in some thirty other libraries, including major historical collections in South Africa. I would be willing to concede that it is what bibliographers call a "ghost" were it not that Toussaint and Adolphe list a pamphlet by R. Deixonne on surra (equine trypanosomiasis), published in Port Louis, Mauritius, in 1903 *and* that the library of the Foreign and Commonwealth Office has a pamphlet on surra, also published in Port Louis, Mauritius, in 1903, which contains extensive testimony by R. Deixonne. Since Deixonne's book was published before Laveran's article of May, 1903, it is almost certainly the first *book* to mention East Coast fever. I would therefore be glad to hear from anyone who knows where a copy may be found.

11 [Robert Koch], *Interim Report on Rhodesian Redwater, or "African Coast*

Fever", dated March 26, 1903, Salisbury, Argus, 1903. See chapter 5, n. 10.

12 A. Theiler, Rhodesian Tick Fever.

13 K. F. Meyer, Preliminary Note on the Transmission of East Coast Fever to Cattle by Intraperitoneal Inoculation of the Spleen or Portions of the Spleen of a Sick Animal, *Journal of Comparative Pathology and Therapeutics* 22: 213–217, 1909.

14 For Theiler's confirmation of Meyer's findings see A. Theiler, The Artificial Transmission of East Coast Fever, in *Union of South Africa. Department of Agriculture. Report of the Government Veterinary Bacteriologist for the Year 1909–10*, Pretoria, Government Printing and Stationery Office, 1911. See also A. Theiler, The Artificial Transmission of East Coast Fever, *Journal of Comparative Pathology and Therapeutics* 24: 161–169, 1911, which summarizes the article in Theiler's annual report for 1909–10. For Theiler's attempts to produce immunity by such injections, see A. Theiler, Immunization of Cattle against East Coast Fever, *Journal of Comparative Pathology and Therapeutics* 26: 261–265, 1913, which is based on Theiler's second report as Director of Veterinary Research of the Union of South Africa.

A remarkable sequel to this work was the inoculation of 283,000 cattle in the Transkei between November, 1911 and April, 1914. 3–10 cc of a mixture of "spleen and lymphatic gland pulp" were injected into the jugular vein. Each batch of the mixture was obtained "from a bovine animal suffering from East Coast fever in a well-advanced stage, and killed for the purpose of vaccine production." Some of the animals contracted East Coast fever and died; of the survivors, 70 percent developed full or partial immunity. James Spreull, who directed this program, concluded that "The present method is one which can never be practised in a civilized area, except as a means to immunize or rapidly make an end of the mortality in a location already badly infected." Spreull also noted that he had observed the first outbreak in the Transkei (in the Cape) on March 31, 1910. By early 1914 it had killed 900,000 cattle and "its eradication will not be effected for some years to come even under the most favourable circumstances" (J. Spreull, East Coast Fever Inoculation in the Transkeian Territories, South Africa, *Journal of Comparative Pathology and Therapeutics* 27: 299–304, 1914).

15 S. F. Barnett, Theileriasis, in D. Weinman and M. Ristic (eds.), *Infectious Blood Diseases of Man and Animals*, New York, Academic Press, 1968, vol. II, pp. 269–328.

16 W. O. Neitz, Aureomycin in *Theileria parva* Infection, *Nature* 171: 34–35, 1953.

17 D. E. Radley, C. G. D. Brown, M. J. Burridge, M. P. Cunningham, I. M. Kirimi, R. E. Purnell and A. S. Young, East Coast Fever: Chemoprophylactic Immunization of Cattle against *Theileria parva* (Muguga) and Five Theilerial Strains, *Veterinary Parasitology* [Netherlands] 1: 35–41, 1975.

18 J. K. H. Wilde, The Control of Theileriosis, in J. B. Henson and M. Campbell (eds.), *Theileriosis: Report of a Workshop Held in Nairobi, Kenya, 7–9 December 1976*, Ottawa, International Development Research Centre, IDRC–086e, 1977. [I.S.B.N. 0–88936–124–X].

19 P. C. Doherty and R. Nussenzweig, Progress on *Theileria* Vaccine, *Nature* 316: 484–485, 1985.

20 *Ibid*. In the opinion of Professor John A. Lawrence, University of Zimbabwe (personal communication, Harare, August 5, 1988) an effective vaccine against East Coast fever might make it possible to lengthen the dipping interval from five days to perhaps two weeks, since less frequent dipping is needed to control other tick-borne diseases of cattle.

For detailed reviews of immunity to East Coast fever see R. E. Purnell, East Coast Fever: Some Recent Research in East Africa, *Advances in Parasitology* 15: 83–131 [esp. 105–119], 1977; see also W. I. Morrison, P. A. Lalor, B. M. Goddeeris and A. J. Teale, Theileriosis: Antigens and Host–Parasite Interactions, in T. W. Pearson (ed.), *Parasite Antigens: Towards New Strategies for Vaccines*, New York and Basle, Dekker, 1986, pp. 167–206; and many articles in A. D. Irvin, M. P. Cunningham and A. S. Young (eds.), *Advances in the Control of Theileriosis*, The Hague, Nijhoff, 1981.

The whole question is complicated by the problem of whether animals that have recovered from East Coast fever or that have been immunized against it are carriers (see chapter 8, especially n. 16).

21 *NAZ* V 1/2/1/1.

22 *Cape of Good Hope. Department of Agriculture. Report of the Government Entomologist for the Year 1902*, Cape Town, Cape Times, Government Printers, 1903 [vi + 41 pp.]. Lounsbury's articles "Ticks and the Rhodesian Cattle Disease" and "Ticks and Malignant Jaundice" are on pp. 16–18 and 18–20 respectively.

23 [L.] G. Neumann, Revision de la Famille des Ixodidés (4e Mémoire, 1), *Mémoires de la Société Zoologique de France* 14: 249–372, 1901. Neumann described *Rhipicephalus appendiculatus (n.p.)* on pp. 270–271, basing his description in part on three male and seven female specimens "du Cap (Coll. Lounsbury)." Gertrud Theiler, who was an eminent entomologist, says that "L. G. Neumann (1846–1930) . . . was the first taxonomist to study ticks from all over the world" (G. Theiler, *Arnold Theiler*). According to A. G. Debus (ed.), *World Who's Who in Science*, Chicago, Marquis, 1968, (Louis) Georges Neumann was born October 22, 1846 and died June 28, 1930. He was a veterinarian; he wrote a well-known text on parasitic diseases of animals and wrote about the history of veterinary medicine. Neumann's textbook was published in English: see L. G. Neumann, *A Treatise on the Parasites and Parasitic Diseases of the Domestic Animals*, translated by G. Fleming, 2nd edition, revised and edited by J. Macqueen, London, Baillière, Tindall and Cox, 1905.

24 C. P. Lounsbury, Ticks and African Coast Fever, *Transvaal Agricul-*

tural Journal 2, no. 5: 4–13, [October] 1903; reprinted in the [Natal] *Agricultural Journal* 6: 773–776 and 818–823, [November 13 and 27] 1903.

25 *Cape of Good Hope. Department of Agriculture. Report of the Government Entomologist for the Year 1903*, Cape Town, Cape Times, Government Printers, 1904 [vi + 46 pp. + 7 plates]. Lounsbury's article "Ticks and African Coast Fever" is on pp. 11–18.

Later reports were published as follows:

Cape of Good Hope. Department of Agriculture. Report of the Government Entomologist for the Half-Year ended June 30th, 1904, Cape Town, Cape Times, Government Printers, 1905. Lounsbury's articles "African Coast Fever" and "Ticks and African Coast Fever" are on pp. 4–7 and 10–13 respectively.

Cape of Good Hope. Department of Agriculture. Report of the Government Entomologist for the Half-Year ended 31st December, 1904, Cape Town, Cape Times, Government Printers, 1906 [iv + 12 pp.]. This report does not deal with East Coast fever.

Report of the Government Entomologist for the Year 1905, in *Cape of Good Hope. Department of Agriculture. Report of the Acting Director of Agriculture (with Appendices) for the Year 1905*. Cape Town, Cape Times, Government Printers, 1906, pp. 95–104. This report contains two paragraphs on East Coast fever (on p. 96 and p. 98) and a full-page tabular summary (on p. 97) of experiments on the transmission of East Coast fever by ticks. Lounsbury's long article cited in n. 31 below was removed from this annual report in accordance with instructions from the government to make the annual report brief.

26 C. P. Lounsbury, Transmission of African Coast Fever, *Agricultural Journal of the Cape of Good Hope* 24: 428–432 + 3 plates, [April] 1904. Reprinted without the first plate, *Rhodesian Agricultural Journal* 2: 174–176 + 2 plates, [June] 1904.

27 *Cape of Good Hope. Department of Agriculture. Report of Proceedings at Inter-Colonial Veterinary Conference (Adjourned from Bloemfontein 5th December, 1903) on Animals' Diseases in South Africa. Held at Cape Town on 25th, 26th, 27th, 28th, 30th and 31st May, 1904*. Cape Town, Cape Times Ltd., Government Printers, 1904 [G. 87–1904].

28 S. F. Barnett, Theileria, in J. P. Kreier (ed.), *Parasitic Protozoa*, Vol. IV, New York, Academic Press, 1977, pp. 77–113. When the nymph or larva feeds on an infected animal it ingests the parasites that are in the animal's red blood cells. Those parasites go through several stages of their cycle within the nymph or larva and finally, after the process of moulting, appear in the salivary glands of the next stage of the tick, which is then an infectious larva or an infectious mature tick. Even then, infectious larvae or infectious mature ticks do not normally infect cattle until they have fed upon them for three or four days; a final maturation of the parasite in the salivary glands of the tick is required. It is possible that the tick, while feeding, actually ingests cells attracted to the feeding site, which are infected within the tick and reinjected

into the animal. (C. G. D. Brown, personal communication, Centre for Tropical Veterinary Medicine, University of Edinburgh, December 9, 1988).

29 A. Theiler, Report of the Veterinary Bacteriologist, in *Report of the Transvaal Department of Agriculture. 1st July, 1903 to 30th June, 1904*, Pretoria, Government Printing and Stationery Office, 1905.

Theiler's detailed documentation of the work he had done on East Coast fever through the middle of 1904 takes up some fifty pages of this annual report, which is dated August 12, 1904. The portion of the annual report devoted to East Coast fever contains twelve charts or tables and thirty-eight pages of text in small print, i.e. about 23,000 words of text (Koch's four reports had come to about 16,000 words). The report is divided into sections or articles, most of which were also published separately, although not always in identical form. The following is a list of those articles or sections, both as part of this report and as separate publications:

(a) A. Theiler, The Piroplasma bigeminum of the Immune Ox, in *Report*, pp. 116–126 + tables on pp. 127–132. Also, with four charts replacing the tables, in *Journal of the Royal Army Medical Corps* 3: 469–488, 1904.

(b) A. Theiler, East Coast Fever, in *Report*, pp. 133–135. Also in *Journal of the Royal Army Medical Corps* 3: 599–601, 1904.

(c) A. Theiler, The Transmission of East Coast Fever by Ticks. In *Report*, pp. 135–150 + tables on pp. 151–156. Also, without tables, in *Journal of the Royal Army Medical Corps* 3: 602–620, 1904. Also, without tables, in *Transvaal Agricultural Journal* 3: 71–86, [October] 1904.

(d) A. Theiler [and S. Stockman], Experiments to Show How Long an Area, Which Was at One Time Infected, Will Remain Infected, in *Report*, pp. 157–158.

(e) A. Theiler [and S. Stockman], Inoculation Experiments According to the Methods of Professor Kock [*sic*], in *Report*, pp. 158–161.

(f) A. Theiler [and S. Stockman], Dipping Experiments, in *Report*, pp. 161–163.

(g) A. Theiler [and S. Stockman], Results with the (Non-Sprayed) Control Animals exposed at the Same Date, in *Report*, pp. 163–165.

(h) A. Theiler [and S. Stockman], Possible Influence of the Different Seasons on the Outbreaks of East Coast Fever, in *Report*, pp. 165–166.

Item (d) begins with a footnote reading "These experiments and the following were planned and conducted in collaboration with Mr. Stockman, Principal Veterinary Surgeon." Items (d)–(h) were combined as A. Theiler and S. Stockman, Some Observations and Experiments in Connection with Tropical Bovine Piroplasmosis (East Coast Fever or Rhodesian Redwater), *Journal of Comparative Pathology and*

Therapeutics 17: 193–203, 1904 (also in *Transvaal Agricultural Journal* 3: 49–58, [October] 1904).

30 Barnett, Theileriasis (see n. 15 above).

31 C. P. Lounsbury, Ticks and African Coast Fever, *Agricultural Journal of the Cape of Good Hope* 28: 634–654, 1906.

32 *Report of the Proceedings of the Conference on Diseases Among Cattle and other Animals in South Africa held on the 3rd, 4th and 5th December, 1903,* Bloemfontein, Argus, 1904.

33 This letter to Orpen was published in the joint report by C. E. Gray and W. Robertson, *Report upon Texas Fever or Redwater in Rhodesia,* Cape Town, Argus, 1902.

34 *TAD* LTG 54/69/9. There is an extensive correspondence about the Lydenburg outbreak in *TAD* CS 175/14939; *TAD* CS 190/16087; *TAD* CS 194/16332; and *TAD* CS 202/16961.

35 *Cape of Good Hope. Department of Agriculture. Report of the Colonial Veterinary Surgeon and the Assistant Veterinary Surgeons for the year 1902.* Cape Town, "Cape Times", Government Printers, 1902, pp. 4–7.

36 D. Hutcheon, The new form of Redwater in the Transvaal. *Transvaal Agricultural Journal* 1, No. 3: 45–57 [April], 1903. The original typed report, in the form of a 47 page long letter addressed to the Secretary of the Transvaal Repatriation Department, is in *TAD* LTG 54/69/5.

37 In his annual report for 1903, Hutcheon says that he left for the Transvaal on January 29, 1903 and that he wrote the special report that appeared in April, 1903, "before I left Pretoria." He presumably wrote his preliminary report at the same time. See *Cape of Good Hope. Department of Agriculture. Reports of the Colonial Veterinary Surgeon and the Assistant Veterinary Surgeons for the Year 1903.* Cape Town, Cape Times, Government Printers, 1904.

38 *TAD* LTG 54/69/9.

39 [Koch], *Interim Report on Rhodesian Redwater* (see n. 11 above).

40 [R. Koch], The Rhodesian Cattle Disease: Dr. Koch's First Report, *Agricultural Journal of the Cape of Good Hope* 23: 33–39, [July] 1903. D. Hutcheon, Virulent Redwater in the Transvaal, *Agricultural Journal of the Cape of Good Hope* 23: 39–60, [July] 1903.

41 A. Theiler, Rhodesian Tick Fever (see n. 4 above).

42 Lounsbury, Ticks and African Coast Fever (see n. 24 above). Lounsbury's remarks are mild compared to Alexander's. They are also mild compared to some much later remarks by Nuttall (G. H. F. Nuttall, Biographical Notes Bearing on Koch, Ehrlich, Behring and Loeffler, with their Portraits and Letters from Three of Them, *Parasitology* 16: 214–238, 1924). Nuttall, who had, overall, a very high opinion of Koch, was unsparing in his description of the authoritarian side of Koch and even claimed that Koch had appropriated the credit for the original observation of *Piroplasma bigeminum* in German East Africa in 1897:

when Koch or members of his school had been given the opportunity of confirming the work of others, there was a decided tendency to arrogate to themselves undue credit in discovery. This resulted in ill-feeling which was none the less bitter because it did not always find its way into print ... Koch was in a position to push others aside and he often did so. Thus, *to my knowledge, when an obscure but observing young veterinarian in German East Africa had found Piroplasma bigeminum in cattle suffering from redwater and had shown the parasites to Koch, we only hear of Koch's work thereon afterwards* [emphasis added].

After some further criticism of Koch's attitudes towards various investigators of malaria, Nuttall said "The instances I have cited might be multiplied ... I presume that constant appeals to him for his opinion may have adversely affected his judgement on some matters, in which case there are obvious disadvantages in being too great an authority in the eyes of one's fellow-men."

That Koch's character had a dark side has been widely recognized. Brock cites Nuttall's comments at length, and speaks of Koch having, in his later years, turned into "a crusty and opinionated tyrant." Brock also refers to Koch's "self-confident arrogance" and says "He was accused of pugnacity, arrogance, failure to give credit for ideas borrowed from others, and reluctance to admit mistakes. All of these criticisms were certainly true" (T. D. Brock, *Robert Koch*, Madison, Science Tech Publishers; Berlin, Springer, 1988, pp. 4, 287 and 291). Dolman (*Dictionary of Scientific Biography*, vol. VII, New York, Scribner, 1973, pp. 420–435) brilliantly captures the contradictions in Koch's character, and closes his article with an allusion to Koch's Faustian qualities, to which earlier writers had also called attention (see R. Bochalli, *Robert Koch*, Stuttgart, Wissenschaftliche Verlagsgesellschaft, 1954, p. 184). Dolman also calls attention to Koch's letters "as collected by K. Kolle" as providing evidence of "marked adolescent emotional turbulence."

The brilliance of Koch's work on anthrax, his creation of fundamentally important bacteriological methods and techniques, his discovery of the tubercle bacillus and of the cause of cholera (in a ten-year period!), were followed by twenty-six years of work that was much less inspired. Koch's genius, his drive to succeed, the dark side of his character, and the decline in his creativity in his later years, may have been linked to a streak of melancholia that emerged with considerable clarity on his sixtieth birthday. A hint of that melancholia (and more than a hint of his love of Africa) are seen in the letter that he wrote to thank his daughter for her birthday greetings (see B. Möllers, *Robert Koch: Persönlichkeit und Lebenswerk, 1843–1919*, Hannover, Schmorl und Seefeld, 1950, pp. 276–277).

Kleine, who was with Koch in Bulawayo, touched on this in an article that has escaped the attention of many later students of Koch, perhaps because it was published in Germany in 1943 (F. K. Kleine, Mit Robert Koch in Afrika und in der Heimat, *Zeitschrift für Hygiene und Infektions Krankheiten* 125: 265–286, 1943). Kleine described the many splendid evenings that he and other members of Koch's party had enjoyed at the Grand Hotel in Bulawayo – evenings accompanied by music, magnificent colored lights and the scent of roses.

Having described those gala evenings, Kleine turned to a particular evening – that of Koch's sixtieth birthday, December 11, 1903. During that evening Koch, Kleine and Neufeld found themselves together for a few moments. During those moments Koch spoke in an impressive way about his life and about the hardships he had suffered as a country doctor in Wollstein. He also spoke of his plans and hopes for future travels – travels full of danger. He did not, Koch said, want to have a "straw death," a term that Kleine says the old German mercenaries used to describe dying in bed. If he did die in bed, then his corpse should be burned and the ashes strewn in the sea – then he might finally find peace.

Only that morning, Kleine went on, Koch had startled him and Neufeld by telling them that he had submitted his resignation as Director of the Institute for Infectious Diseases. In response to the horrified *"Why?"* of Kleine and Neufeld, Koch replied "I want to be free at last." To the objection that he indeed was free and need only request a leave of absence for his scientific travels, Koch rejoined "I do not even want to ask. I want to be entirely free and dependent on nobody, with no need to ask anyone for anything. That is what I yearned for, even in Wollstein." – "Das ist schon in Wollstein meine Sehnsucht gewesen." – Koch officially retired from government service in 1904, twenty-five years after he had left Wollstein for Berlin. Free at last? I doubt it.

43 Typed copy, *NAZ* LO 4/1/14; published version, *Southern Rhodesia. Report of the Department of Agriculture for the Year Ended 31st March, 1903*, Salisbury, Argus, 1903.
44 See L. E. W. Bevan, Autobiography, n.p., n.d., typed (*NAZ* Historical Manuscripts BE 11/7/1). According to Pattison, McFadyean's course in pathology and bacteriology was "specially adapted to the requirements of Officers of the Army Veterinary Department, Colonial Veterinary Surgeons, and Veterinary Inspectors" (I. Pattison, *John McFadyean*, London, J. A. Allen, 1981). McFadyean's first postgraduate course was given in January and February, 1904. It was presumably the second course, given in October and November, 1904, that was attended by Gray and Bevan, since it was during that course that Gray persuaded Bevan to join the Rhodesian Veterinary Service. Gray and Bevan sailed together to Rhodesia, leaving on December 24, 1904. Much to Bevan's regret, Gray almost immediately resigned to become Government Veterinary Surgeon of the Transvaal.
45 A. Theiler, Rhodesian Tick Fever (see n. 4 above).
46 A. Theiler, Piroplasma bigeminum of the Immune Ox (see item a, n. 29 above).
47 A. Theiler, East Coast Fever (see item b, n. 29 above).
48 Du Toit and Jackson, Sir Arnold Theiler (see n. 1 above).

8   THE FIGHT AGAINST EAST COAST FEVER

1   *NAZ* LO 1/2/16. See chapter 3, n. 16.
2   *NAZ* LO 1/2/16. See chapter 3, n. 22 and n. 24.
3   *NAZ* LO 1/2/16.
4   A. Theiler, Rhodesian Cattle Disease and Rabies, *Transvaal Agricultural Journal* 1, no. 1: 37–44, [October] 1902.
5   *Cape of Good Hope. Department of Agriculture. Report of Proceedings at Inter-Colonial Veterinary Conference (Adjourned from Bloemfontein 5th December, 1903) on Animals' Diseases in South Africa. Held at Cape Town on 25th, 26th, 27th, 28th, 30th and 31st May, 1904*, Cape Town, Cape Times Ltd., Government Printers, 1904 [G.87–1904].
6   Letter from Stockman to F. B. Smith dated May 25, 1904 (*TAD* TAD 341/36507).
7   *Report of the Proceedings of the Conference on Diseases Among Cattle and other Animals in South Africa held on the 3rd, 4th and 5th December, 1903*, Bloemfontein, Argus, 1904.
8   S. Stockman, Report of the Work of the Veterinary Division, in *Report of the Transvaal Department of Agriculture. 1st July, 1903 to 30th June, 1904*. Pretoria, Government Printing and Stationery Office, 1905, pp. 37–76.
9   A. Theiler, Report of the Veterinary Bacteriologist, in *Report of the Transvaal Department of Agriculture. 1st July, 1903 to 30th June, 1904*. Pretoria, Government Printing and Stationery Office, 1905, pp. 79–248. This note is on pp. 157–158. For another publication of this brief note see chapter 7, n. 29, item (d).
    Stockman wrote a letter to Watkins-Pitchford as early as December 23, 1903 to say that "we have nearly settled to our satisfaction that the time necessary to purify infected ground in the absence of cattle, lies between one year and fifteen months" (*TAD* TAD 342/36510).
10 Theiler, Report of the Veterinary Bacteriologist, 1903–4. The section on inoculation is on pp. 158–161 of the report; the section on dipping is on pp. 161–163. For other publications of these sections see chapter 7, n. 29, items (e) and (f).
    The final section of the 1904 report was entitled "Possible influence of the different seasons on the outbreaks of East Coast fever" (pp. 165–166 of the report and see chapter 7, n. 29, item (h)). It concluded that the shortest period required to wipe out a herd occurs during January and February and is about twenty-three days. Only a day or two more may be required in March and April. A much greater delay begins in June and is noticeable to the end of the year.
    That the disease dies down during the winter, i.e. during July, August and September, is certainly correct. It does not, however, necessarily remain suppressed during October, November and December. Theiler's study was conducted on fields that had been burnt off during the winter so that the grass was still very short in October. Theiler concluded that infection occurs more readily when the grass is

long. If the grass is not burnt off, the disease resumes in October or November.

East Coast fever certainly flourishes and spreads in January and February, which is why the Australian cattle could not have been the source of the original outbreak. They died in Umtali in January, 1901. Had they died of East Coast fever, conditions would have been ideal for its spread. That it did not spread, as shown by the many healthy head of cattle seen at the Umtali Agricultural Show in April, 1901, is proof that it was not East Coast fever that killed the Australian cattle.

In their next annual report, Theiler and Stockman returned to the question of how long it takes an infected field to purify itself. Almost in passing, that article made a pointed attack on Koch by reminding the reader that, at the Bloemfontein conference, Koch had been of the opinion "that the disease was bound to go all over the country, and that therefore the wisest and most expeditious policy was to let it go, and trust to a method of immunization which had then received but a short trial." See A. Theiler [and S. Stockman], Further Experiments to Note How Long an Area Remains Infected with East Coast Fever, in Report of the Veterinary Bacteriologist, *Transvaal Department of Agriculture. Annual Report of the Director of Agriculture. 1904–1905.* Pretoria, Government Printing and Stationery Office, 1906, pp. 88–92. Also, A. Theiler and S. Stockman, Further Experiments to Determine How Long an Area Remains Infected with East Coast Fever, *Journal of Comparative Pathology and Therapeutics* 18: 163–169, 1905. In both publications a short article follows entitled "Do Salted Cattle Contain the Piroplasma Parvum in Their Blood?" (*Report*, pp. 92–94; *Journal*, pp. 169–171).

11 Letter from Stockman to F. B. Smith dated May 9, 1904 (*TAD* TAD 341/36507).
12 Typed copy in *TAD* TAD 341/36507 and in *PRO* CO 417/392/25248.
13 Letter from Macdonald to Smith dated May 18, 1904 (*TAD* TAD 341/36507).
14 See n. 6 above.
15 *Proceedings at Inter-Colonial Veterinary Conference, Cape Town.*
16 The delegates representing German South West Africa at the Bloemfontein meeting were Dr. von Lindequist (presumably Friedrich von Lindequist, then German Consul-General in Cape Town and soon to become Governor of German South West Africa) and the veterinarian Dr. W. Rickmann.

The preface to the report of the Bloemfontein conference stated that "owing to the disturbed condition of German South West Africa [the Herero uprising] no corrected copy had been received from Herr Rickmann." Probably because of the Herero uprising, Rickmann did not attend the Cape conference, at which German South West Africa was represented by the German Vice-Consul in Cape Town, Dr. F. Keller.

As far as I know East Coast fever never reached German South West

Africa but the authorities there were very alert to the risk. The veterinary files in the Windhoek archives (*SAW* ZBU/1321/0.III.h.z.) contain a long manuscript extract from Gray's letter to Hutcheon of April 11, 1902 (see chapter 3, n. 11) as well as a manuscript German translation of that letter. They also contain a copy of the Transvaal ordinance of August 22, 1902 restricting the movement of cattle, and a copy of a letter from Hutcheon, dated April 1, 1903 on redwater in the Cape, which ends by saying "What is termed the Rhodesian Redwater does not exist in the Cape." In an interesting echo of Milner's approach to Hopetoun, there is a letter from the Colonial Office in Berlin, dated November 10, 1902, reporting on information received from the German Consul in Brisbane on methods for immunizing cattle against redwater and including a pamphlet on that subject by C. J. Pound. In 1908 Rickmann published a book on animal diseases in South West Africa in which he included an excellent discussion of East Coast fever under the heading "Bisher in unserer Kolonie nicht bekannte Tierseuchen" (W. Rickmann, *Tierzucht und Tierkrankheiten in Deutsch-Südwestafrika*, Berlin, Schoetz, 1908, pp. 233–241).

17 *TAD* TAD 341/36507.
18 *CAD* CVS 1/57; the letter to Lyttelton is also in *PRO* CO 417/392/25248.
19 For the text of the legislation see *Transvaal Agricultural Journal* 3, no. 10, 410–417, 1904–5 [January, 1905].
20 Letter to William Macdonald from F. B. Smith dated Savile Club, December 19, 1905 (*TAD* TAD 474/G512). Smith remained on good terms with Stockman: in 1908, in London again, he called on him to supply some cattle to Theiler (see chapter 10, and chapter 10, n. 13).
21 At the Bloemfontein conference of December 1903 Stockman had objected to Koch's inoculation plan on the grounds that it might create immune carriers, a probability conceded by Koch himself. Stockman returned to that question in 1905, saying that if animals are only partially resistant, the importation of cattle from the East Coast would result in "permanent infection of the pastures, and the impossibility of importing [non-immune] cattle from elsewhere, or exporting to other districts which are clean" (S. Stockman, Some Points to be Considered in Connection with Rhodesian Redwater, *Journal of Comparative Pathology and Therapeutics* 18: 64–72, 1905).

From then on, until the end of the 1970s it was widely believed that carriers were rare and that immunity is sterile, but it is now believed that "immune carriers are common" (see A. S. Young, B. L. Leitch and R. M. Newson, The Occurrence of a *Theileria Parva* Carrier State in Cattle from an East Coast Fever Endemic Area of Kenya, in A. D. Irvin, M. P. Cunningham and A. S. Young (eds.), *Advances in the Control of Theileriosis*, The Hague, Nijhoff, 1981, pp. 60–62; see also other articles in the same volume). There appear to be several reasons why earlier studies failed to demonstrate the existence of immune carriers. Immune carriers have the piroplasms in only about 1 percent of their red blood cells, whereas animals suffering from frank East Coast fever may have the piroplasm in 50 percent or more of their red blood.cells. As a result ticks that feed on immune carriers may ingest relatively few or no piroplasms. According to Young *et al.* "the infection rates of *T. parva* in the adult ticks fed as nymphs ... were normally about 2%." Nor is it clear that all cattle that recover from East Coast fever do become carriers. Lounsbury, as always, hit the mark when he said in 1905 "owing, however, to our ignorance of the nature of African Coast fever infection, and the shortness of the period in which the disease has been under careful observation, it seems to be rash to definitely conclude from present evidence that ticks never become infective through feeding on recovered animals" (C. P. Lounsbury, Ticks and African Coast Fever, *Agricultural Journal of the Cape of Good Hope* 28: 634–654, 1906).

The existence of immune carriers means, as Stockman suggested, that cattle cannot be imported into areas where the disease is endemic unless they are previously immunized or otherwise protected against the disease and that cattle cannot be exported to "clean" areas even if they have been immunized. That does not, of course, mean that immunization would not be of value in areas where the disease is endemic, since it would greatly reduce the loss of cattle and improve their general health.

In 1924 C. R. Edmonds wrote a 23,000-word long essay arguing for the existence of carriers of East Coast fever (C. R. Edmonds, East Coast Fever, 67 pp. + 17 charts. Typed copy in the library of the National Archives of Zimbabwe, shelf mark GEN/EDM). Edmonds, whose apparently unpublished report was dated September 1, 1924, was convinced that the constant recurrence of East Coast fever in Rhodesia was caused by the presence of immune carriers. He also argued that the cattle imported from East Africa in 1901 may have been immune carriers. His report gives many examples of opposition to his views and he says that the only person who had given them any credence up to that time was John McFadyean. It now seems that Edmonds was right; the most influential opponent of the view that there are immune carriers was Arnold Theiler! Edmonds compared "relapses" of East Coast fever with relapses of malaria and recalled an occasion when he visited Koch's laboratory in Bulawayo in 1903 and found that Koch "appeared to be very pleased with himself, was extra communicative and dilated on the similarity he found between this [East Coast fever] organism and the malarial parasite." The suggestion that East Coast fever had become (or might become) established on an endemic basis in Rhodesia or South Africa was naturally a very unpopular one, but the existence of immune carriers presumably explains why the final steps in the eradication of the disease in both countries had to include the slaughter of herds. Edmonds pointed to the fact that Mozambique had eradicated the disease by the slaughter of herds as a strong argument for the existence of carriers. Writing in 1973, D. A.

Lawrence said "the Rhodesian Chief Veterinary Surgeons and their field staff, right up to the time that the disease was finally eradicated in 1954, were never convinced that carriers were not responsible for persistence or recrudescence of infection" (D. A. Lawrence, Southern Rhodesia (Rhodesia), in *A History of the Overseas Veterinary Services*, pt. II, London, British Veterinary Association, 1973, pp. 267–268).

22 A. Theiler, The Rhodesian Tick Fever, *Transvaal Agricultural Journal* 1, no. 4: 93–110, + 1 plate facing p. 104, [July] 1903.

23 A. Theiler, Rhodesian Tick Fever, in *Report of the South African Association for the Advancement of Sciences: Second Meeting held at Johannesburg, April 1904*, Published by the Association [n.p.], 1904, pp. 201–220. Also in *Transvaal Agricultural Journal* 2, no. 9: 421–438, [April] 1904.

24 Stockman, Report of the Work of the Veterinary Division (see n. 8 above).

25 When Stockman spoke of "ocular demonstration" as one of the methods used to convince farmers that the disease was new and serious he had in mind a demonstration in which a farmer named D. J. Erasmus had been asked to bring two healthy cattle to their Agricultural Department stables in Pretoria where "the oxen were infected by ticks supplied by Dr. Theiler. Both animals became infected and died. Farmers had the opportunity of seeing them during the progress of the disease and after death at the post-mortem examination." The results were reported at a public meeting on March 30, 1904, at which "Mr. Erasmus stated that he was present at the first post-mortem referred to. He had come to the conclusion that the disease had come from the tick, and was not the ordinary redwater . . . " See the *Transvaal Agricultural Journal* 2, no. 7: 394–395, [April] 1904.

26 *TAD* LTG 55/69/12.

27 *NAZ* LO 11/2/4/14, vol. 1.

28 *NAZ* A 1/5/5. (My copy is marked A/15/5 but A 1/5/5 is probably correct.)

29 T. W. Baxter, *Guide to the Public Archives of Rhodesia*, Salisbury, National Archives of Rhodesia, 1969, p. xxvii.

30 General [W.] Booth, *In Darkest England and the Way Out*, London, The Salvation Army, 1890. Booth was concerned with the unemployed and marginally employed; for a picture of the conditions of some of the *employed* in 1936, see G. Orwell, *The Road to Wigan Pier*, London, Victor Gollancz, 1937; New York, Harcourt Brace & World, 1958.

31 See A. Davidson, *Cecil Rhodes and His Time*, Moscow, Progress Publishers, 1988, p. 36.

32 *NAZ* LO 3/2/28.

33 S. P. Hyatt, *The Old Transport Road*, London, Andrew Melrose, 1914; reprint: Bulawayo, Books of Rhodesia, 1969; and S. P. Hyatt, *The Diary of a Soldier of Fortune*, London, T. Werner Laurie, 1910.

Hyatt was born on January 2, 1877, in Streatham Hill, London, and attended Dulwich College. In the last few years of his life he became sufficiently successful as a novelist to warrant an entry in *Who's Who* and an obituary in *The Times*. The latter (July 1, 1914, p. 10) says that Hyatt worked on a sheep station in New South Wales, returned home and then went to Matabeleland where he helped erect mining machinery. He began trading at the age of 22; with his brother Amyas he explored the rubber jungles of central Mozambique and, on his return, found his ox-transport business ruined by African Coast fever. He then started writing, for the Allahabad *Pioneer* and for some London financial papers. In 1904 he and his brother started wandering in the East and fought through the 1904–5 campaign in the Philippines. After his brother died, Hyatt returned to England, where he worked "on the press" at night and as an "electric light wireman" by day, while writing his first novel. That novel was an immediate success in 1907 and was followed by several other books, the last of which was *The Old Transport Road*. His death certificate in the General Register Office, St. Catherines House, London, shows that he died at 16 Longton Grove, Sydenham, on July 30, 1914. The causes of death were given as "(1) Pulmonary tuberculosis 17 years, (2) Exhaustion." In *Who's Who* Hyatt listed his recreations as "Fighting the tubercle bacillus, socialism."

34 K. Fairbridge, *The Autobiography of Kingsley Fairbridge*, London, Oxford University Press, 1927, gives a vivid picture of life in "frontier" Rhodesia in the 1890s. Whatever one may think about the colonization of Africa, Fairbridge's autobiography makes marvelous reading. Fairbridge quotes from a speech that he gave in 1909 in which he spoke of "over sixty thousand 'dependent' children . . . who have no parents, and no one standing in any such relation to them. What have they before them that can be called a future?" Fairbridge hoped to create his farm schools in Rhodesia, but they were instead created in Australia, where the first children arrived in January, 1913. The passage about their condition and clothing is found in R. Fairbridge, *Pinjarra, the Building of a Farm School*, London, Oxford Univeristy Press, 1937, as quoted in [K. Fairbridge] *Kingsley Fairbridge: His Life and Verse*, Bulawayo, Books of Rhodesia, 1974, p. 205. For some biographical notes on Fairbridge see L. W. Bolze's preface to the latter work.

35 The Fairbridge family home, Utopia, preserved as the Fairbridge Museum in Mutare (Umtali), is a striking example of the kind of "frontier" house and furniture mentioned in the text.

36 See the *Standard Encyclopaedia of South Africa*, vol. VI, p. 17 and vol. VIII, p. 57

37 J. M. Sinclair was Acting Chief Veterinary Surgeon in late 1904 while Gray was on leave in London; he succeeded Gray in 1905 when Gray succeeded Stockman as Chief Veterinary Surgeon of the Transvaal.

38 *CAD* CVS 1/59. Sinclair enclosed a copy of an article in the *Bulawayo Chronicle* of August 27, 1904 reporting a meeting held the week before to demand government action. There had been strong support ex-

pressed for the control of the movement of cattle but it had been far from unanimous.

39 J. M. Sinclair, A Short History of the Infective Diseases Amongst the Domestic Animals of Southern Rhodesia Since the Occupation: African Coast Fever, *Rhodesia Agricultural Journal* 19: 10–16, 1922. For an earlier version see chapter 3, n. 7. (The title of this journal varied; sometimes *Rhodesia*, sometimes *Rhodesian*.)

40 The new ordinance appeared in the *British South Africa Company Government Gazette* of August 5, 1904, as Government Notice no. 183 of 1904. Later Government Notices implementing the new ordinance also appeared in the *Government Gazette*. All such notices also appeared as paid announcements in the newspapers and were reprinted in the *Rhodesia Agricultural Journal*.

41 Stirling was born in Kirkintulloch, Scotland, on October 15, 1886, studied at the Royal Veterinary College in Dublin and qualified by becoming a member of the Royal College of Veterinary Surgeons in 1907. He had a relatively short but brilliant career. At the time of his death in India on August 16, 1935, at the age of 48, he was a Major in the Indian Army Reserve, Director of Veterinary Services of the Central Provinces of India, and a leading force in his field in the whole of India. See the *Veterinary Record* N.S. 15: 1130–1132 and 1165, 1935. For the thesis see R. F. Stirling, East Coast Fever in Rhodesia and its Control, 1912; typed copy in the library of the Royal College of Veterinary Surgeons, London.

42 In spite of Stirling's strictures, Portuguese East Africa became the first country in southern Africa to eradicate East Coast fever. It did that by the ruthless slaughter of infected herds. By 1917 the disease was extinct; it recurred briefly in 1923 but was again wiped out by slaughter (see Diesel, n. 56 below).

43 The *Rhodesia Civil Service List* (see chapter 2, n. 23) confirms Stirling on all of these points. As of September 30, 1904, 1905 and 1906 there were four men on the veterinary staff. As of April 30, 1908 and December 31, 1909, there were seven veterinarians attached to the service. Six more were hired during 1910 and eight more during 1911. Some people left, including Stirling, but, on December 31, 1910 there were 12 staff veterinarians and on December 31, 1911 there were 16.

44 Testimony, *NAZ* ZAB 2/1/1; depositions, *NAZ* ZAB 2/2/1. Published report: *Southern Rhodesia. Report of Committee of Enquiry on African Coast Fever*, Salisbury, Government Printer, 1910.

45 *NAZ* A 11/2/2/14, vol. 2.

46 L. E. W. Bevan, Autobiography, n.p., n.d., typed (*NAZ* Historical Manuscripts BE 11/7/1).

47 *NAZ* V 1/2/12/1.

48 *Transvaal Department of Agriculture. Report of the Proceedings of the Pan-African Veterinary Conference*. Pretoria, Government Printing and Stationery Office, 1909.

49 J. Spreull, East Coast Fever Inoculation in the Transkeian Territories,

South Africa, *Journal of Comparative Pathology and Therapeutics* 27: 299–304, 1914. For Spreull's immunization of 283,000 cattle in the Transkei, see chapter 7, n. 14. The Transkei was an area reserved to Africans, and, as Spreull says, East Coast fever spread through it in an all but uncontrolled fashion as it had earlier done in the African-occupied parts of Natal. (See also chapter 9, n. 28.)

A 1,000 mile-long fence had been built in 1896 to stop the spread of rinderpest into the Cape; it too failed. The construction of the fences to keep cattle out of the Cape and Bechuanaland was begun in 1904 and was a direct result of the failure of the Transvaal to adopt the recommendation that infected herds be slaughtered (see n. 18 above).

50 Herbert Watkins-Pitchford (June 6, 1865–June 25, 1951) did his studies on dipping in Natal. He published four articles on the subject. Professor John Lawrence has told me that Watkins-Pitchford's contribution was the development of arsenical dips that were strong enough to kill ticks without harming the cattle, even when used at intervals as short as three to five days, and the demonstration that short-interval dipping would control East Coast fever. See H. Watkins-Pitchford, Dipping and Tick-destroying Agents [same overall title for all articles], *Natal Agricultural Journal* 12: 436–459, 1909; Second Report, *Natal Agricultural Journal*, 15: 312–329, 1910; Part III, *Agricultural Journal of the Union of South Africa* 2: 33–79, 1911; Part IV, Union of South Africa Department of Agriculture, Pretoria, Government Printing and Stationery Office 1912, 31 pp.

51 The 1914 ordinance made dipping mandatory, but not in all parts of the country. For the battle against ticks in Rhodesia see J. A. Lawrence and R. A. I. Norval, A History of Ticks and Tick-borne Diseases of Cattle in Rhodesia, *Rhodesian Veterinary Journal* 10: 28–40, 1979. According to Lawrence and Norval, the "counts and smears" policy was begun in Rhodesia as early as 1927, and, "finally, in 1944, a policy of intensive supervision was introduced, with Cattle inspectors attending every dipping and smears being submitted from every dead animal."

52 *Report of the Rhodesian Redwater Commission*, Pretoria, Government Printing and Stationery Office, 1905, xx + 116 pp.

53 *Southern Rhodesia. Report of the Committee of Enquiry on African Coast Fever, Quarter-Evil and Epizootic Diseases of Cattle, 1917* [38 pp.]. Followed by a dissenting report: *Southern Rhodesia. Supplementary Report by the Chairman and a Member of the Committee Appointed on 19th August, 1917, to enquire into African Coast Fever, Quarter-Evil and Epizootic Diseases of Cattle* [18 pp.]. Salisbury, Government Printer, 1917.

54 *Southern Rhodesia. Report of the Committee of Enquiry in Respect of African Coast Fever, 1920.* Salisbury, Government Printer, 1920.

55 [*Union of South Africa*] *Report from the Select Committee on the Spread of East Coast Fever in the Union.* Cape Town, 1920.

56 A. M. Diesel, The Campaign Against East Coast Fever in South Africa, *Onderstepoort Journal of Veterinary Science and Animal Industry* 23: 19–31, 1948. See also A. M. Diesel and G. C. van Drimmelen, The

Diagnosis of East Coast Fever in South Africa: A Review, *Journal of the South African Veterinary Medical Association* 19: 81–88, 1948.

57 J. K. H. Wilde, The Control of Theileriosis, in J. B. Henson and M. Campbell, (eds.), *Theileriosis: Report of a Workshop held in Nairobi, Kenya,* 7–9 December 1976, Ottawa, International Development Research Centre, IDRC–086e, 1977. [I.S.B.N. 0–88936–124–X].

58 Personal communication, Harare, August 5, 1988.

59 T. Lees-May, Diseases of Stock in Rhodesia: African Coast Fever, *C.S.C. [Cold Storage Commission] News,* vol. 1 (no pagination), March, 1966. In 1966, Lees-May was the Director of Veterinary Services of Rhodesia.

60 *Southern Rhodesia. Committee of Enquiry on African Coast Fever, 1917.*

61 J. A. Lawrence, East Coast Fever: One of the Great Cattle Plagues of Africa, *Zimbabwe Science News* 16: 14–18, 1982.

62 Stockman, Report of Work of the Veterinary Division (see n. 8 above).

63 See W. Trager, *Living Together: The Biology of Animal Parasitism,* New York, Plenum, 1986, p. 214.

64 P. C. Doherty and R. Nussenzweig, Progress on *Theileria* vaccine, *Nature* 316: 484–485, 1985.

65 Douglas M. Parham, personal communication, Brechin Estates, Norton (Zimbabwe), August, 1986; J. P. Fraser-McKenzie, personal communication, Harare, August, 1987; Conrad E. Yunker, personal communication, Harare, August 30, 1988 and letter to P. F. Cranefield, September 5, 1988. I owe the estimate that there are about 5.5 million cattle in Zimbabwe today to Professor J. A. Lawrence (letter dated January 4, 1989). According to J. P. Fraser-McKenzie, large numbers of cattle are moved annually from one part of Zimbabwe to another, which makes dipping of great importance. Morrison *et al.* offer a comparable estimate of the cost of dipping in Kenya; those authors point out that it is very difficult to obtain reliable figures on the number of cattle that die of East Coast fever in countries where it is endemic. But they estimate that 50 percent to 80 percent of the ten million adult cattle in Kenya are at risk and that at least 1 percent of them die of East Coast fever annually. More importantly, perhaps 10 to 12 percent of heifer calves die before they reach calving age. Morrison *et al.* add that without dipping "the disease would undoubtedly have a catastrophic effect on the cattle population" (W. I. Morrison, P. A. Lalor, B. M. Goddeeris and A. J. Teale, Theileriosis: Antigens and Host–Parasite Interactions, in T. W. Pearson (ed.), *Parasite Antigens: Towards New Strategies for Vaccines,* New York and Basle, Dekker, 1986, pp. 167–206, in particular pp. 174–175). Several articles on the economic cost of East Coast Fever in areas in which it is endemic appear in A. D. Irving, M. P. Cunningham and A. S. Young (eds.), *Advances in the Control of Theileriosis,* The Hague, Nijhoff, 1981 (see pp. 1–3 and 393–415). As things stand, East Coast fever is second only to trypanosomiasis ("tse-tse fly disease") as a threat to the cattle of Africa.

9 THE AFRICAN-OWNED CATTLE IN RHODESIA

1 R. F. Stirling, East Coast Fever in Rhodesia and its Control, thesis for Fellowship of the Royal College of Veterinary Surgeons, 1912, typed copy in the library of the Royal College of Veterinary Surgeons, London.

2 *NAZ* A 11/2/2/14, vol. 2.

3 C. E. Gray and W. Robertson, Report upon Texas Fever or Redwater in Rhodesia, Cape Town, Argus, 1902.

4 *NAZ* LO 4/1/16.

5 A. Keppel-Jones, *Rhodes and Rhodesia: The White Conquest of Zimbabwe 1884–1902*, Pietermaritzburg, University of Natal Press, 1983 (also Kingston and Montreal, McGill–Queen's University Press, 1983).

6 A. H. Croxton, *Railways of Zimbabwe*, Newton Abbot and London, David and Charles, 1982.

7 *NAZ* LO 4/1/11 to *NAZ* LO 4/1/20, for the years 1902–4.

8 *NAZ* LO 4/1/11.

9 *NAZ* LO 4/1/14.

10 *NAZ* A 11/2/12/11.

11 *NAZ* LO 4/1/16.

12 Wankie, now Hwange, is the center of one of the largest deposits of coal in all of southern Africa and the home of a coal-fired electric power station that makes a vital contribution to the economy of Zimbabwe.

13 *NAZ* V 4/1/1.

14 See chapter 8, n. 39 and n. 40.

15 S. P. Hyatt, *The Old Transport Road*, London, Andrew Melrose, 1914 p. 174; reprint, Bulawayo, Books of Rhodesia, 1969.

16 *NAZ* V 1/2/12/1.

17 C. E. Gray, Inoculation for African Coast Fever, *Rhodesian Agricultural Journal* 2: 8–9, 1904; *Journal of Comparative Pathology and Therapeutics* 17: 203–205, 1904.

18 Joseph B. Loudon, personal communication, Savile Club, London, April 27, 1987. Age was not reckoned by year but by age groups or "regiments," which were defined both by when boys reached puberty and by when they had served as herd boys.

19 Joseph B. Loudon, personal communication, London, November, 1988. Dr. Loudon tells me there is a Zulu saying "where the children are, the cattle are not," which means that the children are with their mother and father, whereas the cattle that were used to pay the bride price are at the home of the mother's parents.

20 Parts of Tanzania are free of East Coast fever, and in parts it is present in an endemic (enzootic) form. But in parts where the level of immunity is low, severe outbreaks occur from time to time. Sukumaland includes areas of all three types. A study of the movement of cattle in those areas revealed that

  In the epizootic zone the stockowners had less children than owners in the enzootic zone. Even though bride price requirements seemed to be less exacting in the epizootic zone, it was thought that the shortage of bridewealth in these areas led to the late marriages of male persons, and that this was reflected by the differences in the populations of children.

In addition, "It seemed that the bulk of all transactions were directly or indirectly associated with bride price payments. It was thought that these exchanges greatly aggravated the spread of the disease." On the other hand, "the impression was gained that while control of [East Coast fever] could result in an increase in cattle population, the bulk of the benefit would be absorbed in the social structure of the Sukuma-land community by, for example, increased bride price demands" (B. McCulloch, B'Q. J. Suda, R. Tungaraza and W. J. Kalaye, A Study of East Coast Fever, Drought and Social Obligations, in Relation to the Need for the Economic Development of the Livestock Industry in Sukumaland, Tanzania, *Bulletin of Epizootic Diseases of Africa* 16: 303–326, 1966).

In a more recent study, Beinart has examined the role of cattle in the economy and society of Pondoland and has reviewed the effects on the Mpondo society of the introduction of East Coast fever in 1912. Pondoland is part of what is now called the Transkei. Beinart examines, among other things, a period of resistance to dipping, the effects of East Coast fever on bride price, the collapse of the cattle industry caused by East Coast fever and the gradual recovery of the cattle population (see W. Beinart, *The Political Economy of Pondoland*, Cambridge, Cambridge University Press, 1982).

21 *NAZ* LO 4/1/21.
22 See n. 10 above.
23 Hyatt, *Old Transport Road*, p. 166.
24 D. N. Beach, *War and Politics in Zimbabwe 1840–1900*, Gweru, Mambo Press, 1986, p. 128.
25 See Keppel-Jones, *Rhodes and Rhodesia*, p. 497.
26 See *Africa News*, vol. 29, no. 8, April 18, 1988, p. 12; *New York Times*, September 18, 1988; and *Africa News*, vol. 30, no. 7, October 3, 1988, pp. 1–2.
27 According to the *Bulawayo Chronicle* of September 6, 1902, the Chief Native Commissioner for Matabeleland, several Native Commissioners, and the Assistant Veterinary Surgeon (C. R. Edmonds), met in the Chief Native Commissioner's office in Bulawayo with Chiefs Gambo, Mazwi, Samvubu, Dakamala, Nyangazonke, Nhlukalao, Holi and several other chiefs to discuss the epidemic. The chiefs "fully realize the danger of the visitation, and are very anxious to cooperate . . . [they] unanimously agreed to destroy all dogs at the kraals with the exception of a few favourites, which they agreed to tie up." The *Chronicle* added that it was hoped that the Europeans would follow suit!

According to the *Chronicle* of September 20, 1902, Chief Gambo "says his father told him that a disease similar to this one had been known previous to their coming to this country, so that to some of the

natives its occurrence was not very surprising." This is a fascinating
fragment of unintentional oral history, since, according to Rasmussen,
Chief Gambo Sitole, or Gampu Sithole (c. 1840s–1916) was the son of
Makegeni (d. 1870) who was one of Mzilikazi's original followers in
Zululand (R. K. Rasmussen, *Historical Dictionary of Zimbabwe/Rho-
desia*, Metuchen, N.J. and London, Scarecrow, 1979). Taken at face
value, this means that Chief Gambo's father had told him, prior to
1870, of having seen rabies in Zululand prior to 1821 (or, at the latest,
in the Transvaal prior to 1838). A memory of having been told of
rabies during Chaka's reign in Zululand may thus have coincided with
the summoning of Pasteur's nephew to come from Paris to cope with
the outbreak. If what Makageni remembered really was rabies, the
whole story is even more interesting since rabies is believed to have
been very rare in southern Africa before 1850 and we have only isolated
reports of it.

28 African-owned cattle in other places did not escape East Coast fever,
perhaps because the population density was much greater. The disease
ran out of control in Natal during the 1906 uprising; in the Transkei,
900,000 African-owned cattle died between 1910 and 1914 (see J.
Spreull, East Coast Fever Inoculation in the Transkeian Territories,
South Africa, *Journal of Comparative Pathology and Therapeutics*, 27:
299–304, 1914). Rhodesia was large (about 150,000 square miles) and
its African population was between 500,000 and 750,000. Natal occupied some 35,000 square miles and had an African population of nearly
one million, of whom 250,000 were in the 10,000 square miles of
Zululand. The Transkei was also far more densely populated than
Rhodesia.

10 TWO MORE PARASITES AND ANOTHER NEW DISEASE

1 R. Koch, *Second Report on African Coast Fever*, Salisbury, Argus, 1903;
Robert Koch, *Third Report on African Coast Fever*, Salisbury, Argus,
1903. See chapter 5, n. 10 for republications.

2 *Report of the Proceedings of the Conference on Diseases Among Cattle and
Other Animals in South Africa held on the 3rd, 4th and 5th December, 1903*,
Bloemfontein, Argus, 1904.

3 A. Theiler, The Piroplasma bigeminum of the Immune Ox, in *Report
of the Transvaal Department of Agriculture. 1st July, 1903 to 30th June,
1904*, Pretoria, Government Printing and Stationery Office, 1905, pp.
116–132.

4 A. Theiler, Report of the Government Veterinary Bacteriologist
[dated November 12, 1906] in *Report of the Transvaal Department of
Agriculture. 1st July, 1905 to 30th June, 1906*. Pretoria, Government
Printing and Stationery Office, 1907, pp. 81–109 (see especially pp.
81–83 and 89).
  A. Theiler, Piroplasma mutans (N. spec.) of South African Cattle,

Journal of Comparative Pathology and Therapeutics 19: 292–300, 1906; Further Notes on Piroplasma mutans – a New Species of Piroplasma in South African Cattle, *Journal of Comparative Pathology and Therapeutics* 20: 1–18 + 1 plate, 1907; Further Notes on Piroplasma mutans, *Journal of Comparative Pathology and Therapeutics*, 22: 115–133, 1909.

5 C. M. Wenyon, *Protozoology*, New York, William Wood, vol. II, 1926, pp. 1001–1002 and 1035.

6 R. Koch, *Fourth Report on African Coast Fever*, Salisbury, Argus, 1904 (see chapter 5, n. 10 for republications); Theiler, Piroplasma bigeminum.

7 E. Dschunkowsky and J. Luhs, Die Piroplasmen der Rinder, *Centralblatt für Bakteriologie, Parasitenkunde and Infektionskrankheiten* 35: 486–492, + 3 plates, 1904.

In a later article (E. Dschunkowsky, Einige Bemerkungen über "Anaplasma", *Archiv für Schiffs- und Tropen-Hygiene* 31: 563–573, 1927), Dschunkowsky pointed out that he and Luhs had done this work in 1901 and 1902 and had published their results in a Russian journal in 1903. None of the many later authors (including myself) who cite this fact has located the original publication. Koch referred to the 1904 publication in his fourth report, which was dated February 29, 1904. In the article that appeared in 1904, Dschunkowsky and Luhs actually mentioned the work of Koch, Edington, Gray, Robertson, Watkins-Pitchford and Theiler.

8 Both *Theileria parva lawrencei* and *Theileria parva bovis* were described by D. A. Lawrence of the Southern Rhodesia Veterinary Service. Lawrence's son, Professor John A. Lawrence, tells me that Lawrence's reports of the new parasite (*T.p. lawrencei*) were published only in his annual reports; when Neitz identified that parasite as the cause of "corridor disease" he gave Lawrence credit for his earlier studies (W. O. Neitz, A. S. Canham and E. B. Kluge, Corridor Disease: A Fatal Form of Bovine Theileriosis Encountered in Zululand, *Journal of the South African Veterinary Medical Association* 26: 79–87, 1955).

For a full bibliography of D. A. Lawrence's publications on this subject see W. O. Neitz, Theileriosis, Gonderioses and Cytauxzoonoses: A Review, *Onderstepoort Journal of Veterinary Research* 27: 275–430, 1957, in which the citations of Lawrence's work are on pp. 380–381; and W. O. Neitz, Theileriosis, *Advances in Veterinary Science* 5: 241–297, 1959, in which the citations of Lawrence's work are on p. 292. In the opinion of Professor John Lawrence corridor disease is rarely, if ever, transmitted within a herd of cattle because the parasite is so lethal that an infected animal usually dies before the parasite can complete its life cycle and produce the form of the parasite in the red blood cell that is able to infect the tick. Corridor disease, transmitted from buffalo to cattle, thus does not cause epidemics among cattle. Professor Lawrence also tells me that, in Zimbabwe, a few hundred cattle a year are found to be infected with *Theileria parva bovis* which causes "a disease distinguishable from East Coast fever" (J. A. Lawrence, Bovine Theileriosis in Zimbabwe, in A. D. Irvin, M. P. Cunningham and A. S. Young (eds.), *Advances in the Control of Theileriosis*, The Hague, Nijhoff, 1981, pp. 74–75). See also J. A. Lawrence and R. A. I. Norval, A history of ticks and tick-borne diseases of cattle in Rhodesia, *Rhodesian Veterinary Journal* 10: 28–40, 1979.

9 See W. I. Morrison, P. A. Lalor, B. M. Goddeeris and A. J. Teale, Theileriosis: Antigens and Host–Parasite Interactions, in T. W. Pearson (ed.), *Parasite Antigens: Towards New Strategies for Vaccines*, New York and Basle, Dekker, 1986, p. 168. The existence of three organisms that are morphologically and serologically all but identical and that are distinguished in part by the ease with which they are transferred from one animal to another and in part by the severity of the disease that they cause provides another example of the question discussed earlier in this chapter: how does one show that a disease or a parasite is a new one? The question of cross-immunity has also arisen in the discussion of the nature of these "strains" of *Theileria parva*. Very recent work has shown that there may be one monoclonal antibody that discriminates between *T. parva bovis* and the other two parasites. To add to the complexity of the problem, it is not clear whether *Theileria parva bovis* is or is not identical with a parasite found in Kenya, *Theileria taurotragi*. See H. T. Koch, J. G. R. Ocama, F. C. Munatswa, B. Byrom, R. A. I. Norval, R. P. Spooner, P. A. Conrad and A. D. Irvin, Isolation and Characterization of Bovine *Theileria* Parasites in Zimbabwe, *Veterinary Parasitology* 28: 19–32, 1988. I am indebted to Dr. Conrad E. Yunker for calling my attention to this article. For additional information on the classification of the parasites see chapter 11, n. 1, and n. 17 below.

10 M. W. Henning, *Animal Diseases in South Africa*, 2nd edition, South Africa, Central News Agency, 1949, pp. 393–400.

11 Theiler, Report of the Government Veterinary Bacteriologist, 1905–6, pp. 81–3.

12 Theiler, Further Notes on Piroplasma mutans (1909) (see n. 4 above).

13 See T. Gutsche, *There was a Man: The Life and Times of Sir Arnold Theiler*, Cape Town, Timmins, 1979, p. 246. Smith had joined the Savile in 1905. He was proposed by Basil Williams, author of the *Dictionary of National Biography* entry on Milner and supported by Erskine Childers, author of *The Riddle of the Sands*. Smith, Williams and Childers had served together during the Boer War. For the Savile and the Malaria Committee see chapter 4, n. 40.

14 A. Theiler, Anaplasma marginale (Gen. and spec. nov.). The Marginal Points in the Blood of Cattle Suffering from a Specific Disease, in *Transvaal Department of Agriculture. Report of the Government Veterinary Bacteriologist for the Year 1908–1909*, Pretoria, Government Printing and Stationery Office, 1910, pp. 7–64 + 1 plate. See also A. Theiler, "Anaplasma marginale". A New Genus and Species of the Protozoa, *Transactions of the Royal Society of South Africa* 2: 69–72, 1910, where Theiler specifically says that "The American literature not being avail-

able to me at the beginning of my investigation, I described them as marginal points in my various reports." See also A. Theiler, Gall-sickness of South Africa (Anaplasmosis of Cattle), *Journal of Comparative Pathology and Therapeutics* 23: 98–115, 1910. For a full list of Theiler's publications on *Anaplasma marginale*, see P. J. Du Toit and C. Jackson, The Life and Work of Sir Arnold Theiler, *Journal of the South African Veterinary Medical Association* 7: 135–186, 1936.

15 Lignières had, as early as 1900 (see chapter 3, n. 5), dismissed the small parasites described by Smith and Kilborne as being artefacts and had argued that the mild and severe forms of Texas fever were caused by the same parasite. For Lignières, the mild form resulted when the infection was arrested early in its course and the severe form resulted when the spread of the parasite was rapid and general.

The connection between the "marginal points" and the small cocci described by Smith and Kilborne was pointed out explicitly by Theiler. Having reviewed the work of Smith and Kilborne, Theiler said "The conclusion . . . is: – Texas fever is the name for two diseases, the one due to *Piroplasma bigeminum*, representing Texas fever, *sensu strictu* and identical with our redwater, the other one due to *Anaplasma marginale* and corresponding to Anaplasmosis" (Theiler, Anaplasma marginale (Gen. and spec. nov.), p. 34).

The situation remained controversial in 1926. See Wenyon, *Protozoology*, vol. II, pp. 1053–1056, where the organism is discussed under the heading "Intracellular structures of a doubtful nature." In a series of articles published in 1933, Dikmans agreed with Theiler's views (see, in particular, G. Dikmans, Anaplasmosis. III: A Further Experimental Demonstration of its Identity in Louisiana, *Journal of the American Veterinary Medical Association* 82: 855–861, 1933; Anaplasmosis. IV: The Carrier Problem, *Journal of the American Veterinary Medical Association* 82: 862–870, 1933). But, for Dikmans, the nature of the "parasite" remained an unsolved problem (see G. Dikmans, Anaplasmosis. V: The Nature of Anaplasma, *Journal of the American Veterinary Medical Association* 83: 101–104, 1933).

In 1960, Ristic (M. Ristic, Anaplasmosis, *Advances in Veterinary Science* 6: 111–192, 1960) regarded the organism as being a major challenge to the taxonomists, and remarked that "classification is to a degree, an art . . . it need not be realistic." He was inclined to place *Anaplasma marginale* "between the smallest bacteria and the filterable viruses." In the same review, Ristic documented the fact that Anaplasmosis is "a disease of major economic importance to the cattle industry throughout the tropic and subtropic world." In 1963, Ristic (M. Ristic, Anaplasmosis, in D. Weinman and M. Ristic (eds.), *Infectious Blood Diseases of Man and Animals*, New York, Academic Press, 1968, pp. 474–542) again called attention to the difficulty of classifying the parasite.

In view of the world-wide economic importance of bovine Anaplasmosis and in view of the facts that even today *Anaplasma marginale* presents a challenge to taxonomists, that so many previous workers had seen and misinterpreted Anaplasma marginale, and that Theiler's conclusions were correct but were for so long challenged, Theiler's success in identifying Anaplasma marginale and Anaplasmosis must be regarded as being as impressive as his work on East Coast fever.

16 See T. Smith and F. L. Kilborne, Investigations into the Nature, Causation, and Prevention of Southern Cattle Fever, U.S. Department of Agriculture. Bureau of Animal Industry, Bulletin No. 1, Washington Government Printing Office, 1893; reprinted in [E. C. Kelly], Medical Classics, vol. I, no. 5, Baltimore, Williams and Wilkins, 1937, pp. 341–597. Smith and Kilborne described the parasite as being pear-shaped or "pyriform," and named it Pyrosoma bigeminum. As early as 1895, Wandolleck pointed out that "pyro" refers to fire rather than to pears, that the name Pyrosoma had long before been introduced as the name of a phosphorescent ascidian, and that even pyrisoma or pirisoma would be a combination of a Latin form (pirum, pear) and a Greek form (soma, body). He proposed an all–Greek term, apiosoma, which was not adopted (see B. Wandolleck, Pyrosoma bigeminum, Centralblatt für Bakteriologie und Parasitenkunde, erste Abteilung 17: 554–556, 1895). The change to Piroplasma was proposed in 1895 (W. H. Patton, The Name of the Southern or Splenic Cattle-fever parasite, American Naturalist 22: 498, 1895).

Part of the confusion arose from the fact that the Latin word for pear, pirum, had become pyrum in medieval Latin. However, in both American and English usage of the time, the word meaning pear-shaped (piriform) was commonly spelled pyriform (see the Century Dictionary, first edition, 1890, p. 4874; A New English Dictionary, vol. VII, 1909, p. 1688). Apart from the fact that Piroplasma (pear form) had not been previously used in zoological nomenclature, it was not much of an improvement over Pyrosoma from the point of view of linguistic purists since it was, again, a mixed Latin–Greek form. It was eventually replaced by Babesia; Smithia was suggested and dismissed by Wandolleck in his brief, smug and sarcastic article.

17 It is now known that Theileria mutans is not transmitted by the brown tick. From a historical point of view the importance of the discovery of Theileria mutans was that it led to an explanation of the finding that inoculation of blood could cause small parasites similar to those that cause East Coast fever to appear in the blood of the inoculated animal. Theileria mutans has always occupied a special place because it differs from Theileria parva in many ways. It can easily be transmited by inoculation since the parasite multiplies within red blood cells far more readily than it does within lymphocytes. For that and other reasons Theileria mutans was, for many years, placed in a separate genus (see chapter 11, n. 1). In spite of those differences it was believed for many years that Theileria mutans could be transmitted by the brown tick, and that finding was always attributed to Theiler. In the 1970s, however, it was shown that Theileria mutans cannot be transmitted by the brown

tick, although it can be transmitted by a tick of the *Amblyomma* genus. The name *Theileria mutans* remains in use to describe the parasite that is readily transmitted by inoculation. Two theilerial parasites of relatively low pathogenicity that *can* be transmitted by the brown tick are *Theileria taurotragi* and *Theileria parva bovis* (see G. Uilenberg, Theilerial species of domestic livestock, in A. D. Irvin, M. P. Cunningham and A. S. Young (eds.), *Advances in the Control of Theileriosis*, The Hague, Nijhoff, 1981, pp. 4–37). In addition, it was suggested, as recently as 1988 (see n. 9 above), that what is called *Theileria taurotragi* in Kenya may be very similar to at least some strains of what is called *Theileria parva bovis* in Zimbabwe.

What is puzzling about this is that, as far as I can see, in none of his major articles of 1906, 1907 and 1909 (Theiler, Piroplasma mutans; Theiler, Further Notes on Piroplasma mutans (1907); Theiler, Further Notes on Piroplasma mutans (1909): see n. 4 above) did Theiler claim to have transmitted what he called *Piroplasma mutans* by the brown tick or any other tick. In his annual report for 1905–6 (Theiler, Report of the Government Veterinary Bacteriologist: see n. 4 above) he did say that since so many animals were infected with both *Piroplasma bigeminum* and *Piroplasma mutans* it might be inferred that both infections are introduced at the same time and probably by the same tick (which would be the blue tick). In his articles of 1906 and 1907 he described transmission of *Piroplasma mutans* only by inoculation. In his article of 1907 he concluded that *Piroplasma mutans* is *not* transmitted by the blue tick *and* he said (p. 17) that "another tick is responsible for this piroplasmosis infection," but he did not specify that other tick. In his last major article on the subject (1909), Theiler reported many cases of transmission of *Piroplasma mutans* by inoculation. He also spoke of infesting three animals "with larvae of either [the brown tick] or the [blue tick] collected from animals immune against piroplasma bigeminum and piroplasma mutans and therefore containing those parasites in their blood." Only one of those three animals was infested with the brown tick (heifer no. 639). That is the animal mentioned in my text, which "contracted ordinary redwater and died." That death led Theiler to say that "in one instance we were able to transmit piroplasma bigeminum by larvae of [the brown tick]. This is an exception to the general rule, but the experiments were undertaken in such a way that no other explanation is possible." (Far be it from me to suggest that Arnold Theiler could not diagnose a case of redwater, but redwater cannot be transmitted by the brown tick. Moreover, the course of the illness was not typical of redwater. Fever appeared only on the fifteenth day, a few pear-shaped parasites appeared on the fifteenth day, and the urine was red only on the sixteenth day, the day before the animal died. It sounds more like a relapse of redwater in the course of another fatal illness. In any event, Theiler did not claim to have transmitted *Piroplasma mutans* in this experiment.)

The difficulty arose from a short and unimpressive article, some 700 words long, that also appeared in 1909 (A. Theiler, Transmission des Spirilles et des Piroplasmes par Différentes Espèces de Tiques, *Bulletin de la Société Pathologie Exotique* 2: 293–294, 1909). In that article, which is little more than an abstract, Theiler listed four cases in which he thought he had transmitted *redwater* by the *brown tick*. One of the cases was heifer 638, discussed above. He also listed one case of transmission of *Theileria mutans* by the brown tick and another by the red tick. It is this brief resumé that was later cited by Wenyon, Henning and Uilenberg, among others.

It seems odd that this summary exerted more influence than Theiler's detailed reports of his research, but since he did publish it we cannot claim that all of his statements about the three small parasites have stood the test of time. What is more interesting is the fact that Theiler may indeed have transmitted a relatively non-pathogenic theilerial parasite by the brown tick and by the red tick. If so, then either *Theileria taurotragi* or *Theileria parva bovis* existed in the Transvaal as early as 1907 or 1908, the years in which the experiments were done. (As early as 1910, Richard Gonder remarked that the brown tick "transmit[s] *P. mutans* only in exceptional cases." See R. Gonder, On the Development of *Piroplasma parvum* (Protozoa) in the Various Organs of Cattle, *Transactions of the Royal Society of South Africa* 2: 63–68, 1910.)

What Theiler did *not* do, obviously, was transmit by ticks a parasite that had been proven to be *Theileria mutans* by previous transmission by inoculation: his criteria must simply have been morphology and relative non-pathogenicity. This brief article is not one of Theiler's better efforts.

18 C. P. Lounsbury, Ticks and African Coast Fever, *Transvaal Agricultural Journal*, 2, no. 5: 4–13, [October] 1903.

19 A. Theiler, The Transmission of East Coast Fever by Ticks, in *Report of the Transvaal Department of Agriculture. 1st July, 1903 to 30th June, 1904*, Pretoria, Government Printing and Stationery Office, 1905.

20 J. W. W. Stephens and S. R. Christophers *The Practical Study of Malaria*, London, for the University Press of Liverpool by Longmans, Green & Co., [November] 1903. The relevant passage on African Coast fever is on pp. 331–332, along with a figure taken from Laveran (A. Laveran, Sur la Piroplasme Bovine Bacilliform, *Comptes rendus Académie des Sciences* 136: 648–653, 1903) showing both the tiny cocci and the bacilliform parasites and a statement that "atypical forms have been described by Theiler and, subsequently more fully, by Laveran." Stephens and Christophers even said, as early as November, 1903: "It is important to note that together with the atypical forms typical forms are always found though these may be rare. These atypical forms occur in the severe cases. Similar cocci-like forms, described by Smith and Kilborne in Texas fever, occurred in the *slight* cases."

21 See Wenyon, *Protozoology*, vol. II, p. 1029.

22 K. C. Carter, Koch's Postulates in Relation to the Work of Jacob Henle

and Edwin Klebs, *Medical History* 29: 353–374, 1985; The Koch–Pasteur Dispute on Establishing the Cause of Anthrax, *Bulletin of the History of Medicine* 62: 42–57, 1988.

The viability of Koch's postulates provides an example of a phenomenon to which Professor Hao Wang has called attention: certain insightful hypotheses have a "tolerance" or "flexibility" that permits their formal structure to survive changes in their specific content. (In that connection Wang cites a joke that I told him about the farmer who spoke of "the best ax I ever had, it has lasted through two new heads and three new handles.") See H. Wang, The Formal and the Intuitive in the Biological Sciences, *Perspectives in Biology and Medicine* 27: 525–545, 1984. Koch's postulates have certainly lasted for a long time, although both head and handle have often been replaced.

23 Theiler, Piroplasma bigeminum (see n. 3 above).

24 I am greatly indebted to Professor Maclyn McCarty for several discussions of these problems.

25 R. Koch, *Reise-Berichte über Rinderpest, Bubonenpest in Indien und Afrika, Tsetse-oder Surrakrankheit, Texasfieber, Tropische Malaria, Schwarzwasserfieber*, Berlin, Julius Springer 1898. See chapter 5, n. 4 for republication and translation.

26 A. Laveran, Sur la Piroplasme bovine bacilliform, *Comptes rendus Académie des Sciences* 136: 648–653, 1903.

27 The notion that facts are stubborn things apparently first appeared in E. Budgell, *Liberty and Property*, second part, second edition, London, W. Mears, 1732, pp. 76–77. I have condensed the 97-word long title of Budgell's pamphlet. The *Dictionary of National Biography* (vol. VII, pp. 224–225) would have us believe that Budgell was deranged, but he was certainly sound on the question of facts.

28 Smith and Kilborne, *Investigations*.

29 Koch, *Reise-Berichte*.

11 WHAT IS EAST COAST FEVER?

1 Barnett points out that one reason why Bettencourt and his colleagues separated the *Babesia* from the *Theileria* was that theilerial parasites sometimes look like a Maltese cross under light microscopy (S. F. Barnett, Theileriasis, in D. Weinman and M. Ristic (eds.), *Infectious Blood Diseases of Man and Animals*, New York, Academic Press, 1968, vol. II, pp. 269–328; A. Bettencourt, C. França and I. Borges, Un cas de Piroplasmose bacilliform chez le Daim, *Archivos do Real Instituto Bacteriologico Camara Pestana* 1: 341–349 + 2 plates, 1907). This is correct, but in many ways, as they stated, Bettencourt *et al.* followed Theiler, who, in his 1906 description of *Piroplasma mutans* (A. Theiler, Piroplasma mutans (N. spec.) of South African Cattle, *Journal of Comparative Pathology and Therapeutics* 20: 1–18, 1907) set up three classes of the parasites seen in cattle. One class contained the Texas fever parasite, a second class contained the inoculable parasites (*Pi-*

roplasma mutans and the parasite of "tropical piroplasmosis"), and the third class contained the non-inoculable parasite of East Coast fever. Bettencourt *et al.* proposed two groups, the first of which contained what they called *Babesia*, characterized by the facts that at some stage in their life cycle they are pear-shaped and that they often appear in pairs in the same red blood cell. The second class, which they called *Theileria*, assume the shape of the "baguette," i.e. are bacilliform. The "baguettes" were further divided into inoculable (*Theileria mutans*) and non-inoculable (*Theileria parva*). They thus created a new genus "que nous proposerions d'appeler – *Theileria* – englobant tous les parasites qui présentent la forme en baguette et qui se divisent en originant les formes en croix." The "Maltese cross" that results when a single piroplasm of *Theileria parva* divides into four "merozoites" in a red blood cell was shown clearly in 1986 (P. A. Conrad, D. Denham and C. G. D. Brown, Intraerythrocytic Multiplication of *Theileria parva in vitro*: An Ultrastructural Study, *International Journal for Parasitology* 116: 223–229, 1986). Barnett also states that du Toit later made the distinction rest in part on the fact that theilerial parasites multiply in the lymphocytes, thus placing *Theileria mutans*, which did not appear to do so, into a new genus (*Gonderia*), which was later abandoned (P. J. du Toit, Zur Systematik der Piroplasmen, *Archiv für Protistenkunde* 39: 84–104, 1918). For our purposes the point is that one of the motives for studying the life-cycle of the parasites was (and is) to determine how they should be classified. For reviews of the taxonomic problem as of 1968 and 1977, see Barnett, Theileriasis, pp. 270–278 and S. F. Barnett, Theileria, in J. P. Kreier (ed.), *Parasitic Protozoa*, New York, Academic Press, vol. IV, 1977, pp. 77–113 (in particular, pp. 89–93). See also G. Uilenberg, Theilerial species of domestic livestock, in A. D. Irvin, M. P. Cunningham and A. S. Young (eds.), *Advances in the Control of Theileriosis*, The Hague, Nijhoff, 1981, pp. 4–37.

Members of the *Babesia* genus and members of the *Theileria* genus have many similarities and it is interesting that as early as his interim report, Koch said of Texas Fever and "African Coast fever" that

we may ultimately find that in pyrosomal diseases of cattle, we have to deal with a class of disease[s] related to one another in much the same way as the various types of human malaria, formerly classified as one, but which we now know to be caused by infection with the different parasites of the quartan, tertian and the tropical types of Malarial fever (R. Koch, *Interim Report on Rhodesian Redwater or "African Coast Fever"*, Salisbury, Argus, 1903).

The malarial parasites have remained in a single genus largely because their life cycles are so similar (William Trager, Professor Emeritus, The Rockefeller University, personal communication) whereas the *Babesia* and the *Theileria* have been separated not only because of differences in their life cycle but also because of other differences discovered more recently, including differences in their ultrastructure. Nevertheless, there are many similarities between these kinds of piroplasm (Maria Rudzinska, Professor Emeritus, The Rockefeller University, personal communication).

From the point of view of what constitutes a new disease (see chapter 10), the malarial parasites provide an interesting example, since there is no cross-immunity between the diseases that they cause and because those diseases differ in character and in virulence.

2 Strictly speaking, the animals develop what the hematologist calls an "aleukemic" leukemia, since although there are many lymphoblasts in the tissues, the number of circulating lymphocytes usually falls throughout the course of the disease (C. G. D. Brown, personal communication, Centre for Tropical Veterinary Medicine, University of Edinburgh, December 9, 1988).

3 See Gray's *Annual Report* for 1901–2 and the joint report of Gray and Robertson (C. E. Gray, Annual Report 1901–1902, in *The British South Africa Company. Reports on the Administration of Rhodesia, 1900–1902*, printed for the Information of Shareholders [London, 1903], pp. 224–230; C. E. Gray and W. Robertson, *Report upon Texas Fever or Redwater in Rhodesia*, Cape Town, Argus, 1902).

4 Koch, *Interim Report*.

5 R. Koch, Beiträge zur Entwicklungsgeschichte der Piroplasmen, *Zeitschrift für Hygiene und Infecktionskrankheiten* 54: 1–9 + 3 plates, 1906; also in *Gesammelte Werke von Robert Koch*, Leipzig, Thieme, 1912, vol. II, p. 1, pp. 487–492 + 3 plates. "Koch's blue bodies" are not mentioned in the text of this article but are shown in figs. 48 and 49 and described in the legend to those figures.

6 K. F. Meyer, Preliminary Note on the Transmission of East Coast Fever to Cattle by the Intra-peritoneal inoculation of the Spleen or Portions of the Spleen of a Sick Animal, *Journal of Comparative Pathology and Therapeutics* 22: 213–217, 1909. In this article Meyer had already considered the possibility that "Koch's granules are a stage in the life cycle of the parasite."

7 K. F. Meyer, Notes on the Nature of Koch's Granules and their Rôle in the Pathogenesis of East Coast Fever, in *Union of South Africa. Department of Agriculture. Report of the Government Veterinary Bacteriologist for the Year 1909–1910*. Pretoria, Government Printing and Stationery Office, 1911, pp. 56–68 + 1 plate. This report is often cited as *Report of the Government Veterinary Bacteriologist of the Transvaal 1909–1910*, Pretoria, Government Printing and Stationery Office, 1911. Although most of the work reported in it was done before the Transvaal became part of the Union of South Africa in May, 1910, few if any libraries catalogue this report under Transvaal, so that that citation is singularly unhelpful.

K. F. Meyer, Beiträge zur Genese und Bedeutung der Kochschen Plasmakugeln in der Pathogenese des afrikanischen Küstenfiebers, *Centralblatt für Bakteriologie*, I. Abt. Originale, 57: 415–432 + 3 plates, 1911.

8 R. Gonder, On the Development of *Piroplasma parvum* (Protozoa) in the Various Organs of Cattle, *Transactions of the Royal Society of South*

Africa 2: 63–68, 1910.

R. Gonder, The Life Cycle of Theileria parva: the Cause of East Coast Fever in South Africa, Journal of Comparative Pathology and Therapeutics 23: 328–335, 1910.

R. Gonder, Die Entwicklung von Theileria parva, dem Erreger des Küstenfiebers der Rinder in Afrika, Archiv für Protistenkunde 21: 143–164 + 3 plates, 1911.

R. Gonder, The Development of Theileria parva, the Cause of East Coast Fever of Cattle in South Africa, in Union of South Africa. Department of Agriculture. Report of the Government Veterinary Bacteriologist for the year 1909–1910, Pretoria, Government Printing and Stationery Office, 1911, pp. 69–83 + 5 plates [also usually miscited: see n. 7 above].

R. Gonder, Die Entwicklung von Theileria parva, dem Erreger des Küstenfiebers des Rinder in Afrika. II. Teil, Archiv für Protistenkunde 22: 170–178 + 2 plates, 1911.

R. Gonder, The Development of Theileria parva, the Cause of East Coast Fever of Cattle in South Africa (Part 2), in Union of South Africa. Department of Agriculture. First Report of the Director of Veterinary Research, Pretoria, Government Printing and Stationery Office, [August] 1911, pp. 224–228 + 1 plate.

9 The form of the Theileria parva parasite that appears in the red blood cell is the form that infects the tick. The question of whether that parasite ever multiplies within the red blood cells of the infected animal was debated for many years. Elegant electronmicrographs showing that it can do so were published recently (D. W. Fawcett, P. A. Conrad, J. G. Grootenhuis and S. P. Morzaria, Ultrastructure of the Intra-erythrocytic Stage of Theileria species from Cattle and Waterbuck, Tissue and Cell 19: 643–655, 1987). I am indebted to Dr. Fawcett for calling my attention to this study and to the studies cited in n. 39 and n. 42 below.

10 Barnett, Theileriasis, p. 278.

11 E. V. Cowdry and W. B. C. Danks, Studies on East Coast Fever. II: Behaviour of the Parasite and the Development of Distinctive Lesions in Susceptible Animals, Parasitology 25: 1–63 + 10 plates, 1933.

12 L. Hulliger, J. K. H. Wilde, C. G. D. Brown and L. Turner, Mode of Multiplication of Theileria in Cultures of Bovine Lymphocytic Cells, Nature 203: 728–730, 1964.

13 E. Reichenow, Die Entwicklungsgang des Küstenfiebererregers im Rinde und in der übertragende Zecke, Archiv für Protistenkunde 94: 1–56 + 3 plates, 1940. The quotation is from Barnett, Theileriasis, p. 297. See in particular Reichenow's plate 1, figs. 3–6, and pp. 11–18.

14 I. Tchernomoretz [Tsur], Multiplication in vitro of Koch Bodies of Theileria annulata, Nature 156: 391, 1945.

15 I. Tsur-Tchernomoretz [Tsur], W. O. Neitz and J. W. Pols, The Development of Koch Bodies of Theileria parva in Tissue Culture,

Refuah Veterinarith 14: 53–51 [*sic*], 1957. (The figures are in the Hebrew version of this article, pp. 6–12 of the same volume.)

16 D. W. Brocklesby and F. Hawking, Growth of *Theileria annulata* and *T. parva* in tissue culture, *Transactions of the Royal Society of Tropical Medicine and Hygiene* 52: 414–420, 1958.

17 I. Tsur and S. Adler, Cultivation of Theileria annulata Schizonts in Monolayer Tissue Culture, *Refuah Veterinarith* 19: 225–224 [*sic*], 1962.

18 Hulliger *et al.*, Mode of Multiplication of *Theileria*.

19 L. Hulliger, Cultivation of Three Species of *Theileria* in Lymphoid Cells *in vitro, Journal of Protozoology* 12: 649–655, 1965.

20 See, for example, W. A. Malmquist, M. B. A. Nyindo and C. G. D. Brown, East Coast Fever: Cultivation *in vitro* of Bovine Spleen Cell Lines Infected and Transformed by *Theileria parva, Tropical Animal Health and Production* 2: 139–145, 1970; for further citations see T. J. Kurtti, U. G. Munderloh, A. D. Irvin and G. Büscher, *Theileria parva*: Early Events in the Development of Bovine Lymphoblastoid Cell Lines Persistently Infected with Macroschizonts, *Experimental Parasitology* 52: 280–290, 1981.

21 W. Trager, *Living Together: The Biology of Animal Parasitism*, New York, Plenum, 1966, p. 214.

22 S. F. Barnett, Connective Tissue Reactions in Acute Fatal East Coast Fever (*Theileria parva*) of cattle, *Journal of Infectious Diseases* 107: 253–282, 1960.

23 W. F. H. Jarrett and D. W. Brocklesby, A Preliminary Electron Microscopic Study of East Coast Fever (*Theileria parva* Infection), *Journal of Protozoology* 13: 301–310, 1966.

24 For example, in 1967, Büttner argued against the position of Reichenow and Hulliger and spoke of their "false assumption of a repeated binary fission" ("falschen Auffassung einer wiederholten Zweiteilung"). See D. W. Büttner, Elektronenmikroscopische Studien der Vermehrung von Theileria parva im Rind, *Zeitschrift für Tropenmedizin und Parasitologie* 18: 245–268, 1967.

25 Malmquist *et al.*, East Coast Fever.

26 J. E. Moulton, H. H. Krauss and W. A. Malmquist, Transformation of Reticulum Cells to Lymphoblasts in Cultures of Bovine Spleen Infected with *Theileria parva, Laboratory Investigation* 24: 187–196, 1971. When the macroschizont breaks up into a large number of smaller forms of the parasite (the microschizonts) the lymphocyte dies and releases those microschizonts into the blood, where they invade the red blood cell to become the "bacilliform parasite." This process can be hastened, in cell culture, by increasing the temperature (L. Hulliger, C. G. D. Brown and J. K. H. Wilde, Transition of Developmental Stages of *Theileria parva in vitro* at High Temperatures, *Nature* 211: 328–329, 1966). It may be that it is precipitated in the infected animal by the development of fever (C. G. D. Brown, personal communication, Centre for Tropical Veterinary Medicine, University of Edinburgh, December 9, 1988).

27 J. C. DeMartini and J. E. Moulton, Responses of the Bovine Lymphatic System to Infection by *Theileria parva*. I: Histology and Ultrastructure of Lymph Nodes in Experimentally-Infected Calves, *Journal of Comparative Pathology* 83: 281–298, 1973.
28 D. E. Radley, C. G. D. Brown, M. J. Burridge, M. P. Cunningham, M. A. Peirce and R. E. Purnell, East Coast Fever: Quantitative Studies of *Theileria parva* in Cattle, *Experimental Parasitology* 36: 278–287, 1974.
29 W. I. Morrison, G. Büscher, M. Murray, D. L. Emery, R. A. Masake, R. H. Cook and P. W. Wells, *Theileria parva*: Kinetics of Infection in the Lymphoid System of Cattle, *Experimental Parasitology* 52: 248–260, 1981.
30 W. I. Morrison, P. A. Lalor, B. M. Goddeeris and A. J. Teale, Theileriosis: Antigens and Host–Parasite Interactions, in: T. W. Pearson (ed.), *Parasite Antigens. Towards New Strategies for Vaccines*, New York and Basle, Dekker, 1986, pp. 167–213; see especially pp. 169–173.
31 C. G. D. Brown, W. A. Malmquist, M. P. Cunningham, D. E. Radley and M. J. Burridge, Immunization against East Coast Fever. Inoculation of Cattle with Theileria parva Schizonts Grown in Cell Culture [abstract]. Proceedings of the Second International Congress of Parasitology, in *Journal of Parasitology* 57: no. 4, section II, pt. 1, pp. 59–60, 1971 (often incorrectly cited as 57: 59–60).
32 C. G. D. Brown, M. P. Cunningham, L. P. Joyner, R. E. Purnell, D. Branagan, G. L. Corry and K. P. Bailey, *Theileria parva*: Significance of Leukocytes for Infecting Cattle, *Experimental Parasitology* 45: 55–64, 1978.
33 C. G. D. Brown, personal communication, Centre for Tropical Veterinary Medicine, University of Edinburgh, December 9, 1988.
34 C. G. D. Brown, D. A. Stagg, R. E. Purnell, G. K. Kanhai and R. C. Payne, Infection and Transformation of Bovine Lymphoid Cells *in vitro* by Infective Particles of *Theileria parva*, Nature 245: 101–103, 1973.
35 D. A. Stagg, D. Chasey, A. S. Young, S. P. Morzaria and T. T. Dolan, Synchronization of the Division of *Theileria* Macroschizonts and their Mammalian Host Cells, *Annals of Tropical Medicine and Parasitology* 74: 263–265, 1980.
36 D. A. Stagg, T. T. Dolan, B. L. Leitch and A. S. Young, The Initial Stages of Infection of Cattle Cells with *Theileria parva* Sporozoites *in vitro*, *Parasitology* 83: 191–197, 1981.
37 F. L. Musisi, R. G. Bird, C. G. D. Brown and M. Smith, The Fine Structural Relationship Between *Theileria* Schizonts and Infected Bovine Lymphocytes from Cultures, *Zeitschrift für Parasitenkunde* 65: 31–41, 1981.
38 T. J. Kurtti, U. G. Munderloh, A. D. Irvin and G. Büscher, *Theileria parva*: Early Events in the Development of Bovine Lymphoblastoid Cell Lines Persistently Infected with Macroschizonts, *Experimental Parasitology* 52: 280–290, 1981.

39 D. W. Fawcett, S. Doxsey, D. A. Stagg and A. S. Young, The Entry of Sporozoites of Theileria parva into Bovine Lymphocytes in vitro. Electron microscopic observations, *European Journal of Cell Biology* 27: 10–21, 1982.

40 W. G. Z. O. Jura, C. G. D. Brown and B. Kelly, Fine Structure and Invasive Behavior of the Early Developmental Stages of *Theileria annulata* in vitro, *Veterinary Parasitology* 12: 31–44, 1983.

41 W. G. Z. O. Jura, C. G. D. Brown and A. C. Rowland, Ultrastructural Characteristics of in vitro Parasite–Lymphocyte Behavior in Invasions with *Theileria annulata* and *Theileria parva*, *Veterinary Parasitology* 12: 115–134, 1983.

42 D. Fawcett, A. Musoke and W. Voigt, Interaction of Sporozoites of *Theileria parva* with Bovine Lymphocytes *in vitro*. I: Early Events after Invasion, *Tissue and Cell* 16: 873–884, 1984.

43 D. W. Fawcett and D. A. Stagg, Passive Endocytosis of Sporozoites of *Theileria parva* in Macrophages at 1–2°C, *Journal of Submicroscopic Cytology* 18: 11–19, 1986.

44 For an early review, written just as the role of the lymphocytes in the immune system was beginning to be clear, see J. L. Gowans and D. D. McGregor, The Immunological Activities of Lymphocytes, in P. Kallós and B. H. Waksman, (eds.), *Progress in Allergy* 9: 1–78, 1965. Only eleven years later, volume 20 of *Progress in Allergy* began with a preface that said "The overwhelming preoccupation of the immunological community with lymphocytes . . . is reflected in this volume . . . of the four reviews, three deal exclusively with lymphocytes." The editor added that "These reviews are written against a background of increasing crisis in communication within the field of Immunology. The mass of current research . . . is simply staggering" (B. H. Waksman, Introduction, in: P. Kallós, B. H. Waksman and A. de Weck (eds.), *Progress in Allergy* 20: ix–xii, 1976). Needless to say, I have not attempted to condense the story of the T cell between 1965 and the present into a sentence or two.

45 S. Kasakura and L. Lowenstein, A Factor Stimulating DNA Synthesis Derived from the Medium of Leucocyte Cultures, *Nature* 208: 794–795, 1965; J. Gordon and L. D. MacLean, A Lymphocyte-Stimulating Factor Produced *in vitro*, *Nature* 208: 795–796, 1965.

46 K. A. Smith, T-Cell Growth Factor, *Immunological Reviews* 51: 337–357, 1980.

47 B. J. Poiesz, F. W. Ruscetti, J. W. Mier, A. Woods and R. C. Gallo, T-Cell Lines Established from Human T-Lymphocytic Neoplasias by Direct Response to T-Cell Growth Factor, *Proceedings of the National Academy of Sciences U.S.A.* 77: 6815–6819, 1980.

48 J. E. Gootenberg, F. W. Ruscetti, J. W. Mier, A. Gazdar and R. C. Gallo, Human Cutaneous T Cell Lymphoma and Leukemia Cell Lines Produce and Respond to T Cell Growth Factor, *Journal of Experimental Medicine* 154: 1403–1418, 1981.

49 S. Gillis and J. Watson, Biochemical and Biological Characterization

of Lymphocyte Regulatory Molecules. V: Identification of an Interleukin 2-producing Human Leukemia T Cell Line, *Journal of Experimental Medicine* 152: 1709–1719, 1981. (T-cell growth factor or IL-2 is now produced in useful quantities by recombinant DNA techniques.)

50 M. Pinder, K. S. Withey and G. E. Roelants, *Theileria parva* Parasites Transform a Subpopulation of T Lymphocytes, *Journal of Immunology* 127: 389–390, 1981.

51 W. C. Brown and D. Grab, Biological and Biochemical Characterization of Bovine Interleukin 2. Studies with Cloned Bovine T Cells, *Journal of Immunology* 133: 3184–3190, 1985.

52 W. C. Brown and K. S. Logan, Bovine T-Cell Clones Infected with *Theileria parva* Produce a Factor with IL 2-like activity, *Parasite Immunology* 8: 189–192, 1986.

53 D. A. E. Dobbelaere, T. M. Coquerelle, I. J. Roditi, M. Eichhorn and R. O. Williams, *Theileria parva* Infection Induces Autocrine Growth of Bovine Lymphocytes, *Proceedings of the National Academy of Sciences U.S.A:* 85: 4730–4734, 1988

12 EPILOGUE

1 Halfway through my study of the history of East Coast fever I wrote to E. H. Ackerknecht to say that the story seemed to be the result of both accident and over-determination. That, he replied, is what he had always thought history was. Rather later I remarked to Professor Hao Wang that my story was turning into a tautology: things happened the way they did because they happened the way they did. He replied that in his opinion the end result of any successful intellectual analysis is a tautology in the sense that the real work of the analysis lies in sorting things out until their connections become obvious, inevitable and self-evident.

2 As Ackerknecht said in 1955: "Only those who have followed the slow and painful growth of the art and science of medicine, only those who know how much has been accomplished and how much still remains to be done, only those who know how many centuries and even millennia it took to build up knowledge which is now taken for granted, can see this science in its proper proportion" (E. H. Ackerknecht, *A Short History of Medicine*, New York, Ronald Press, 1955, p. xviii).

3 For two such studies and for citations of others see Worboys' thesis and MacLeod's article on the "moving metropolis" (M. Worboys, Science and British Colonial Imperialism 1895–1940, unpublished D.Phil. thesis, University of Sussex, 1979; R. MacLeod, On Visiting the 'Moving Metropolis': Reflections on the Architecture of Imperial Science, *Historical Records of Australian Science* 5: 1–16, 1982).

4 When speaking of a network of scientists, I use the word "network" in a slightly different sense than MacLeod (see R. MacLeod, The X-Club. A Social Network of Science in Late-Victorian England, *Notes and*

Records of the Royal Society of London 24: 305–322, 1970) and to mean something slightly different from what Cannon calls a "sociological group" (W. F. Cannon, The Role of the Cambridge Movement in Early 19th Century Science, in *Proceedings of the Tenth International Congress of the History of Science*, Paris, Hermann, 1964, pp. 317–320). MacLeod and Cannon examine the importance of "networks" of individuals who knew one another personally and often met to discuss topics of mutual interest.

When I refer to a network, for example the "Texas fever network," I mean a group of experts, widely dispersed throughout the world, who may or may not ever have met each other but who looked on one another as experts on the subject, who read each other's published work, and who probably corresponded from time to time. I also use the word network to refer to a set of interests, e.g. economic, imperial or institutional interests.

5 All of them were British; some were even English.

6 Smith did not actually introduce the extension system into Great Britain but he was an early and influential proponent of it (see chapter 4 and chapter 4, n. 3).

For a brief history of the U.S. Department of Agriculture, see A. P. Chew, *The Response of Government to Agriculture: An Account of the Origin and Development of the United States Department of Agriculture, on the Occasion of its 75th Anniversary*, Washington, United States Government Printing Office, 1937. The Department was created in 1862; the Homestead Act and the Morrill Land-Grant College Act were also passed in 1862. The Hatch Act that created the experimental stations was passed in 1887. The formal act creating the extension system was not passed until 1914, but the land-grant colleges had programs directed at practical farmers that were particularly active between 1880 and 1910 (see W. Rasmussen, *Taking the University to the People*, Ames, Iowa State University Press, 1989).

The head of the Department of Agriculture was given cabinet rank in 1889; the British Board of Agriculture became the Ministry of Agriculture in 1919. For the Ministry, see S. Foreman, *Loaves and Fishes: An Illustrated History of the Ministry of Agriculture, Fisheries and Food 1889–1989*, London, H.M.S.O., 1989

7 I long have thought that a study of which books and articles were, at any given period and in any given country, thought to be important enough to be translated into the language of that country might yield significant insights into what advances seemed important enough to be made widely available. Such insights would provide an index of the structure of scientific interests in the translating country. I have also noticed that very few biographical sketches of scientists tell us which languages those scientists could and did read. Misunderstanding caused by reliance on translations played an important role in the Bell–Magendie controversy (see P. F. Cranefield, *The Way In and the Way Out*, Mount Kisco, Futura, 1974).

8 Scientific journals in Switzerland, Scandinavia and Japan published many articles written in German until 1918 and, in some cases, until 1945. Jacques Loeb, a dedicated socialist who despised Bismarck and post-Bismarck German imperialism, founded the *Journal of General Physiology* in 1918, in part so that biologists in the United States would not have to publish in German journals. Loeb believed that the subsidizing of scientific journals was part of a conscious effort to expand the role of the German empire. See, for example, a letter from Jacques Loeb to W. J. V. Osterhout, dated May 11, 1918 (in the files of the editor of the *Journal of General Physiology*; reprinted with the permission of Professor John N. Loeb):

The more I think about it the more I come to the conclusion that the German scientific periodicals which printed everything that was sent to them, which paid in addition their editors liberal salaries, and which moreover paid every contributor, were secretly subsidized by the government. When Engelmann was in this country in 1912 he amazed me by the statement that Roux's Archiv had only 400 subscribers and that the only one of the scientific journals which was near the line of self-support was Ostwald's Zeitschrift für physikalische Chemie. Now whatever these publishers may be they are not mere philanthropists, and I have an idea that the scheme of making Germany the purveyor of science for the whole world was possibly a part of their idea of world control. Of course, it is hypothetical, but I mention this all because I feel that in this country if we ever wish to make it unnecessary for the next generation to be turned over, gagged and bound again to the German Kultur, we have to offer the scientists at least a possibility of publishing their good work in this country, and the only possibility lies in the creation of sufficient outlet for publications of a high order.

See also P. J. Pauly, *Controlling Life: Jacques Loeb and the Engineering Ideal in Biology*, New York, Oxford University Press, 1987, pp. 150 and 161–162.

9 The implications of the concept of the "moving metropolis" are most easily understood in terms of the debates about historiography that led up to it. The notions of the center or metropolis and the periphery or frontier are descendants of Frederick Jackson Turner's views, as expressed in F. J. Turner, The Significance of the Frontier in American History, *Proceedings, 41st Annual Meeting of the State Historical Society of Wisconsin*, Madison, State Historical Society, 1894, pp. 79–112; reprinted in F. J. Turner, *The Frontier in American History*, New York, Holt, 1920, pp. 1–38.

For Turner the frontier was not the backwoods, cut off from the civilization of the center, but a place of abundant resources and equality of opportunity, the source of individualism, inventiveness and idealism. For Turner, the frontier was a place of great creativity and perennial rebirth. In the hands of Webb (W. P. Webb, *The Great Frontier*, Austin, University of Texas Press, 1951; reissued 1964) the frontier became a world-wide source of unexplored resources, the exploitation of which led to an economic boom that lasted 400 years

and ended between 1890 and 1910. It was that boom that nourished the
development of modern European and Western civilization. For Careless, on the other hand, "what Webb called 'The Age of the Great
Frontier' might just as well be called the 'Age of the Great Metropolis',
when western Europe in general, by spreading out its system of
communication and commerce, organized the world about itself."
Moreover, for Careless, "The frontier's culture, too, originally stems
from a metropolitan community – at root, learning and ideas radiate
from there – and thus is Turner answered . . . when this analysis is
carried through . . . The frontier, far from being essentially independent and self-reliant, is in the largest sense a dependant." For Canadian
history, at least, Careless thought that "Frontierism . . . has had its use
and day – the metropolitan approach . . . provides a new framework."
Careless not only gave pride of place to the metropolis and to "metropolitanism" as against "frontierism," he regarded the metropolis as
multi-centered, a "chain" with links both in the New World and the
Old. Nor did he place much faith in what he called the "Britannic, or
Blood is Thicker than Water" school of Canadian history (see J. M. S.
Careless, Frontierism, Metropolitanism and Canadian History, *Canadian Historical Review* 35: 1–21, 1954).

The "mobile metropolis" of Hancock was first postulated in an
article that Lewis and McGann described as one of "a group of papers
and comment dealing with the 'Great Frontier' concept, that attempt
to generalize from the American frontier experience and give it a
broader application on the world stage in modern times" (A. R. Lewis
and J. F. McGann (eds.), *The New World Looks at its History. Proceedings
of the Second International Congress for the Historians of the United States
and Mexico*, Austin, University of Texas Press, 1963, General introduction, pp. vii–ix).

In Hancock's words,

Turner proclaimed the significance of the frontier in American history. To
Turner the American frontier was a unique thing, to Webb it is one of a class.
Turner emphasized its separateness from the European homelands; Webb links
together Great Frontier and Metropolis within the complex interplay of shared
historical experience.

Hancock also said that

I do not think of the Metropolis as an inert slab of geography – unchanging
Europe confronting the unchanging New World. I think of it as a function –
mobile, flexible and increasingly dispersed throughout the whole western
world, in Europe, in Australia, above all in America, that great powerhouse of
metropolitan energies (K. Hancock, The Moving Metropolis, in A. R. Lewis
and J. F. McGann (eds.), *The New World Looks at its History. Proceedings of the
Second International Congress for the Historians of the United States and Mexico*,
Austin, University of Texas Press, 1963, pp. 135–141).

MacLeod extended Hancock's concept in part to explain his disagreement with Basalla's views on the introduction by "diffusion" of

the science of Western Europe, as developed in the sixteenth and seventeenth centuries, into non-European nations (MacLeod, On Visiting the 'Moving Metropolis'; G. Basalla, The Spread of Western Science, *Science* 156: 611–622, 1967). I agree with MacLeod that, for the purposes of the history of science, the notion of a single source of light radiating from a single center is inadequate. Moreover, although the metropolis is indeed multi-centered and mobile, no map of a single intellectual discipline or set of interests can be sufficient for the historical analysis of any complex phenomenon. One definition of metropolis given by the *Oxford English Dictionary* is "the chief centre or seat of some form of activity." Since each form of activity may have its own center and its own frontiers, the metropolis is not only multi-centered and mobile but multi-layered, i.e. made up of many networks.

I do not know what Turner would have made of all of this. As Hancock mentions, for Turner it was the frontier that was multiple and moving, and, indeed, made up of many networks. In Paxson's words, Turner "traced in his famous essay the spread over the continent of a series of frontiers, of the discoverer and the explorer, the missionary, the soldier, the trapper and the farmer . . . He regarded the frontier less as a place than as a continuous process sweeping the continent" (see F. L. Paxson's biographical sketch of F. J. Turner in *Dictionary of American Biography*, vol. XIX, New York, Scribner, 1936, pp. 62–64).

10 See C. van Onselen, Reactions to Rinderpest in South Africa, *Journal of African History* 13: 473–488, 1972.

11 Kenya often comes to mind when one thinks of British emigration to Africa, but South Africa was developed long before Kenya. As to Rhodesia, there are more persons of European ancestry in Zimbabwe today than there ever were in Kenya. Bulawayo was connected to the South African railway system in 1897 and Umtali was linked to Beira in 1898. By 1902 one could go by rail from Beira to Cape Town, via Umtali, Salisbury and Bulawayo. The railway from Mombasa to Nairobi was not begun until 1898 and the permanent way to Victoria Nyanza was completed only in March 1903. Although settlers soon followed, they arrived in large numbers only some 20 years after the original settlers came to Rhodesia (see E. Huxley, *White Man's Country: Lord Delamere and the Making of Kenya*, London, Macmillan, 1935). Huxley (vol. I, p. 88) remarked that in 1900 "Nairobi's site was a speck of frog-infested swamp and bare veld unmarked by so much as a single hut."

12 In 1985, the mineral production of Zimbabwe was valued (in Zimbabwe dollars, at that time equal to about 60 U.S. cents), as follows: coal: 2,920 million; iron ore, 1,098 million; chrome, 526.5 million; gold, 472 million; asbestos, 173.5 million (D. Berens (ed.), *A Concise Encyclopaedia of Zimbabwe, Harare and Gweru*, Mambo Press, 1988, p. 22). The mining industry is, of course, now wholly independent of

ox transport, although communal farming is not. In 1986 the export of tobacco produced 424 million Zimbabwe dollars; that of gold produced 413 million Zimbabwe dollars and that of ferrochrome, 210 million Zimbabwe dollars (Berens, *Concise Encyclopaedia*, p. 39). Of the some 5.5 million cattle in the country, about half are owned by communal farmers. Most of the rest are raised commercially, for beef; about 100,000 are dairy cattle. There are still areas where the presence of tse-tse flies and nagana makes the raising of cattle impossible and there are areas where heartwater is a threat, but East Coast fever remains absent. Although cattle-raising is flourishing, only a very small part of the total beef produced is exported; the industry largely serves to supply the home market. In 1983, some 513,000 cattle were slaughtered and had a value of about 147 million Zimbabwe dollars. In 1982, 165,000 tons of milk were produced, valued at 46 million Zimbabwe dollars (*Tabex Encyclopaedia Zimbabwe*, Harare, Quest Publishing, 1987, p. 5).

For a detailed study of the economic history of Rhodesia from the beginning to a period just prior to the formation of the Federation of Rhodesia and Nyasaland, see I. Phimister, *An Economic and Social History of Zimbabwe 1890–1948: Capital Accumulation and Class Struggle*. London and New York, Longman, 1988.

13 Many descendants of the early settlers of Rhodesia remain in Zimbabwe today including descendants of Charles Rudd (of the Rudd concession), of Rhys Fairbridge and of Lionel Cripps. The African population of Zimbabwe has increased more than ten-fold since 1902 as has the number of African-owned cattle. The raising of maize and of cattle is an important part of communal farming.

14 It is interesting that East Coast fever, presumably endemic for centuries in East Africa, was not "discovered" until it was introduced into Rhodesia and the Transvaal. Huxley (*White Man's Country*, vol. I, p. 94) comments that the early settlers imported cattle into Kenya between 1900 and 1902 but that "imported animals flourished well enough at first, then, almost invariably, they died, sometimes suddenly, sometimes wastingly, from a strange disease. No one knew, at the start, about East Coast fever; and dipping did not become the practice until just before the war." Lord Delamere's herd of dairy cattle was destroyed by East Coast fever in 1906 (Huxley, vol. I, pp. 145–146). Koch had, of course, seen cases in German East Africa in 1897 and 1898, but he mistook the disease for Texas fever. The loss of non-immune cattle brought into areas where East Coast fever was endemic presumably made much less impression than the death of 95 percent of the cattle that occurred when the disease itself was introduced into a region where none of the cattle were immune. A few interesting comments on East Coast fever were made by Winston Churchill in *My African Journey*, London, Hodder & Stoughton, 1908; *reissued*, New York, Norton, 1989, p. 40 and pp. 45–46.

15 A recent outbreak of foot-and-mouth disease in Zimbabwe has

produced comments reminiscent of those of the Rhodesian press in 1902:

[Harare] *Sunday Mail*, July 23, 1989:

The scourge of the livestock disease foot-and-mouth is costing this country millions of dollars in lost beef exports. The real tragedy is that the current foot-and-mouth disease outbreak could have been contained at the beginning . . . one of the main worries . . . is that Zimbabwe is suffering a serious shortage of experienced veterinary staff.

[Harare] *Sunday Mail*, July 30, 1989:

Due to the recent outbreaks of foot-and-mouth disease and acting upon the instructions and advice of the Department of Veterinary Services, the Zimbabwe Agricultural Society has cancelled all cattle, sheep, goat and pig entries for this year's Harare show.

[Harare] *Herald*, August 30, 1989:

The Department of Veterinary Services is taking stringent measures to control the spread of the disease. But the department says its efforts were being hampered by the lack of discipline by some communal, small scale and commercial farmers who fail to report the presence of the disease on their farms . . . the situation was made worse by the continued illegal movement of cattle . . . and through stock thefts, poaching, fence cutting and stray cattle which roam along railway lines and roads.

16 I am indebted to Lesley Cripps for helping me to arrange this visit. According to Hereward Cripps, the Shona rendering of the cry of the Namaqua dove is "Babanguee, Babe wa Kafa, Mai wa kafa, Hana dzangu dsapera kufa, Ndega, Ndega, Ndega." That lament was echoed in a brief farewell to Zimbabwe's greatest writer since Doris Lessing, Dambudzo Marechera, that appeared in the [Harare] *Herald* on August 22, 1987, five days after Marechera's death at the age of 35.

Index

Note that East Coast fever is often abbreviated as ECF.

Printed in the United States
By Bookmasters